Migraine

AF694459

Shalini Shah
Editor

Migraine

Emerging Innovations and Treatment Options

Springer

Editor
Shalini Shah
Department of Anesthesiology & Perioperative Care
University of California Irvine
Irvine, CA
USA

ISBN 978-3-030-75238-5   ISBN 978-3-030-75239-2 (eBook)
https://doi.org/10.1007/978-3-030-75239-2

© Springer Nature Switzerland AG 2021
This work is subject to copyright. All rights are reserved by the Publisher, whether the whole or part of the material is concerned, specifically the rights of translation, reprinting, reuse of illustrations, recitation, broadcasting, reproduction on microfilms or in any other physical way, and transmission or information storage and retrieval, electronic adaptation, computer software, or by similar or dissimilar methodology now known or hereafter developed.
The use of general descriptive names, registered names, trademarks, service marks, etc. in this publication does not imply, even in the absence of a specific statement, that such names are exempt from the relevant protective laws and regulations and therefore free for general use.
The publisher, the authors and the editors are safe to assume that the advice and information in this book are believed to be true and accurate at the date of publication. Neither the publisher nor the authors or the editors give a warranty, expressed or implied, with respect to the material contained herein or for any errors or omissions that may have been made. The publisher remains neutral with regard to jurisdictional claims in published maps and institutional affiliations.

This Springer imprint is published by the registered company Springer Nature Switzerland AG
The registered company address is: Gewerbestrasse 11, 6330 Cham, Switzerland

To my loving parents, Vishakha and Suresh, none of the spark or accomplishment could have been done without your dedication, support, and constant positivity. Thank you for giving me the vision to see, be, and do more.

Foreword

Migraine is a complex pain condition with intense head pain that is often difficult to treat. Every time a physician encounters a patient with migraine, a complex process of diagnosis and management ensues along with skepticism of effective therapy. However, it is obvious that the physician is expected to precisely diagnose the condition and effectively manage it. Therefore, it is of paramount importance to present all information pertaining to migraine in a book collectively, so the treating physician is better equipped to steer the challenges of managing the most complex condition. Studies have shown that quality of life of patients suffering from migraine compounded by accompanying symptoms including nausea, phonophobia, photophobia, and mood disorders is negatively affected and the daily life is interrupted, reflecting on family and social dynamics.

I must compliment Dr. Shalini Shah for transforming the abstracts and chapters into a much needed complete book focused on migraine, and contributing to the body of literature in pain medicine. Similarly, I compliment all the outstanding authors with exemplary backgrounds for making important contributions to this book.

The book presents a complex condition in a format that is easy to understand with simple but striking illustrations. This book is a capsule of everything you would want to know – pathophysiology, symptomatology, and prophylactic and therapeutic management of migraine, including highly sophisticated evidence-based immunomodulation, neuromodulation therapies, and surgical options as well as emerging innovations. The other highlights include pediatric migraine and dietary modification for migraine relief. This book is a perfect source of complete information for residents, fellows, and pain physicians to understand the pathophysiology, mechanism, and characteristics of headache and diagnose and manage the symptomatology of migraine.

Migraine: Emerging Innovations and Treatment Options is a marvelous example of providing a practical approach to treat patients with migraine. It emphasizes on the steps with a typical and atypical diagnostic certainty based on clinical presentation. The diagnostic acumen, with precise signs and symptoms to treat migraine and status migrainosus, is often challenging and frustrating for the patients and their healthcare providers. This book reflects the distinction and compassion to help physicians provide the best care anywhere for a disabling disease state of migraine.

Sudhir Diwan
President, Advanced Spine on Park Avenue
Associate Clinical Professor
Albert Einstein College of Medicine
Bronx, NY, USA

Former Director and Chief
Tri-Institute Pain Medicine Fellowship
Weill Cornell School of Medicine
New York, NY, USA

Preface

Important advances in the basic science and clinical practice of migraine pain have evolved greatly over the last two decades, with new options and therapeutics being developed at a much needed rapid pace. This text was written both for the clinician community as well as a comprehensive "go to" reference guide for patients interested in learning more about migraine etiology and treatments.

In this edition, the reader will find the latest scientific mechanistic principles that demonstrate how migraine develops and in whom, as well as various treatment options, from medications to injection therapy to surgical options for pain. We are fortunate to include a special chapter specifically dedicated to those children who suffer from disabling migraine pain, with promising treatment options for this vulnerable population. We have also included a comprehensive chapter on integrative and complementary treatment options for migraine disorder, as often patients and physicians alike are interested in pursuing simple daily dietary modifications that may have an enormous impact on pain and suffering. Understanding the science behind dietary changes, we hope, will be tremendously valuable to both patients and the medical community. Finally, a quick reference guide to pharmacotherapeutics was included to guide residents, fellows, physicians, and clinicians in the busy clinic setting.

The book reflects the seasoned medical opinion of expert physicians and scientists in headache and migraine pain management, many of whom rely on the clinical experience at the University of California Irvine. The purpose of this work is to serve as a handbook for the medical community as well as the educated patient who is motivated to learn more about the treatment journey ahead.

I gratefully acknowledge the dedication and scholarship that my colleagues have put into their contributions. In particular, a grateful thanks to Ms. Margaret Burns for her editorial assistance. In addition, I am indebted to all of my mentors throughout my career; some of you may not know the indelible contribution you have had on me personally and professionally. Above all, my deepest appreciation goes to all of the contributors' families whose understanding, patience, and encouragement have made this book possible.

Irvine, CA, USA — Shalini Shah

Contents

Contributors

Natasha Acosta Diaz, MD Department of Neurology, Pediatric Neurology and Epilepsy, Southeastern Regional Medical Center, Lumberton, NC, USA

Lilian Au, ND, MPH Susan Samueli Integrative Health Institute, University of California Irvine Health, Costa Mesa, CA, USA

Michael-David Calderon, BS Department of Anesthesiology and Perioperative Care, University of California Irvine Health, Orange, CA, USA

Rakhi Dayal, MD Department of Anesthesiology, University of California Irvine Health, Orange, CA, USA

Nathaniel Dusto, MD Department of Physical Medicine and Rehabilitation, University of California Irvine, Orange, CA, USA

Jihan Grant, MD Department of Neurology, Headache Medicine, Mount Sinai Hospital, New York, NY, USA

Antoinette Green, BS Department of Neurology, Cincinnati Children Hospital Medical Center (CCHMC), Cincinnati, OH, USA

Amitabh Gulati, MD Department of Anesthesiology and Critical Care, Memorial Sloan Kettering Cancer Center, New York, NY, USA

Kim Hecht, DO Susan Samueli Integrative Health Institute, University of California Irvine Health, Costa Mesa, CA, USA

Diana Heringer, MD Department of Pain Management, University of California Irvine, Irvine, CA, USA

Rohan Jotwani, MD, MBA Department of Anesthesiology, Pain Management, New York-Presbyterian/Weill Cornell Medical College, New York, NY, USA

Marielle Kabbouche, MD, FAHS Department of Neurology, Cincinnati Children Hospital Medical Center (CCHMC), Cincinnati, OH, USA

Melissa Kanack, MD Department of Plastic Surgery, University of California Irvine, School of Medicine, Irvine, CA, USA

Lynn Kohan, MD Department of Anesthesiology, University of Virginia, Charlottesville, VA, USA

Clarence Li, MD Department of Anesthesiology, University of Virginia, Charlottesville, VA, USA

Ojas Mainkar, MD Department of Anesthesiology, Pain Management, New York-Presbyterian/Weill Cornell Medical College, New York, NY, USA

Neel Mehta, MD Department of Anesthesiology, Pain Management, New York-Presbyterian/Weill Cornell Medical College, New York, NY, USA

Bridget Mueller, PhD, MD Department of Neurology, Headache Medicine, Mount Sinai Hospital, New York, NY, USA

Samer N. Narouze, MD, PhD Center for Pain Medicine, Western Reserve Hospital, Cuyahoga Falls, OH, USA

Danielle Perret Karimi, MD Department of Physical Medicine and Rehabilitation and Department of Anesthesiology, University of California Irvine Health, Orange, CA, USA

Department of Physical Medicine and Rehabilitation, University of California Irvine Health, Orange, CA, USA

Sharoon Qaiser, MBBS, MD Department of Neurology, Cincinnati Children Hospital Medical Center (CCHMC), Cincinnati, OH, USA

Shalini Shah, MD Department of Anesthesiology & Perioperative Care, University of California Irvine, Irvine, CA, USA

Stephen D. Silberstein, MD, FACP Jefferson Headache Center, Thomas Jefferson University, Philadelphia, PA, USA

Adrian Darryll Sulindro, MD Biohealth Pain Management, Lawndale, CA, USA

Pranamya Suri, MD Department of Physical Medicine and Rehabilitation, University of California Irvine Health, Orange, CA, USA

Brett Toimil, MD Department of Anesthesiology, University of Virginia, Charlottesville, VA, USA

Raj M. Vyas, MD, FACS Department of Plastic Surgery, University of California Irvine, Orange, CA, USA

Jennifer Wu, MD, PhD Department of Physical Medicine and Rehabilitation, University of California Irvine Health, Orange, CA, USA

Department of Pediatric Rehabilitation, Spaulding Rehabilitation Hospital, Boston, MA, USA

Bi-Ying Yeh, MD Department of Physical Medicine and Rehabilitation, University of California Irvine Health, Orange, CA, USA

Hyerin Yoon Department of Anesthesiology, University of Virginia, Charlottesville, VA, USA

Hsiangkuo Yuan, MD, PhD Jefferson Headache Center, Thomas Jefferson University, Philadelphia, PA, USA

Migraine Diagnosis and Symptomatology

1

Brett Toimil, Hyerin Yoon, Clarence Li, and Lynn Kohan

Migraine continues to be a prevalent and disabling condition worldwide [1, 2]. The 1-year prevalence rate overall is approximately 10%, ranging from 4.5 to 6% in men and from 14.5 to 18% in women [3–5]. Most patients develop migraines within the first three decades of life; however, it may also develop later into the fourth and fifth decades in some patients. Traditionally, most descriptions of migraine have emphasized three features, including unilateral distribution of the headache, the presence of a warning symptom (often visual), and nausea or vomiting [6]. Migraine headaches were formerly divided into two categories: classic and common; [7] however, the diagnostic criteria have evolved over time to include several different types of migraine classifications.

Migraine has recently been theorized as a continuum of episodic to chronic migraine, with variations in headache days and symptoms and with an estimated 3% of patients progressing from episodic migraine (EM) to chronic migraine (CM) each year [8]. There may be natural variation in headache day frequency within patients, meaning individual patients can fluctuate between EM and CM [9]. Given the prevalence of migraine disease, it is imperative that it is properly diagnosed; however, it has been reported that less than half of migraine cases are properly diagnosed [10]. Underdiagnosis can lead to deficiencies in treatment. Undertreatment can lead to increased headache-related disability and poor health-related quality of life (HRQoL) [11]. This chapter will discuss the most updated diagnostic criteria for migraine headaches, as well as both typical and atypical symptoms associated with the disease.

B. Toimil · H. Yoon · C. Li · L. Kohan (✉)
Department of Anesthesiology, University of Virginia, Charlottesville, VA, USA
e-mail: LRK9G@hscmail.mcc.virginia.edu

© Springer Nature Switzerland AG 2021

S. Shah (ed.), *Migraine*, https://doi.org/10.1007/978-3-030-75239-2_1

Migraine Characteristics

There are numerous causes of headache classified as either primary (no underlying cause) or secondary (i.e. due to underlying cause). Migraine is classified as a primary headache disorder. Patients presenting with headache should be evaluated thoroughly to rule out a secondary cause of headache. This can be done by performing a careful history and examination [12]. The presence of red flag symptoms (thunderclap headache, positional headache, worsening with valsalva, sidelocked headache, new headache in age > 50, neurologic symptoms, systemic symptoms, or immunosuppression) should warrant further investigation with neuroimaging and investigative studies [13].

Classic migraine symptoms typically include a throbbing, unilateral, or bilateral headache with photophobia, phonophobia, and/or osmophobia. Patients typically prefer to lay down in a dark room until their symptoms subside [14]. There is typically a premonitory phase that occurs hours to days before the onset of a migraine as well as a postdrome that occurs after the headache itself. Migraines are classified into subtypes, including migraine with and without aura, hemiplegic migraine, migraine with brainstem aura, retinal migraine, vestibular migraine, and chronic migraine [15]. Migraines are more common in women than in men, with about two-thirds of patients with migraine being women. On average, patients with migraine experience one to two attacks per month [16]. Migraines typically last between 4 and 72 hours, and a duration of headache beyond 72 hours is referred to as status migrainosus.

Migraines are often associated with triggers suggesting an interaction between the environment and a susceptible host. Triggers include exertion, diet, sleep disturbances, hormonal influences, medications, and trauma [14]. Additionally, migraines are associated with comorbid conditions, including mitral valve prolapse, Raynaud phenomenon, stroke, epilepsy, and several psychiatric conditions (i.e. depression, anxiety, bipolar disorder, and social phobias) [17].

Migraine is a recurrent disorder often associated with sensory symptoms such as photo- or phonophobia, nausea/vomiting, and high rates of disability. Migraines can be classified as episodic (occurring <15 days/month) or chronic (occurring >15 days/month) [15]. Patients with migraines may appear normal in between episodes; however, abnormalities in brain function as measured by contingent negative variation and transcranial magnetic stimulation have been documented [14].

Premonitory Symptoms

The premonitory (prodromal) phase occurs hours to days prior to the onset of a migraine and consists of a heterogeneous group of non-painful symptoms. Because many of the studies looking at the premonitory phase have been conducted retrospectively, the prevalence of these symptoms in adults and children has been quoted as ranging from 9% to 88% [18]. One prospective multicenter study using an electronic diary found that premonitory symptoms were followed by a migraine headache within 72 hours on 72% of occasions [19]. The symptoms described are often non-specific and can be divided into three broad categories associated with cognition, sensation, and homeostasis [18]. Of these, the most commonly reported symptom is fatigue in both adults and children [19–21]. Additional symptoms include difficulty concentrating, irritability, depression, yawning, craving, stress, sleep disturbance, neck stiffness, photophobia, phonophobia, and nausea [22]. Because the premonitory symptomatology overlaps with that of the headache, clinical timing is important and a patient diary can help distinguish this phase from a migraine attack.

Aura Symptoms

Migraine may occur with or without aura. Aura is not an ideal term since it can occur before or during the headache, in the absence of a headache, and can be associated with some non-migraine headaches [14]. Migraine with aura accounts for 10.7–46.6% of migraine patients [23]. The most common aura manifestation is visual. Visual symptoms may present as enlarging scotoma with a shimmering edge or other visual disturbances such as the appearance of stars, dots, wavy lines, complex patterns or shapes, or visual distortions. Sensory auras are less common. Somatosensory auras are typically positive, begin gradually, and progress slowly, which is in contrast to the abrupt onset of a cerebrovascular event or the rapid tempo of a seizure. An example of a somatosensory aura includes the cherio-oral aura in which paresthesia begins in the hand and slowly ascends to the shoulder and ipsilateral face, inside of the mouth and tongue [14]. This "slow march" is thought to correlate with the rate of "cortical spreading depression," which is an initially excitatory wave of depolarization, followed by an inhibitory depolarization then repolarization. Typically, migraine auras are positive phenomena, but negative symptoms do occur. Auras causing hemiplegias or hemiparesis are uncommon as are auras involving the frontal or temporal lobes resulting in possible speech disturbances [14].

Postdromal Symptoms

The postdromal period following a migraine headache is the least-studied phase of the disease and is not characterized in commonly used migraine diagnostic criteria. The postdrome is defined as the time period between resolution of headaches to return to baseline. However, there is no clear marker for the end of the migraine and the start of the postdrome, and it can be difficult to distinguish from a low-level headache. The range of postdrome symptoms vary from study to study; however, fatigue was reported as the most common symptom, and is experienced in 88% of patients (Table 1.1). Similar to premonitory symptoms, other common postdromal symptoms include in order of frequency: difficulty with concentration (67%), head pain (33.1%), irritability (22%) [20], cognitive difficulties (11.7%), hangover (10.7%), gastrointestinal symptoms (8.4%), mood change (6.8%), and weakness

Table 1.1 Characteristic symptoms for each migraine phase

Prodrome (hours to days)	Aura (minutes)	Headache (hours to days)	Postdrome (hours to days)
Fatigue	Visual symptoms	Unilateral headache	Fatigue
Difficulty concentrating	Somatosensory changes	Pulsatile headache	Difficulty concentrating
Irritability	Hemiplegia	Moderate/severe intensity	Head pain
Depression	Hemiparesis	Photophobia	Irritability
Yawning	Speech disturbance	Phonophobia	Cognitive difficulty
Craving	Vertigo	Nausea	Hangover
Stress	Tinnitus	Vomiting	GI symptoms
Sleep disturbance	Hearing changes	Aggravated by physical activity	Mood change
Neck stiffness			Weakness
Photophobia			
Phonophobia			
Nausea			

(6.2%) [24]. It has been shown that 80% of migraine attacks are followed by non-headache symptoms. Severity of migraine does not seem to correlate with duration of the postdrome. The average duration of the postdrome was 25.2 hours, with 56% having postdrome for <12 hours, 32% for 12–24 hours, and 12% for >24 hours [24].

Patients with postdrome tend to have more stereotyped and more frequent migraines than patients without postdrome. Additionally, they have a greater percentage of headaches with aura, greater headache intensity, and more throbbing and stabbing qualities to their headache. Disability tends to be greater in migraine patients with postdrome, and the headaches are more easily triggered [24]. Given the similarity between premonitory and postdromal symptoms, a shared neural activation pathway for these phases has been postulated. Though migraine sufferers typically return to their clinical baseline between attacks, functional brain imaging has shown a widespread reduction in blood flow in the postdromal period [25].

Migraine Without Aura

The International Classification of Headache Disorders (ICHD) is an instrumental resource for criteria for the diagnosis of migraine. This classification system has evolved over time, reflecting a growing understanding of heterogeneity of migraine and their variable clinic presentations. The ICHD is available online and is routinely updated. The ICHD 3rd edition is the most recent iteration of this classification system. Migraine is a diagnosis of inclusion, requiring meeting a set of specific features, as well as exclusion, since secondary headaches have to be excluded. The diagnostic criteria for migraine without aura are shown in Table 1.2. Two statements in the criteria serve to exclude secondary headaches: at least five lifetime attacks are required and the explicit statement that secondary headache must be excluded based on a normal neurological examination and, if necessary, diagnostic testing [15].

Table 1.2 Diagnostic criteria: migraine without aura

1. At least 5 attacks fulfilling criteria B–D
2. Headache attacks lasting 4–72 hours (untreated or unsuccessfully treated)
3. Headache has at least two of the following four characteristics
   A. Unilateral location
   B. Pulsating quality
   C. Moderate or severe pain intensity
   D. Aggravation by or causing avoidance of routine physical activity (e.g. Walking or climbing stairs)
4. During headache at least one of the following:
   1. Nausea and/or vomiting
   2. Photophobia and phonophobia
5. Not better accounted for by another ICHD-3 diagnosis

From: Headache Classification Committee of the International Headache Society (HIS) [15], with permission

In migraines without aura, in which 15% of the population is affected, there are four categories of symptoms: visual, language, sensory, and motor. Accompanying symptoms of nausea, vomiting, photophobia, and phonophobia are more present in migraine without aura than migraine with aura. In addition, double vision, inverted 2- and 3-D vision, and altered perception of body weight and size were found more often in migraines without aura [26]. Mean age of the migraine without aura onset is about 19 years, with more likelihood of onset between childhood and 35 years of age, and resolves spontaneously after age 50. The pain score was also rated higher and the average duration of the headache phase recorded longer in migraines without aura [27]. The difference between migraine without aura and migraine with aura is that the headache is the most prominent characteristic of migraine without aura, while migraine with aura can be characterized with either a migraine or non-migraine.

Migraine With Aura

The classification of migraine with aura has transformed over time, becoming more specific with newer versions of the ICHD. Recently, the ICHD-3 criteria were shown to be more specific than the ICHD-3 beta criteria for distinguishing migraine with aura from a transient ischemic attack [28]. In the ICHD-3, migraine with aura is divided into several different categories, including migraine with typical aura, typical aura with headache, typical aura without headache, migraine with brainstem aura, hemiplegic migraine, several types of familial hemiplegic migraine, sporadic hemiplegic migraine, and retinal migraine [15]. Migraine with aura is a transient neurological symptom that most commonly involves the visual fields, but can present with other sensory, language, or motor disturbances. It includes hemispheric symptoms but no motor aura. Furthermore, migraine with aura affects 8% of the population [29]. Mean age at MA varies widely, but has onset more frequently in early adulthood [30]. Aura symptoms of sensory, motor, or speech disturbances often occur with coexisting visual disturbances [31]. Although many patients manifest a combination of phenomena, the majority with migraine aura manifested only visual phenomenon. Most patients had visual auras that last from 1 to 30 minutes, which can start either in the periphery or the center of the visual fields [32]. The most common visual phenomena are small bright dots (42%), flashes of light (39%), blind spots (32%), and foggy vision (27%) [33]. The prevalent symptoms of migraine with aura include photophobia (86.5%), nausea (75.6%), phonophobia (70.5%), and vomiting (40.4%), and are more pronounced in females [27]. There was a correlation between the intensity of headache and associated symptoms.

Currently, cortical-spreading depression is accepted to be responsible for the reversible cerebral cortical dysfunction in migraine aura. A disruption of cell membrane ion gradients caused by elevations in extracellular potassium leads to depolarization followed by a prolonged inhibition of the neuronal activity [34]. Propagation of CSD releases pro-inflammatory and excitatory mediators such as nitric oxide, glutamate, and adenosine triphosphate, and subsequently activates trigeminal nociceptors that trigger the pain associated with migraine [35]. However, the exact trigger for the initial change in extracellular potassium concentration in migraine is unclear. It has also been found that the pathophysiology of persistent visual auras may be attributable to N-methyl-D-aspartate (NMDA)-receptor hyper-excitability or central inhibitory dysfunction [36].

It remains unclear whether the structural changes cause migraines with aura; however, it has been speculated that certain features such as higher neuron-to-astrocyte ratio and its distinct columnar organization increase the occurrence of migraines. Furthermore, migraine patients with visual aura have been found to have a small reduction in volume of the left fusiform gyros relative to healthy controls. They also have reduced volume in the left temporal pole and rostral middle frontal cortex compared to patients with somatosensory and dysphasia aura.

In addition to genetic influences of migraine, hormonal changes increase the risk of migraine with aura. In particular, estrogens affect migraine by interacting with vascular endothelium, modulating neuronal excitability through dopamine, endorphins, and serotonin, and increasing excitatory glutamatergic tone via NMDA channels. The diagnostic criteria for migraine with aura are shown in Table 1.3.

Migraine With Aura Subtypes

A new diagnosis in the ICHD-3 is migraine with brainstem aura, which was previously classified as a basilar migraine in the ICHD-1 and basilar type migraine in ICHD-2. The terms basilar artery migraine was first described in 1961 by Bickerstaff [37]. The original criteria in ICHD-1 for basilar migraine included migraine that was characterized by aura symptoms originating in the brainstem or simultaneously from both cerebral hemispheres, including vertigo, ataxia, diplopia, dysarthria, tinnitus, decreased hearing, visual symptoms, in both the temporal and nasal fields of both eyes, bilateral paresis, bilateral paresthesia, and decreased level of consciousness. At that time, it was felt that these characteristic symptoms were secondary to

Table 1.3 Diagnostic criteria: migraine with aura

1. At least two attacks fulfilling criteria B and C
2. One or more of the following fully reversible aura symptoms
   1. Visual
   2. Sensory
   3. Speech and/or language
   4. Brainstem
   5. Retinal
3. At least three of the following six characteristics
   A. At least one aura symptom spreads gradually over ≥5 minutes
   B. Two or more aura symptoms occur in succession
   C. Each individual aura symptom lasts 5–60 minutes
   D. At least one aura symptom is unilateral
   E. At least one aura symptom in positive
   F. The aura is accompanied, or followed within 60 minutes, by headache
4. Not better accounted for by another ICHD-3 diagnosis

From: Headache Classification Committee of the International Headache Society (HIS) [15], with permission

spasm or constriction of the basilar artery. However, no evidence was found to support vasospasm of the basilar artery and this migraine subtype was reclassified. The ICHD revised the criteria in 2004 by removing the symptom of bilateral paresis from the criteria to differentiate hemiplegic migraine from basilar type migraine. The distinguishing feature of this subtype of migraine with aura in ICHD-3 is that symptoms originate in the brainstem and do not include motor weakness, which occurs in hemiplegic migraine [38]. More specifically, ICHD-3 criteria for migraine with brainstem aura include migraine attack fulfilling criteria for migraine with aura and at least two brainstem aura symptoms consisting of ataxia, decreased level of consciousness, vertigo, diplopia, dysarthria, tinnitus and hyperacusis in the decreasing order of frequency, but not motor or retinal symptoms. Additionally, bilateral visual disturbances and bilateral sensory symptoms were prevalent [37].

A rare form of migraine, retinal migraine, has been reintroduced in the ICHD-3. It is described as repeated attacks of reversible monocular visual disturbances which may include positive features such as scintillations or fortification spectra or negative features including scotomata or blindness [15]. Contrary to ICHD-3 criteria, the majority have a history of migraine with aura. Typically, monocular visual features consist of partial or complete visual loss lasting <1 hour [39]. These symptoms need to be verified during the headache attack by confirming either or both clinical visual field examination or the patient's drawing of the monocular visual disturbance. One needs to rule out other causes of transient monocular blindness in order to establish the diagnosis [15]. Retinal migraine describes patients with episodes of transient and permanent monocular visual impairment, specifically in the absence of migraine headache. It is typically characterized by negative monocular visual phenomena lasting less than 1 hour. Reported cases of recurrent transient monocular visual loss subsequently experienced permanent monocular visual loss. The duration of the transient visual symptoms varied from a few seconds to 1 hour. This disorder is 16 times more likely to be found in women than in men.

Hemiplegic migraine is largely distinguished by motor weakness, muscle weakness, and paralysis in one side. Characteristics of hemiplegic migraine auras are (1) motion aura and (2) complex aura symptoms that include any of the aura symptoms of migraine with aura, such as vision, speech, and sensation, or basilar-type migraine [29]. Visual symptoms in hemiplegic migraine consist of positive features (flickering spots or zigzag lines) with or without a negative feature (scotoma). Sensory symptoms combine positive (pins and needles, painful or cold sensations) and negative (numbness) features [29]. Attacks include severe headache, scintillating scotoma, visual field defect, numbness, paresthesia, unilateral weakness, aphasia, fever, lethargy, coma, and seizures, and last for hours to days with resolution of symptoms. There are two types of hemiplegic migraine – familial hemiplegic migraine (FHM) and sporadic hemiplegic migraine (SHM). FHM is divided into four categories based on identified specific genes in familial hemiplegic migraine (FHM) [38]. One-third of patients with hemiplegic migraine experience severe attacks with impairment of consciousness with full recovery [40]. This subtype of migraine with aura is classified as fulfilling the criteria for migraine with aura in which the aura is fully reversible and motor weakness also exists that is fully reversible [40]. Hemiplegic migraine is classified as sporadic if no first- or second-degree family members have headaches with similar motor symptoms.

Familial hemiplegic migraine (FHM) is an autosomal dominant disorder of migraines occurring in two or more family members in the same family with unilateral motor deficits during the aura. This type of migraine only occurs in 0.01% of the population and is characterized by an aura with either fully-reversible motor weakness or fully-reversible visual, sensory, speech, and language symptoms [41]. Attacks of transient hemiparesis, followed by a migraine headache, are further divided into pure familial hemiplegic migraine (80%) and familial hemiplegic migraine with permanent cerebellar signs (20%). The hemiparesis during the aura is always associated with sensory, language, and visual symptoms [40]. However, one-fourth of the patients with FHM do not have visual symptoms and only one-third of patients demonstrate bilateral motor signs. Gene mutations in familial hemiplegic migraine have been understood to increase neuronal excitability and reduce the threshold for cortical spreading depression. Genetic studies have implicated that mutations in the ion transportation genes, *CACNA1A*, *ATP1A2*, and *SCN1A*, all cause the FHM phenotype [29]. The *CACNA1A* missense mutation, Thr666Met substitution contributed to 40% of FHM and induces gain-of-function effects with enhanced calcium ion influx and increased neurotransmitter release. It also has an increased probability of excitatory glutamate release. The mutation in SCN1A decreased glutamate uptake. The *ATP1A2* exhibits loss of function, impairing glial reuptake of potassium and glutamate from the synaptic cleft with slow recovery from the neuronal excitation. The *SCN1A* mutation results in hyper-excitability due to the inhibitory effect of interneurons. However, other genes responsible for this phenotype are still to be identified as at least a quarter of the large families affected do not have a mutation in the three genes [29].

Sporadic hemiplegic migraine (SHM) shares all the clinical symptoms with familial hemiplegic migraine, but SHM affects only one individual and none of the family members. A de-novo mutation in the three genes that were involved in the familial hemiplegic migraine has been understood to cause the SHM; however, these do not play a big role in SHM because no *SCN1A* mutation has been found and only a few *CACNA1A* and *ATP1A2* mutations [29]. Another possible explanation of the etiology is inheritance of a gene mutation from an asymptomatic parent with FHM. Population with sporadic hemiplegic migraine usually presents all four aura symptoms: sensory (98%), visual (91%), aphasic (81%), and motor, and at least two symptoms were portrayed by each patient during the SHM attacks. Specifically, visual aura symptoms consist of unilateral visual aura symptoms, flickering light, scotoma, zigzag/fortification lines, and without preserved central vision. Difficulty with finding the right word and impaired production of language or comprehension of language were categorized under the aphasic aura symptoms. Finally, both sensory and motor aura symptoms were primarily localized in the arm and hand, along with the face, tongue, foot, and leg. Upper limb symptoms were experienced most often. Bilateral motor signs are observed in 1/3 of patients whose both sides are affected either in succession or simultaneously. The unilateral hemiplegic migraine switches sides between or during attacks. The duration of SHM's aura symptom was longer and bilateral motor symptoms were more frequent in comparison to migraine with typical aura [29].

Vestibular migraine is characterized by episodic attacks of positional vertigo, head motion-induced vertigo, and visual vertigo that last from 5 minutes to 3 days. The neural mechanisms of vestibular migraine are still unclear as the variability of symptoms suggests that migraine interacts with the vestibular system at various levels [42]. One possible explanation for the pathophysiology of vestibular migraine is spreading depression, which is a cortical mechanism that produces vestibular symptoms when it reaches the multisensory vestibular cortex [42]. Another possible contributor of the pathogenesis of vestibular migraine includes neurotransmitters, such as calcitonin-gene related peptide, serotonin, noradrenaline, and dopamine, that modulate the activity of central and peripheral vestibular neurons. A human experimental model of vestibular migraine demonstrated that those with migraine had a lower threshold for crosstalk between the neighboring brainstem structures when trigeminal activation produced spontaneous nystagmus in migraine patients [42].

Chronic Migraine

Patients presenting with a history of chronic headache should also undergo a careful history and physical examination. If no causes of secondary headache are identified, patients with chronic headache should be assessed for a primary headache disorder, which can include chronic tension-type headache, new daily persistent headache, hemicrania continua, and chronic migraine (CM) [12, 15]. The diagnostic criteria according to the ICHD-3 for chronic migraine can be seen in Table 1.4. Chronic daily migraine is a disabling condition that impacts approximately 0.5–5% of the general population [43]; however, the true incidence is difficult to ascertain

Table 1.4 Diagnostic criteria: chronic migraine

A. Headache (migraine-like or tension-like) on ≥15 days/month for >3 months, and fulfilling criteria B and C
B. Occurring in a patient who has had at least five attacks fulfilling criteria B–D for 1.1 *Migraine without aura* and/or criteria B and C for 1.2 *Migraine with aura*
C. On ≥8 days/month for >3 months, fulfilling any of the following: Criteria C and D for 1.1 *Migraine without aura* Criteria B and C for 1.2 *Migraine with aura* Believed by the patient to be migraine at onset and relieved by a triptan or ergot derivative
D. Not better accounted for by another ICHD-3 diagnosis

From: Headache Classification Committee of the International Headache Society (HIS) [15], with permission

secondary to heterogeneous data collection instruments and patient recall bias. Compared to episodic migraine, CM is less common but is associated with greater headache-related disability, diminished physical, social, and occupational functioning, and worse health related quality-of-life [44]. Patients with CM also have a higher incidence of co-morbid psychiatric and medical conditions, which can result in complex cases of multidimensional migraine [44].

Notable differences exist between ICHD-3 and its predecessor. Revisions include changes to the criteria for chronic migraine, specifically under the ICHD-2 criteria patients needed to have 15 migraine headache days per month in the absence of medication overuse headache to qualify for a diagnosis of chronic migraine, while in the ICHD-3 beta classification states that patients have to have 15 headache days per month but only 8 of those need to have migraine-associated features. In addition, medication overuse can concurrently occur with chronic migraine [45].

Even with these guidelines, it may be difficult to accurately diagnose migraine because patients may not be able to report an accurate number of headache days per month, especially without the use of a "headache diary." Patients may also tend to report their severe headache days but fail to mention/record milder headache days [46]. Risk factors for the chronification of episodic migraine to chronic migraine include obesity (especially when comorbid with depression or anxiety), a history of frequent headache (>1 headache/week), caffeine consumption, and overuse of as-needed headache-analgesics (>10 days/month), ergots, and triptans [12, 47]. Approximately 3% of patients with EM progress to CM each year [8].

Additional Considerations

Many migraines do not fit the traditional definition of migraine without or with aura, so the ICHD-3 incorporates additional presentations into the classification system. Probable migraine can occur with or without aura, and is defined as meeting all but one of criteria A–D for migraine without aura or A–C of migraine with aura [15]. In order to be considered a probable migraine, other headaches that better explain the symptoms should be ruled out first.

The connection between gastrointestinal inflammatory disorders and migraine are starting to become established, as it is postulated the autonomic nervous system plays a role in the pathophysiology of several conditions involving abdominal pain, nausea, and vomiting [48]. Recognizing this association, the ICHD-3 created the new term recurrent gastrointestinal disturbance and defined it as five or more episodes of severe abdominal pain or nausea and vomiting that occur in the presence of a normal gastrointestinal evaluation and cannot be attributed to other disorders. Predominantly thought to affect children, cyclic vomiting syndrome and abdominal migraine are subtypes of gastrointestinal disturbance. Cyclic vomiting syndrome is more narrowly thought of as self-limiting episodic vomiting that occurs in a predictable manner with complete resolution of symptoms between attacks, whereas abdominal migraine is more broadly defined as attacks of abdominal pain that last 2–72 hours untreated with complete symptom resolution between attacks. Both of these conditions have been established as highly associated with concurrently experiencing migraines or predisposing to migraine attacks in the future [48, 49].

Conclusion

Migraine continues to be a difficult disease to diagnose despite its high prevalence. The ICHD has developed migraine diagnostic criteria, which continues to expand and improve specificity for distinguishing migraine from secondary headache disorders. Migraine is currently thought of as a continuum between episodic attacks and chronic attacks that can occur without or with an aura, and the latest version of ICHD now includes a new classification of brainstem aura. Given the heterogeneity of migraine symptoms, using a headache diary can be useful for improving diagnostic accuracy. Because of the debilitating nature of this disease and its impact on health-related quality of life, continued efforts to improve diagnosis and prevent delay to treatment are needed.

References

1. GBD 2015 Disease and Injury Incidence and Prevalence Collaborators. Global, regional, and national incidence, prevalence, and years lived with disability for 310 diseases and injuries, 1990–2015: a systematic analysis for the Global Burden of Disease Study 2015. Lancet. 2016;388:1545–602.
2. GBD 2016 Disease and Injury Incidence and Prevalence Collaborators. Global, regional, and national incidence, prevalence, and years lived with disability for 328 diseases and injuries for 195 countries, 1990–2016: a systematic analysis for the Global Burden of Disease Study 2016. Lancet. 2017;390:1211–59.
3. Rasmussen BK, Olesen J. Symptomatic and non-symptomatic headaches in a general population. Neurology. 1992;42(6):1225–31.
4. Steiner TJ, Scher AI, Stewart WF, Kolodner K, Liberman J, Lipton RB. The prevalence and disability burden of adult migraine in England and their relationships to age, gender and ethnicity. Cephalalgia. 2003;23(7):519–27.

5. Stewart WF, Lipton RB, Celentano DD, Reed ML. Prevalence of migraine headache in the United States. Relation to age, income, race, and other sociodemographic factors. JAMA. 1992;267(1):64–9.
6. Walter CT, Grogan MA. Migraine with tardy pleocytosis. Neurology. 1986;36(5):733.
7. Silberstein SD. Treatment of headache in primary care practice. Am J Med. 1984;77(3):65–72.
8. Aurora SK, Brin MF. Chronic migraine: an update on physiology, imaging, and the mechanism of action of two available pharmacologic therapies. Headache. 2017;57(1):109–25.
9. Serrano D, Lipton RB, Scher AI, Reed ML, Stewart WBF, Am A. Fluctuations in episodic and chronic migraine status over the course of 1 year: implications for diagnosis, treatment and clinical trial design. J Headache Pain. 2017;18(1):101.
10. Lipton RB, Diamond S, Reed M, Diamond ML, Stewart WF. Migraine diagnosis and treatment: results from the American Migraine Study II. Headache. 2001;41(7):638–45.
11. Lipton RB, Scher AI, Kolodner K, Liberman J, Steiner TJ, Stewart WF. Migraine in the United States: epidemiology and patterns of health care use. Neurology. 2002;58(6):885–94.
12. Dodick DW. Clinical practice: chronic daily headache [published correction appears in N Engl J Med. 2006;354(8):884]. N Engl J Med. 2006;354(2):158–65.
13. Micieli A, Kingston W. An approach to identifying headache patients that require neuroimaging. Front Public Health. 2019;7:52.
14. Ward TN. Migraine diagnosis and pathophysiology. Continuum. 2012;18(4):753–63.
15. Headache Classification Committee of the International Headache Society (HIS). The international classification of headache disorders, 3rd edition (beta version). Cephalgia. 2013;33(9):629–808.
16. Foxhall K. Migraine: a history [Internet]. Baltimore: Johns Hopkins University Press; 2019.
17. Lipton RB, Silberstein SD. Why study the comorbidity of migraine? Neurology. 1994;44(10 suppl 7):S4YS5.
18. Karsan N, Bose P, Goadsby P. The migraine premonitory phase. Continuum. 2018;24(4):996–1008.
19. Giffin N, Ruggiero L, Lipton R, Silberstein S, Tvedskov J, Olesen J. Premonitory symptoms in migraine: an electronic diary study. Neurology. 2003;60(6):935–40.
20. Cuvellier J, Mars A, Vallée L. The prevalence of premonitory symptoms in paediatric migraine: a questionnaire study in 103 children and adolescents. Cephalalgia. 2009;29(11):1197–201.
21. Karsan N, Prabhakar P, Goadsby P. Premonitory symptoms of migraine in childhood and adolescence. Curr Pain Headache Rep. 2017;21(7):34.
22. Schoonman G, Evers D, Terwindt G, Dijk J, Ferrari M. The prevalence of premonitory symptoms in migraine: a questionnaire study in 461 patients. Cephalalgia. 2006;26(10):1209–13.
23. Wang SJ, Fuh JL, Young YH, Lu SR, Shia BC. Prevalence of migraine in Taipei,Taiwan: a population-based survey. Cephalalgia. 2000;20(6):566–72.
24. Kelman L. The postdrome of the acute migraine attack. Cephalalgia. 2005;26:214–20.
25. Bose P, Karsan N, Goadsby PJ. The migraine postdrome. Continuum. 2018;24(4):1023–31.
26. Jurgens TP, Schulte LH, May A. Migraine trait symptoms in migraine with and without aura. Neurology. 2014;82(16):1416–24.
27. Russel MB, Rasmussen BK, Fenger K, Olesen J. Migraine without aura and migraine with aura are distinct clinical entities: a study of four hundred and eighty-four male and female migraineurs from the general population. Cephalalgia. 1996;16:239–45.
28. Göbel CH, Karstedt SC, Münte TF, Göbel H, Wolfrum S, Lebedeva ER. ICHD-3 is significantly more specific than ICHD-3 beta for diagnosis of migraine with aura and with typical aura. J Headache Pain. 2020;21(1):2.
29. Russell MB, Ducros A. Sporadic and familial hemiplegic migraine: pathophysiological mechanisms, clinical characteristics, diagnosis, and management. Lancet Neurol. 2011;10:457–70.
30. Manzoni GC, Torelli P. Migraine with and without aura: a single entity? Neurol Sci. 2008;29:40–3.
31. Rasmussen BK, Olesen J. Migraine with aura and migraine without aura: an epidemiological study. Cephalalgia. 1992;12(4):221–8.

32. Thomsen LL, Elsebet O, Olesen J, Russell MB. Evidence for a separate type of migraine with aura. Neurology. 2003;60:595–601.
33. Queiroz LP, Friedman DI, Rapoport AM, Purdy RA. Characteristics of migraine visual aura in southern Brazil and northern USA. Cephalalgia. 2011;31:1651.
34. Bolay H, Reuter U, Dunn AK. Intrinsic brain activity triggers trigeminal meningeal afferents in a migraine model. Nat Med. 2002;8:136–42.
35. Fraser CL, Hepschke JL, Jenkikns B, Prasad S. Migraine aura: pathophysiology, mimics, and treatment options. Semin Neurol. 2019;39:739–48.
36. Chen WT, Wang SJ, Fuh JL, Lin CP, Ko YC, Lin YY. Persistent ictal-like visual cortical excitability in chronic migraine. Pain. 2011;152(2):254–8.
37. Yamani N, Chalmer MA, Olesen J. Migraine with brainstem aura: defining the core syndrome. Brain. 2019;142(12):3868–75.
38. Ashina S, Oelsen J, Lipton R. How well does the ICHD 3 (Beta) help in real-life migraine diagnosis and management? Curr Pain Headache Rep. 2016;20(12):66.
39. Grosberg BM, Solomon S, Lipton RB. Retinal migraine. Curr Pain Headache Rep. 2005;9:268–71.
40. Ducros A, Denier C, Joutel A, Cecillion M, Lescoat C, Vahedi K, et al. The clinical spectrum of familial hemiplegic migraine associated with mutations in a neuronal calcium channel. N Engl J Med. 2001;345(1):17–24.
41. Trahan EM, Mercado JM. Familial hemiplegic migraines and baseline neuropsychological testing: a case report. Headache. 2019;59(6):917–23.
42. Lempert T. Vestibular migraine. Semin Neurol. 2013;33:212–8.
43. Natoli J, Manack A, Dean B, Butler Q, Turkel C, Stovner L. Global prevalence of chronic migraine: a systematic review. Cephalalgia. 2010;30(5):599–609.
44. Buse D, Manack A, Serrano D, Reed M, Varon S, Turkel C. Headache impact of chronic and episodic migraine: results from the American Migraine Prevalence and Prevention study. Headache. 2012;52(1):3–17.
45. Charles A. The pathophysiology of migraine: implications for clinical management. Lancet Neurol. 2018;17:174–82.
46. Lipton RB. Chronic migraine, classification, differential diagnosis, and epidemiology. Headache. 2011;51(suppl 2):77–83.
47. Dodick DW, Silberstein SD. Migraine prevention. Pract Neurol. 2007;7(6):383–93.
48. Hindiyeh N, Aurora SK. What the gut can teach us about migraine. Curr Pain Headache Rep. 2015;19(33):33.
49. Irwin S, Barmherzig R, Gelfand A. Recurrent gastrointestinal disturbance: abdominal migraine and cyclic vomiting syndrome. Curr Neurol Neurosci Rep. 2017;17(3):21.

2 Pathophysiology of Migraine Disorder

Bridget Mueller, Natasha Acosta Diaz, and Jihan Grant

Despite migraine being described for thousands of years, the pathophysiology of this disorder is still not completely understood. Migraine is a form of sensory dysfunction, with many manifestations [1, 2]. Migraineurs exhibit photic allodynia and dysfunctional baseline central sensory processing indicating the brain of a migraineur differs from a nonmigraineur even at baseline [3, 4]. Genetics are known to play a part in migraine as there is a statistically higher incidence of migraine amongst first degree relatives and in identical twins with migraine [5]. Studies examining the potential mode of inheritance have been conflicting indicating the etiology of migraine likely stems from a complex interaction between genes and the environment [1]. There is a consistent correlation of migraine with aura with disorders such as familial hemiplegic migraine illustrating the importance of genetics [1]. In addition, environmental triggers such as changes in weather and different food are known to play a significant role in migraine generation. This chapter will review the current knowledge of the pathophysiology of migraine through an examination of the four major phases of a migraine: premonitory, aura, headache, and postdrome.

B. Mueller · J. Grant (✉)
Department of Neurology, Headache Medicine, Mount Sinai Hospital, New York, NY, USA
e-mail: jihan.grant@mssm.edu

N. A. Diaz
Department of Neurology, Pediatric Neurology and Epilepsy, Southeastern Regional Medical Center, Lumberton, NC, USA

© Springer Nature Switzerland AG 2021
S. Shah (ed.), *Migraine*, https://doi.org/10.1007/978-3-030-75239-2_2

Premonitory Phase

The migraine premonitory phase is characterized by nonpainful symptoms affecting arousal, homeostasis, and sensitivity to stimuli that precede the headache or aura phase by up to 72 hours. Prevalence of premonitory symptoms in adult migraineurs ranges from 30% to 90% [6, 7]. The premonitory phase is similarly prevalent in pediatric patients; 42% of migraineurs 4–18 years of age reported a reliable prodrome before headache onset [8]. Aura, baseline anxiety, autonomic symptoms, and a higher migraine burden are significantly associated with the presence of a premonitory phase [8, 9].

While the premonitory phase of migraine was described decades ago, significant challenges have impeded its full characterization [10]. Premonitory symptoms are frequently confused with migraine triggers. Did the piece of chocolate trigger a migraine? Or were food cravings part of a premonitory phase of a migraine already in process? Premonitory symptoms often continue through headache and the other post-ictal phases further obscuring accurate recall [10]. While complicating the establishment of clear temporal relationships, the inter-connectedness of symptoms occurring in the premonitory, aura, and headache phases suggests an underlying shared neural network and provides a framework for studying the pathophysiology of the prodrome [11]. Common premonitory symptoms include fatigue, food cravings, and hypersensitivity to stimuli. Disturbances in homeostatic function (e.g. urination, constipation, nausea) also reliably predict an impending migraine [7, 12]. Understanding the neuroanatomy and neurochemistry involved in the generation of these seemingly disparate symptoms may shed light on the neural networks underlying the premonitory phase.

Sleep

Fatigue and sleep disturbances are common premonitory symptoms [6, 9]. The sleep-wake cycle has been shown to originate in the suprachiasmatic nucleus (SCN), a small region of the hypothalamus [13]. The SCN is synchronized to ambient light through input from photosensitive retinal ganglion cells (ipRGCs) and has been shown to regulate (1) arousal through projections to hypothalamic nuclei involved in the sympathetic nervous system, (2) emotion via communication to the hypothalamic pituitary adrenal (HPA) axis, and (3) appetite through effects on the dorsomedial hypothalamus [14]. The dorsomedial hypothalamus projects to the paraventricular nucleus of the hypothalamus which subsequently modulates activity of the spinal trigeminal nucleus. Therefore this nucleus acts to ingrate signals regulating food intake, sleep, emotion, and trigeminal pain processing [15].

Disturbed sleep cycle and fatigue may also be linked to the headache phase through orexins, neuropeptides released by the hypothalamus that are involved in regulating wakefulness and the sleep wake cycle [16, 17]. Orexinergic projections have been shown to directly activate the locus coeruleus (LC), a nucleus involved in trigeminal pain processing [18]. A functional magnetic resonance imaging (fMRI) study showed increased connectivity between the hypothalamus and locus coeruleus in migraineurs compared to controls interictally [19]. It is unclear if these differences in connectivity develop from repeated migraine attacks, or baseline differences in connectivity that increase vulnerability to develop migraine. The LC also has important connections to centers of pain modulation in the brainstem, including the rostroventral medulla (RVM), ventral tegmental area (VTA), and the periaqueductal gray (PAG) [18]. During sleep, "off" neurons in the PAG and RVM actively inhibit response to sensory input and decrease pain sensation. Conversely, "on" neurons in the PAG and RCM facilitate sensory input from the periphery and are active during waking hours [20]. Therefore a network involving orexins may connect premonitory symptoms involving sleep disturbances and reduced arousal with the painful headache phase of migraine.

Food Cravings

Food cravings and appetite changes are reported by a significant number of migraineurs; estimates range from 10% to 40%. Nearly 25% of migraineurs report that specific foods reliably trigger migraine [7, 11, 21]. Appetite and feeding behavior are controlled by circuitry involving the hypothalamus, the nucleus tractus solitaire (NTS), the ventral tegmental area (VTA) and several brainstem nuclei. Leptin, a hormone influenced by alteration in sleep-wake cycles, stress, and meal timing, acts on the arcuate nucleus to either stimulate or inhibit feeding [22]. The NTS and VTA are connected to the hypothalamus, and are critical to the regulation of appetite. The hypothalamus, NTS, and VTA connect directly with nuclei involved in pain processing, including the periaqueductal grey (PAG), locus coeruleus (LC), and spinal trigeminal nucleus. Further, neurons in the anterior, posterior, ventromedial, and supraoptic hypothalamic nuclei, and paraventricular hypothalamic nuclei have been shown to be activated by noxious dural stimulation [22]. This evidence suggests that crosstalk between the hypothalamus and pain processing regions underlies the relationship between changes in food intake/appetite to generation of pain during the headache phase of migraine.

Hypersensitivity to Sensory Input

In a retrospective questionnaire study completed by 1800 migraineurs, prevalence of photophobia and phonophobia preceding headache by more than 2 hours occurred in approximately 35% of migraineurs. Osmophobia occurred in approximately 25% [11]. In these cases, light, sound, or smell are perceived as unusually intense or unpleasant. Patients with photo- phono- or osmo- phobia preceding migraines are more likely to report these stimuli as migraine triggers [12]. The pathophysiology for this increased sensitivity to stimuli in the premonitory phase is not completely understood, but emerging evidence suggests the thalamus, a major integrator of sensory stimuli, plays an important role [23]. However, it is possible that this hypersensitivity to sensation persists interictally, to some degree, in migraineurs. A Positron Emission Tomography (PET) study showed lower light luminance activated the visual cortex in migraineurs but not controls. This visual cortex activation was further increased by trigeminal pain [24].

Hypersensitivity to Sensory Input

Functional imaging studies have provided direct insight into the neural networks involved in the premonitory stage of migraine. In 2014, a PET study utilizing nitrogylcerine to induce a migraine identified specific brain regions active during the premonitory phase of a migraine. Brain regions showing an increase in blood flow during premonitory symptoms without pain included the hypothalamus, PAG, and cortical areas, including the prefrontal and temporal cortex [25]. The importance of the hypothalamus was again highlighted in a study that used daily fMRIs on a migraineur for 30 days. Imaging captured three spontaneous and untreated migraines. Hypothalamic activation was consistently seen in the 24 hours preceding the headache phase of migraine. During the premonitory phase, the hypothalamus showed high functional connectivity to the spinal trigeminal nucleus. The following day, during the headache phase, hypothalamic connectivity shifted to the dorsal rostral pons, elucidating how alterations in neural connections originating from the hypothalamus may underlie the transition from premonitory symptoms to headache [26].

In conclusion, a neural network with the hypothalamus at the hub, modulating and integrating external stimuli appears to drive the premonitory phase of migraine. Orexogenic efferent pathways appear to link many common premonitory signs with the generation of headache. A greater understanding of the pathophysiology underlying the premonitory phase may lead to the identification of novel targeted therapies to abort migraines before the headache phase.

Aura Phase

Migraine aura has been documented as far back as 400 BCE in excerpts from Hippocrates manuscripts. He wrote, " Most of the time he saw something shining before him like a light, usually in part of the right eye, at the end of a moment a violent pain in the right temple, then in all the head," which is presumed to be aura followed by migraine headache. It is estimated that about 30% of migraineurs experience an aura [1, 27]. Aura is a complex of transient focal neurological features that usually occur before the headache, but may begin after the headache phase has commenced, continue into the headache phase, and may occur in absence of a headache [28, 29]. There are various presentations of aura, which may include visual, sensory, language, or motor symptoms, or a combination of these. The most common presentation, however, is visual aura. The International Classification of Headache Disorders –3 (ICHD-3) delineates that auras develop over 5 minutes or more with each deficit typically lasting 5 to 60 minutes [28]. However, in auras such as motor aura deficits have been known to last longer (up to 72 hours) [2].

Cortical Spreading Depression

Aura correlates with a phenomenon known as cortical spreading depression. In 1941, Karl Lashley mapped his own visual aura as it was progressing and inferred that it was a cortical process propagating at a rate of 2–3 mm/min [30]. In 1944, while studying electroencephalograms of lisencephalic animals, a physiologist known as Aristides Leão noted a phenomenon of neuronal depolarization followed by suppression of activity and gradual recovery which occurred centrifugally at roughly 3 mm/min and could be triggered by protons, electrical stimulation, or mechanical stimulation [31]. Later this phenomenon, termed cortical spreading depression (CSD), was noted to correspond to migraine aura and be the most likely pathophysiological process underlying migraine aura [32, 33]. This correlation was made through blood oxygenation level-dependent (BOLD) functional magnetic resonance imaging studies which showed spreading suppression of initial neuronal activation and increased occipital cortex oxygenation in patients after triggered aura [34]. CSD moves across contiguous parenchyma without respecting the neurovascular boundaries of functional cortex [35].

The initial depolarization of neural and glial membranes corresponds with an increase in cerebral blood flow, which is then followed by CSD and a decrease in blood flow due to decreased metabolic demands of the neurons [33, 36]. CSD leads to the release of protons, nitric oxide, glutamate, eicosanoids, potassium, and adenosine triphosphate (ATP) which may activate meningeal and perivascular nociceptive neurons [37, 38]. Glutamate is particularly important in maintaining a state of neuronal hyperactivity [38]. Activated trigeminovascular neurons cause a sterile inflammatory response leading to the release of substance P, calcitonin gene-related peptide (CGRP), neurokinin A and may also cause oxidative stress of trigeminal afferents triggering pain response [37]. This is evidence that migraine aura may be a trigger for headache or may allow for prolongation of headache. The trigger for CSD in migraineurs is unknown [39]. Interestingly, CSD may also be seen outside of the migraine setting in patients with head trauma, ischemic stroke, and hemorrhage [40].

Hemiplegic Migraine

Hemiplegic migraine is different from other forms of migraine aura in that it includes motor weakness. People with hemiplegic migraine do still experience typical aura (visual, sensory, language disturbances) [28]. Hemiplegic migraine has variable genetic penetrance and mechanisms. There are sporadic forms and there are three known familial forms of familial hemiplegic migraine (FHM) with specific, associated gene mutations. Recent studies, however, support that FHM is likely polymorphic with theses specific gene mutations being genes with high effect size rather than the sole cause of the disorder [41]. Gormerly et al. assessed polygenic risk scores (PRS) from recent genome-wide associated studies and assessed the contribution of common polygenic and rare variation to migraine in a large cohort of 1589 Finnish families with migraine, including FHM subtype. Familial cases had an overall increased risk in PRS compared to population cases and controls [41].

FHM 1 has associated genetic mutations in the CACN A1A gene located at 19p13.1 which encodes a neuronal calcium channel. This is a gain of function mutation and leads to increased calcium presynaptically at the glutaminergic synapses causes increased glutamate release and resultant hyperexcitability and a decreased threshold for cortical spreading depression [42]. FHM 2 is associated with a mutation in ATP1A2 located on chromosome 1q21-q23 that encodes a subunit of a glial sodium/potassium pump. This is a loss of function mutation and causes a decreased sodium electrochemical gradient resulting in a failure of passive astrocyte membrane transporters leading to a decrease in glutamate uptake and increased glutamate leading to a lower threshold for CSD [42]. FHM 3 is associated with mutations in SCN1A located at 2q24 which encodes a neuronal voltage gated sodium channel subunit. This is a gain of function mutation and leads to faster recovery of sodium channels after axonal depolarization, increased action potentials per unit time, and increased glutamate at the synapse leading to hyperexcitability [43]. The FHM mutations linked migraine aura to ionopathies and has resulted in studies of different pharmacological targets attempting to prevent CSD [1, 5].

Headache Phase

The most striking and disabling symptom of a migraine attack for most patients is the headache. The International Headache Society defines migraine headache as unilateral, pulsating, moderate, or severe in intensity, aggravated by routine physical activities and associated with at least two out of three of the following symptoms: nausea, photophobia, and phonophobia [28]. The headache phase typically lasts from 4 hours to up to 72 hours. Migraine duration, however, may be shorter in the pediatric population. Headache phase can vary from person to person and from incident to incident, with some migraine attacks causing mild pain, while others are debilitating [5]. The pathophysiology of migraine incorporates several anatomical locations of brain leading to the complex pattern of dysfunction seen during a migraine attack.

Migraine headache is now viewed as an intricate neurological disorder that affects multiple cortical, subcortical, and brainstem areas that regulate autonomic, affective, cognitive, and sensory functions that account for the pain and the wide constellation of symptoms [44]. The trigeminovascular system has been studied to evaluate the peripheral component of the migraine attack and to possibly identify the mechanism of action of migraine-aborting drugs [45].

Trigeminovascular Pathway

In 1979, Moskowitz and colleagues introduced the trigeminovascular hypothesis of migraine in *The Lancet*, calling attention to the key role of the trigeminal nerve and its vasoactive neuropeptide containing axonal projections to the meninges and its blood vessels [46]. The trigeminovascular pathway conveys nociceptive information from the meninges to the central areas of the brain, and subsequently to the cortex. Nociceptive fibers originating from the trigeminal ganglion innervate the meninges and large cerebral arteries, pial vessels, large venous sinuses, and dura mater [47, 48].

Activation of these structures by mechanical, electrical, or chemical (proinflammatory molecules, blood, or infection) stimulation gives rise to headaches that are remarkably similar to the pain of migraine and its most common associated symptoms: nausea, pulsating pain, photophobia, and phonophobia [48]. The sensory innervation of these structures arises mainly through the ophthalmic branch of the trigeminal nerve (V1) and to a lesser extent through the maxillary (V2) and mandibular (V3) divisions, mainly from unmyelinated C-fibers, and thinly myelinated Aδ-fibers, which have their cell bodies in the trigeminal ganglion in the posterior fossa and are in close proximity to the cervical afferents of the upper cervical dorsal roots at what is termed the trigeminocervical complex (TCC) [48]. Nociceptive activation of the trigeminal fibers is referred to as "trigeminovascular activation." The trigeminal fibers that transmit sensory information from such intracranial structures synapse on second-order neurons within the trigeminocervical complex (TCC; trigeminal nucleus caudalis TNC, C1, and C2 spinal levels) [49]. These trigeminal neurons give rise to the main ascending trigemino-thalamic pathway that relays sensory information to third order neurons, mainly in the contralateral thalamus, before processing the information to higher cortical areas [49]. Thalamic neurons project to the somatosensory cortex, but also to areas of the limbic system. The TNC also has polysynaptic connections to the parasympathetic superior salivatory nucleus (SSN) in the pons. This nucleus runs through the sphenopalatine (pterygopalatine) ganglion via the greater superficial petrosal nerve and innervates meningeal vessels and the contents of the nasal sinuses and eyes [50].

Trigeminal fibers innervating cerebral vessels arise from neurons in the trigeminal ganglion that contain substance P and calcitonin gene-related peptide (CGRP), both of which can be released when the trigeminal ganglion is stimulated [51]. These neuropeptides are thought to play a role in causing and maintaining headache.

Peripheral and Central Sensitization

When activated in the altered molecular environment, peripheral trigeminovascular neurons become sensitized (their response threshold decreases and their response magnitude increases) and they begin to respond to dural stimuli to which they showed minimal or no response at baseline [44]. The pulsating nature of migraine headache and the exacerbation of headache by activities that increase cranial pressure (e.g. walking stairs or coughing) are caused by a process of peripheral sensitization [52].

Another common symptom is cutaneous allodynia (perception of pain when a non-noxious stimulus is applied to normal skin). This is thought to be due to central sensitization of second-order neurons in the trigeminal nucleus caudalis (TNC), which receive input from dura and periorbital skin [52]. Extracephalic allodynia must be mediated by neurons that process sensory information they receive from all levels of the spinal and medullary dorsal horn [53].

Neurogenic Inflammation

Plasma extravasation and vasodilation are both important components of the neurogenic inflammatory response, and substantial additional evidence suggests a role for other signaling markers of inflammation in migraine. Neurogenic inflammation can be evoked experimentally by noxious stimulation of nociceptors that innervate a given tissue and the subsequent release of vasoactive neuropeptides such as substance P, neurokinin A, and CGRP from innervating fibers, and this release of neuropeptides might also occur in extracranial pain sensitive structures [46, 53].

CGRP acts indirectly in the periphery to cause plasma extravasation by allowing for vasodilation and further increasing substance P release (although the relevance of this action is unclear in migraine), and CGRP acts centrally within the trigeminal ganglion, where it may be involved in signaling between trigeminal ganglion neurons [47]. Support for the role of neurogenic inflammation in migraine comes from evidence that plasma protein extravasation and mast cell degranulation can be blocked in the rat by acute migraine drugs, such as ergot alkaloids and triptans, and by non-steroidal anti-inflammatory agents, such as indomethacin and acetylsalicylic acid [53]. Blockade of neurogenic plasma protein extravasation (PPE) is not predictive of antimigraine efficacy in humans, as evidenced by the failure in clinical trials of substance P, neurokinin-1 receptor antagonists, specific PPE blockers, CP122,288 and 4991w93, an endothelin antagonist, a neurosteroid and an inhibitor of the inducible form of nitric oxide synthase (iNOS) [54].

The Hypothalamus

The reciprocal anatomical connections between the hypothalamus and the presence of neurons expressing c-fos in several hypothalamic nuclei after dural stimulation support the role of the hypothalamus in different aspects of migraine [48].

The Thalamus

The thalamus is a nociceptive relay station where inputs from the dura mater as well as cutaneous regions are conveyed through second-order trigeminovascular neurons. It is a central area for the processing and integration of pain stimuli and its connection to a wide variety of cortical areas such as the somatosensory, motor, visual, auditory, olfactory, and limbic regions can explain part of the complexity of migraine features [55].

Processing of vascular nociceptive signals in the thalamus occurs in the ventroposteromedial (VPM) thalamus, medial nucleus of the posterior complex, and in the intralaminar thalamus. Application of capsaicin to the superior sagittal sinus activates trigeminal projections with a high degree of nociceptive input that is processed in neurons, particularly in the VPM thalamus and in its ventral periphery. These neurons in the VPM can be modulated by activation of $GABA_A$ inhibitory receptors, and perhaps of more direct clinical relevance, by propranolol though a β_1-adrenoceptor mechanism [54].

Brainstem

The notion that the periaqueductal gray matter (PAG) is a "migraine generator" has been adopted since the first published report describing delayed migraine-like pain in patients undergoing electrodes implantation near the periaqueductal gray matter and the first imaging study that followed it showing activation of the brainstem in spontaneous migraine. However, evidence supporting the role of PAG as a headache generator is lacking [48].

PAG and other neuromodulator structures, including the rostral ventromedial medulla, locus coeruleus, and raphe nucleus, are primarily involved in modulation of nociception. Imaging studies have shown that PAG is a part of the descendent pathway in high cortical control in pain modulation. PAG has a great role in nociceptive pathways in connections coming from the thalamus, hypothalamus, and autonomic nervous system [56].

The locus coeruleus, the major noradrenergic nucleus, has a critical role in the regulation of cortical function and is known to modulate responses to afferent traffic. Its connections are widely distributed throughout the neocortex. In positron emission tomography (PET) studies investigating acute migraine attacks, activation of an area of the dorsolateral brainstem that includes the locus coeruleus has been shown, although there is some remaining uncertainty regarding the exact anatomical location of this activation because of the limited spatial resolution of PET [54].

Postdrome Phase

The postdrome phase typically occurs after the end of the headache phase. It is defined as the period between the resolution of the headache phase and the patient returning to baseline. The migraine postdrome is the least understood phase of migraine and has not been studied specifically with brain imaging [49]. Even fewer studies have been dedicated to this phase in children and adolescents. It is unknown whether every person with migraine suffers from postdrome.

Migraineurs commonly relate symptoms of the postdrome phase to the medication that successfully abolished their headache, indicating that these symptoms appear or reappear after the headache phase has ended while they seem to play a negligible role during the headache phase. However, a meta-analysis of a clinical trial revealed that postdrome symptoms are seen in the placebo arm most prominently when pain is relieved.

The postdrome, while disabling for many patients, has not been yet defined in the ICHD-3 [57]. Historically, the postdrome phase was referred to in 1872 by Liveing who documented that sleep resolved migraine attacks. Selby also described the postheadache phase as the anticlimactic act of the migraine drama in which pain and nausea has settled down, but patients are left with a difficult to describe prostration and malaise yet typical of migraine. Blau suggested that the postdrome may be due to a slow decline in migraine processes and also hypothesized that it could be the converse process of the premonitory phase [58].

Postdrome symptoms have been reported to impact the ability to work, to affect family interactions and social life, and to cause cognitive impairment [57]. The clinical presentation can include neuropsychiatric, sensory, gastrointestinal, and systemic symptoms. Tiredness, concentration difficulty, and neck stiffness are the most typically reported postdrome symptoms. These symptoms are common and occur in 81–94% of patients. No dominant role appears to exist for comorbidities such as anxiety and depression in the occurrence or absence of the postdrome. The average duration of the postdrome reported in different studies varies from 18 to 25.2 hours [58]. There is some overlap between premonitory symptoms and postdromal symptoms, raising the possibility that the postdromal symptoms have been present throughout the attack but simply overshadowed by headache, nausea, or aura symptoms [59].

Blau proposed that the postdrome might reflect a slow decline in migraine processes and that the diversity of postdrome symptoms could be accounted for by an involvement of the whole brain, notably the frontal lobes and the hypothamus. Thus the multitude of symptoms reported by patients in this phase could be explained by a diffuse cortical and subcortical involvement [60]. Bose et al. have proposed that postdrome symptoms might be explained by widespread vasoconstriction mediated by an alpha2-adrenoreceptor mechanism mediated by activation of the brainstem nuclei, with the locus courules playing a pivotal role in this process [60].

There are few studies regarding postdrome symptoms in the pediatric population. Cuvellier et al. studied 100 children and adolescents, with an age range of 4–17 and a mean age of 10.5 years. Patients reported two groups of symptoms occurring during the resolution phase of the headache: symptoms with onset before headache cessation that persisted after it (persistent symptoms), and symptoms with onset after headache cessation (true postdromes). Nearly 91% of patients reported persistent symptoms (asthenia, pallor, cognitive difficulties, anorexia, somnolence, and nausea). True postdromes were reported by 82% of patients (thirst, somnolence, visual disturbances, food craving, paraesthesias, and ocular pain [60]. Griffin et al. conducted a prospective study over 3 months, using electronic diaries. Nonheadache symptoms before, during, and after headache were collected on a daily basis. Visual analogue scales were used to capture the overall level of functioning and the severity of the headache. Of 120 evaluable patients, 97 (81%) reported at least one nonheadache symptom in the postdrome. Postdrome symptoms, in order of frequency, included feeling tired/weary and having difficulty concentrating and stiff neck [61]. Keiman studied 827 consecutives headache clinic patients. Postdrome frequency, duration, and characteristics were analyzed. Nearly 68% of 827 patients reported postdrome with an average of 25.2 hours. The most common symptoms were tiredness (71.8%), head pain (33.1%), cognitive difficulties (11.7%), 'hangover' (10.7%), gastrointestinal symptoms (8.4%), mood change (6.8%), and weakness (6.2%). Compared with patients who do not experience postdrome, patients with postdrome have more characteristic and more frequent migraine features [62]. Further research is needed to better characterize the postdrome as well as to offer solutions that may limit the disability it can cause.

Conclusion

Migraine disorder is a complex sensory dysfunction incorporating several areas of the brain and the peripheral nervous system with strong genetic and environmental involvement. It is a common and potentially disabling disorder throughout each of its stages. The premonitory, aura, headache, and postdrome phases all have the capacity to negatively impact a migraineur's function, although all phases are not always present. In addition, migraineurs have been observed to also have interictal hypersensitivity and sensory dysfunction compared to nonmigraineurs.

Despite many years of investigation and major advances in our understanding, the complete pathophysiology of migraine remains an enigma. This incomplete understanding of the pathophysiology has made it a particularly hard disorder to treat. However, with each advancement in our understanding, new potential treatment targets arise, which illustrates the utmost importance of continued research in the subject matter.

References

1. Pathophysiology and Genetics of Migraine. Headache. p. 88–99.
2. Goadsby PJ, Holland PR, Martins-Oliveira M, Hoffmann J, Schankin C, Akerman S. Pathophysiology of migraine: a disorder of sensory processing. Physiol Rev. 2017;97(2):553–622.
3. Kim JH, Kim S, Suh SI, Koh SB, Park KW, Oh K. Interictal metabolic changes in episodic migraine: a voxel-based FDG-PET study. Cephalalgia. 2010;30(1):53–61.
4. Vanagaite J, Pareja JA, Støren O, White LR, Sanc T, Stovner LJ. Light-induced discomfort and pain in migraine. Cephalalgia. 1997;17(7):733–41.
5. Goadsby PJ, Holland PR. An update: pathophysiology of migraine. Neurol Clin. 2019;37(4):651–71.
6. Becker WJ. The premonitory phase of migraine and migraine management. Cephalalgia. 2013;33(13):1117–21.
7. Giffin NJ, Ruggiero L, Lipton RB, Silberstein SD, Tvedskov JF, Olesen J, et al. Premonitory symptoms in migraine: an electronic diary study. Neurology. 2003;60(6):935–40.
8. Jacobs H, Pakalnis A. Premonitory symptoms in episodic and chronic migraine from a pediatric headache clinic. Pediatr Neurol. 2019;97:26–9.
9. Kelman L. The premonitory symptoms (prodrome): a tertiary care study of 893 migraineurs. Headache. 2004;44(9):865–72.
10. Lipton RB, Pavlovic JM, Haut SR, Grosberg BM, Buse DC. Methodological issues in studying trigger factors and premonitory features of migraine. Headache. 2014;54(10):1661–9.
11. Schulte LH, Jurgens TP, May A. Photo-, osmo- and phonophobia in the premonitory phase of migraine: mistaking symptoms for triggers? J Headache Pain. 2015;16:14.
12. Karsan N, Bose P, Goadsby PJ. The migraine premonitory phase. Continuum (Minneap Minn). 2018;24(4, Headache):996–1008.
13. Watts AG, Swanson LW. Efferent projections of the suprachiasmatic nucleus: II. Studies using retrograde transport of fluorescent dyes and simultaneous peptide immunohistochemistry in the rat. J Comp Neurol. 1987;258(2):230–52.
14. Zhang C, Truong KK, Zhou QY. Efferent projections of prokineticin 2 expressing neurons in the mouse suprachiasmatic nucleus. PLoS One. 2009;4(9):e7151.
15. Robert C, Bourgeais L, Arreto CD, Condes-Lara M, Noseda R, Jay T, et al. Paraventricular hypothalamic regulation of trigeminovascular mechanisms involved in headaches. J Neurosci. 2013;33(20):8827–40.
16. Zurak N. Role of the suprachiasmatic nucleus in the pathogenesis of migraine attacks. Cephalalgia. 1997;17(7):723–8.
17. Cai XJ, Evans ML, Lister CA, Leslie RA, Arch JR, Wilson S, et al. Hypoglycemia activates orexin neurons and selectively increases hypothalamic orexin-B levels: responses inhibited by feeding and possibly mediated by the nucleus of the solitary tract. Diabetes. 2001;50(1):105–12.
18. Jahangirvand M, Yazdi F, Moradi M, Haghparast A. Intra-accumbal orexin-1 receptors are involved in antinociception induced by stimulation of the lateral hypothalamus in the formalin test as an animal model of persistent inflammatory pain. Iran J Pharm Res. 2016;15(4):851–9.
19. Moulton EA, Becerra L, Johnson A, Burstein R, Borsook D. Altered hypothalamic functional connectivity with autonomic circuits and the locus coeruleus in migraine. PLoS One. 2014;9(4):e95508.
20. Mason P. Ventromedial medulla: pain modulation and beyond. J Comp Neurol. 2005;493(1):2–8.
21. Waelkens J. Warning symptoms in migraine: characteristics and therapeutic implications. Cephalalgia. 1985;5(4):223–8.
22. Benjamin L, Levy MJ, Lasalandra MP, Knight YE, Akerman S, Classey JD, et al. Hypothalamic activation after stimulation of the superior sagittal sinus in the cat: a Fos study. Neurobiol Dis. 2004;16(3):500–5.
23. Okamoto K, Tashiro A, Chang Z, Bereiter DA. Bright light activates a trigeminal nociceptive pathway. Pain. 2010;149(2):235–42.

24. Boulloche N, Denuelle M, Payoux P, Fabre N, Trotter Y, Geraud G. Photophobia in migraine: an interictal PET study of cortical hyperexcitability and its modulation by pain. J Neurol Neurosurg Psychiatry. 2010;81(9):978–84.
25. Maniyar FH, Sprenger T, Monteith T, Schankin C, Goadsby PJ. Brain activations in the premonitory phase of nitroglycerin-triggered migraine attacks. Brain. 2014;137(Pt 1): 232–41.
26. Schulte LH, May A. The migraine generator revisited: continuous scanning of the migraine cycle over 30 days and three spontaneous attacks. Brain. 2016;139(Pt 7):1987–93.
27. Manzoni GC, Stovner LJ. Epidemiology of headache. Handb Clin Neurol. 2010;97:3–22.
28. Headache Classification Committee of the International Headache Society (IHS) The International Classification of Headache Disorders, 3rd edition. Cephalalgia. 2018;38(1):1–211.
29. Olesen J, Friberg L, Olsen TS, Iversen HK, Lassen NA, Andersen AR, et al. Timing and topography of cerebral blood flow, aura, and headache during migraine attacks. Ann Neurol. 1990;28(6):791–8.
30. Lashley KS. Patterns of cerebral integration indicated by the scotomas of migraine. Arch Neurol Psychiatr. 1941;46(2):331–9.
31. Leao AA. Spreading depression of activity in the cerebral cortex. J Neurophysiol. 1944;7(6):359–90.
32. Tfelt-Hansen PC. History of migraine with aura and cortical spreading depression from 1941 and onwards. Cephalalgia. 2009;30(7):780–92.
33. Lauritzen M. Pathophysiology of the migraine aura: the spreading depression theory. Brain. 1994;117(1):199–210.
34. Cao Y, Welch KM, Aurora S, Vikingstad EM. Functional MRI-BOLD of visually triggered headache in patients with migraine. Arch Neurol. 1999;56(5):548–54.
35. Lauritzen M, Olesen J. Regional cerebral blood flow during migraine attacks by Xenon-133 inhalation and emission tomography. Brain. 1984;107(Pt 2):447–61.
36. Hadjikhani N, Sanchez Del Rio M, Wu O, Schwartz D, Bakker D, Fischl B, et al. Mechanisms of migraine aura revealed by functional MRI in human visual cortex. Proc Natl Acad Sci U S A. 2001;98(8):4687–92.
37. Bolay H, Reuter U, Dunn AK, Huang Z, Boas DA, Moskowitz MA. Intrinsic brain activity triggers trigeminal meningeal afferents in a migraine model. Nat Med. 2002;8(2):136–42.
38. Dodick DW, Silberstein SD. Migraine. Migraine pathogenesis. Oxford University Press; New York, NY, 2016.
39. DeLange JM, Cutrer FM. Our evolving understanding of migraine with aura. Curr Pain Headache Rep. 2014;18(10):453.
40. Hartings JA, Watanabe T, Bullock MR, Okonkwo DO, Fabricius M, Woitzik J, et al. Spreading depolarizations have prolonged direct current shifts and are associated with poor outcome in brain trauma. Brain. 2011;134(Pt 5):1529–40.
41. Gormley P, Kurki MI, Hiekkala ME, Veerapen K, Happola P, Mitchell AA, et al. Common variant burden contributes to the familial aggregation of migraine in 1,589 families. Neuron. 2018;99(5):1098.
42. Moskowitz MA, Bolay H, Dalkara T. Deciphering migraine mechanisms: clues from familial hemiplegic migraine genotypes. Ann Neurol. 2004;55(2):276–80.
43. Dichgans M, Freilinger T, Eckstein G, Babini E, Lorenz-Depiereux B, Biskup S, et al. Mutation in the neuronal voltage-gated sodium channel SCN1A in familial hemiplegic migraine. Lancet. 2005;366(9483):371–7.
44. Burstein R, Noseda R, Borsook D. Migraine: multiple processes, complex pathophysiology. J Neurosci. 2015;35(17):6619–29.
45. Buzzi MG, Moskowitz MA. The pathophysiology of migraine: year 2005. J Headache Pain. 2005;6(3):105–11.
46. Ashina M, Hansen JM, Do TP, Melo-Carrillo A, Burstein R, Moskowitz MA. Migraine and the trigeminovascular system-40 years and counting. Lancet Neurol. 2019;18(8):795–804.

47. Dodick DW. A phase-by-phase review of migraine pathophysiology. Headache. 2018;58(S1):4–16.
48. Noseda R, Burstein R. Migraine pathophysiology: anatomy of the trigeminovascular pathway and associated neurological symptoms, cortical spreading depression, sensitization, and modulation of pain. Pain. 2013;154(Suppl 1):S44–53.
49. Andreou AP, Edvinsson L. Mechanisms of migraine as a chronic evolutive condition. J Headache Pain. 2019;20(1):117.
50. Ward TN. Migraine diagnosis and pathophysiology. Continuum (Minneap Minn). 2012;18(4):753–63.
51. Goadsby PJ. Pathophysiology of migraine. Ann Indian Acad Neurol. 2012;15(Suppl 1):S15–22.
52. Silberstein SD. Migraine pathophysiology and its clinical implications. Cephalalgia. 2004;24(Suppl 2):2–7.
53. Bernstein C, Burstein R. Sensitization of the trigeminovascular pathway: perspective and implications to migraine pathophysiology. J Clin Neurol (Seoul, Korea). 2012;8(2):89–99.
54. Sprenger T, Goadsby PJ. Migraine pathogenesis and state of pharmacological treatment options. BMC Med. 2009;7:71.
55. Puledda F, Messina R, Goadsby PJ. An update on migraine: current understanding and future directions. J Neurol. 2017;264(9):2031–9.
56. Boran HE, Bolay H. Pathophysiology of migraine. Noro Psikiyatr Ars. 2013;50(Suppl 1):S1–7.
57. Ng-Mak DS, Fitzgerald KA, Norquist JM, Banderas BF, Nelsen LM, Evans CJ, et al. Key concepts of migraine postdrome: a qualitative study to develop a post-migraine questionnaire. Headache. 2011;51(1):105–17.
58. Bose P, Goadsby PJ. The migraine postdrome. Curr Opin Neurol. 2016;29(3):299–301.
59. Charles A. The evolution of a migraine attack – a review of recent evidence. Headache. 2013;53(2):413–9.
60. Cuvellier JC. Pediatric vs. adult Prodrome and postdrome: a window on migraine pathophysiology? Front Neurol. 2019;10:199.
61. Giffin NJ, Lipton RB, Silberstein SD, Olesen J, Goadsby PJ. The migraine postdrome: an electronic diary study. Neurology. 2016;87(3):309–13.
62. Kelman L. The postdrome of the acute migraine attack. Cephalalgia. 2006;26(2):214–20.

3 Acute Migraine Interventions and Evidence

Jennifer Wu, Pranamya Suri, Danielle Perret Karimi, and Bi-Ying Yeh

The history of migraine and its treatment is nearly as old as the history of the written word, with the first descriptions of migraine headache documented nearly 6000 years ago [1]. Caffeine has been recommended for headache treatment for several hundred years and, likely, represents the initial advance in mechanistic headache therapy [2]. Later, novel applications of ergotamine for acute migraine treatment in the twentieth century would lay the groundwork in identifying the serotonergic pathway underlying migraine pathophysiology and lead to the subsequent discovery of triptans for migraine-specific abortive therapy. In the modern era, a multitude of medications targeting multiple pathways are available for acute migraine treatment [3]. Although substantial evidence supports the use of many migraine medications, individual response to treatment is idiosyncratic, with results varying with respect to severity, symptomatology, onset, duration, and differences in drug metabolism. Tailoring of acute migraine treatment is then further complicated by medical comorbidities and related contraindications to specific pharmacotherapy. The following chapter provides an overview of the major classes of acute migraine pharmacotherapy, including a discussion of the indications, limitations, and contraindications for specific agents. Although the discussion is not comprehensive, there is a deliberate emphasis on the most frequently prescribed and recommended medications, while highlighting seminal advances in acute migraine management.

J. Wu
Department of Physical Medicine and Rehabilitation, University of California Irvine Health, Orange, CA, USA

Department of Pediatric Rehabilitation, Spaulding Rehabilitation Hospital, Boston, MA, USA

P. Suri · D. P. Karimi (✉) · B.-Y. Yeh
Department of Physical Medicine and Rehabilitation, University of California Irvine Health, Orange, CA, USA
e-mail: dperret@hs.uci.edu

© Springer Nature Switzerland AG 2021

S. Shah (ed.), *Migraine*, https://doi.org/10.1007/978-3-030-75239-2_3

Abortive Therapy

NSAIDs and Acetaminophen

Non-steroidal anti-inflammatory drugs (NSAIDs) are a drug class which include common over-the-counter (i.e., aspirin, ibuprofen, and naproxen) and prescription medications. NSAIDs are inhibitors of cyclooxygenase (COX) enzymes involved in biochemical pathways for inflammation and blood clotting. In the context of human physiology, COX-1 enzymes are involved in the maintenance and protection of the gastrointestinal system, while COX-2 enzymes are responsible for regulation of inflammation and pain and also involved in the suppression of thromboxane. All NSAIDs lie on a spectrum from COX-1 selective, COX-2 selective, to COX non-selective, with COX-specific selectivity having significant implications on adverse effect profiles. Given their predilection for the gastrointestinal system, selective COX-1 inhibitors are associated with a higher risk for gastrointestinal bleeding. Conversely, disproportionate activity of selective COX-2 inhibitors within blood vessels results in decreased risk of gastrointestinal bleeding, but a higher risk for cardiovascular side effects and stroke due to thrombosis [4]. Frequent or high-dose NSAID use also has a risk of renal injury, especially in individuals with advanced age, chronic kidney disease, co-prescription of nephrotoxic medications, and volume depletion [5].

While previously considered to only act within the central nervous system, recent studies demonstrate acetaminophen (also known as paracetamol, APAP, or N-acetyl-para-aminophenol) to be both a centrally- and peripherally-acting analgesic. As with NSAIDs, acetaminophen demonstrates activity on both COX-1 and COX-2 enzymes, with a slight predominance of COX-2 activity. Additionally, acetaminophen is shown to stimulate descending serotoninergic pathways in the brain responsible for modulating pain, as well as to exert an indirect stimulatory activity on the endogenous cannabinoid system of the brain and spinal cord [6].

Acetaminophen is considered an extremely safe medication under normal circumstances, with a wide therapeutic window up to 4 grams per day. Since its clinical introduction in the United States as Tylenol in 1950, acetaminophen is the most common treatment of pain and fever in the western world and is listed among the World Health Organization's essential medications [7]. It can be safely used in adults with conditions such as renal disease, cardiovascular disease, and gastrointestinal disorders that prevent them from using NSAIDs. It is safe during pregnancy, with breastfeeding, and in children. It is also safe for use by people with liver disease when given in adjusted doses.

Unfortunately, due to widespread prevalence of acetaminophen, overdose is relatively common and can lead to liver failure [8]. A common scenario leading to unintentional overdose results from co-administration of multiple acetaminophen-containing medications; for example, a combination of acetaminophen-hydrocodone for pain with cold medication that also contains acetaminophen. In order to protect consumers, the Food and Drug Administration now requires all manufacturers to include clear labeling on acetaminophen-containing products and have limited acetaminophen dosage in combination drugs to 325 mg per dose [9].

There is a substantive literature supporting the use of nonsteroidal anti-inflammatory drugs (NSAIDs) for abortive therapy in mild-to-moderate acute migraine [2, 10]. Specifically, ibuprofen, acetylsalicylic acid (ASA), naproxen sodium, and diclofenac potassium represent the core placebo-controlled evidence demonstrating NSAID efficacy for acute migraine treatment [11–14]. In patients with contraindications to NSAID use, acetaminophen has demonstrated similar efficacy for acute migraine treatment in both placebo-controlled studies and comparative studies against NSAIDs [15, 16]. Dose-finding studies generally report a dose-dependent effect with greater benefit from higher doses and with combination therapy [11, 16–18].

Pharmacokinetic differences across the group (Table 3.1), particularly with respect to differing available formulations, have implications for efficacy, onset, and indication in any specific patient. Ibuprofen and diclofenac potassium have special formulations for rapid absorption with demonstrated faster efficacy compared to standard oral tablet formulations [17, 19]. Similarly, effervescent ASA also

Table 3.1 Pharmacokinetics of NSAIDs in acute migraine treatment

Drug	Recommended dosing	Repeat interval	Onset to efficacy	Half-life (hrs)	Max daily dose (mg)
ASA	PO: 320–1000 mg	4 to 6 hrs	Nonenteric-coated: 60 min Enteric-coated: 3–4 hrs	Low dose (300–600 mg): 3 hrs High dose (1000 mg): 5 to 6 hrs	4000 mg
Ibuprofen	PO: 200–800 mg IV: 400–800 mg	PO: 6–8 hrs IV: 6 hrs	PO: 30–60 min IV: 60 min	PO: 2 hrs IV: 2 hrs	PO: 3200 mg IV: 3200 mg
Naproxen sodium	PO: 250–500[a] mg	6–8 hrs	30–60 min	12–17 hrs	1250 mg
Diclofenac potassium	PO solution: 50 mg powder	Not applicable, recommended for single dosing only	15 min	2 hours	100 mg
Ketorolac	IM: 60 mg as a single dose or 30 mg every 6 hrs IV: 30 mg as a single dose or 30 mg every 6 hrs PO: 10–20 mg	IM: 6 hrs IV: 6 hrs PO: 4–6 hrs	IM: 30 min IV: 30 min PO: 30–60 min	2–9 hrs	IM: 120 mg IV: 120 mg PO: 40 mg
Acetaminophen	PO: 325–650 mg	4–6 hrs	60 min	2–3 hrs	4000 mg

Data from Refs. [2, 10, 159–169]

Abbreviations: *ASA*acetylsalicylic acid, *PO* by mouth or orally, *IM* intramuscularly, *IV* intravenously, *hrs* hours, *min* minutes, *mg* milligrams

[a]Recommended loading dose for naproxen sodium is 750 mg

demonstrated faster absorption compared to regular tablets [20]. While mostly limited to use in emergency room settings, parenteral NSAIDs, including ASA and ketorolac, have been shown to be highly effective in acute migraine treatment [21, 22]. Some studies report parenteral NSAIDs to be more effective and better tolerated than subcutaneous sumatriptan [23], the gold standard of acute migraine treatment. NSAIDs are generally safe and well tolerated, with some practice guidelines recommending initiation of all acute migraine algorithms with NSAIDs for first line treatment [24]. However, high dose and repeated NSAID use in migraine is typically limited, particularly for patients with renal disease and in certain trimesters of pregnancy [25].

Triptans

Serotonin (5-HT) was first identified as a potential target for migraine therapy in the 1960s, with subsequent drug development yielding the triptans as the first targeted drug class for migraine treatment. Triptans are agonists of serotonin 5-HT_{1B} 5-HT_{1D}, and 5-HT_{1F} receptors in the central nervous tissue and overlying meningeal vessels, resulting in vasoconstriction and inhibition of pro-inflammatory neuropeptides release [26]. Specifically, triptans relieve migraine symptoms by binding to 1B and 1D receptors within the vessels of the central nervous system and 1F receptors within the cranial nerves and nervous system peripherally [27]; unfortunately, the presence of 1B and 1D receptors within both coronary and extremity arteries is currently believed to be the cause of the primary triptan side effects (stroke, arrhythmia, myocardial infarction, Raynaud phenomenon) and has led to the introduction of a 1F selective agonist Lasmiditan classified as the first "ditan" medication [28], which will be discussed separately.

In 1992, Sumatriptan was the first triptan to gain FDA approval for treatment of acute migraine. It continues to be the most widely prescribed within the class. The initial large-scale randomized, placebo-controlled studies were performed in thousands of patients across four continents and reported excellent efficacy in the treatment of acute migraine [29]. In patients presenting to hospitals, specialist headache clinics, and in general practitioners' clinics with acute migraine symptoms resulting in functional impairment, subcutaneously delivered sumatriptan was found to substantially decrease or completely relieve headache intensity and improve symptoms of clinical disability [30, 31]. Similar results were noted for orally-dosed sumatriptan [32]. Dose-ranging studies reported an overall dose-dependent effect for both therapeutic benefit and development of adverse events, with maximum therapeutic benefit and minimal adverse effects noted at a 6 mg dose given subcutaneously [33] and a 100 mg dose given orally [34]. Pharmacokinetic studies comparing subcutaneous and oral sumatriptan formulations reported significantly higher bioavailability following subcutaneous [96%] compared to oral [14%] administration [35]. These differences may underlie results from comparative studies demonstrating greater headache relief, increased improvement of clinical disability, and superior alleviation of secondary symptoms such as nausea, photophobia, and phonophobia with subcutaneous compared to oral sumatriptan [36]. For the approximately 50% of patients with incomplete relief after a single oral or subcutaneous dose, studies on multiple-dose regimens found that, although repeat dosing was not effective at preventing or delaying headache recurrence, repeat dosing was both well tolerated and highly effective for treating headache recurrence [37, 38]. In cross-over studies comparing sumatriptan and NSAIDs, sumatriptan was routinely found to outperform NSAIDs for acute migraine relief, while dual therapy in which sumatriptan was combined with an NSAID was superior to sumatriptan monotherapy [39, 40]. More recent studies also detail promising results with intranasal [41] and transdermal delivery systems [42].

Following sumatriptan, the FDA has since approved six additional triptans for the treatment of acute migraine: zolmitriptan, naratriptan, rizatriptan, almotriptan, frovatriptan, and eletriptan. Although the seven triptans differ with respect to dosing and formulations (Table 3.2), multiple randomized controlled studies have demonstrated good efficacy of all seven FDA-approved triptans in placebo-controlled

Table 3.2 Formulations and recommended dosing of tripans

Triptan	Brand name	Year of FDA approval	Route of administration	Formulations	Repeat interval	Daily maximum dose (mg)
Sumatriptan	Imitrex Imigran Onzetra Xsail Sumavel Zembrace	1992	PO Nasal (0.1 mL) SC (0.5 mL) PO Nasal powder Nasal powder SC SC	PO 25, 50, 100 mg Nasal: 5, 20 mg SC: 4, 6 mg 50, 100 mg 11 mg 11 mg 6 mg/0.5 mL 3 mg/0.5 mL	PO: 2 hrs Nasal: 2 hrs SC: 1 hr. 2 hrs 2 hrs 2 hrs 1 hr. 1 hr	PO: 200 Nasal: 40 SC: 12 mg 200 mg 44 mg 44 mg 12 mg 12 mg
Zolmitriptan	Zomig Zomig ZMT	1997	PO Nasal (0.1 mL) ODT	PO: 2.5, 5 mg Nasal: 2.5, 5 mg 2.5, 5 mg	2 hrs	10 mg
Naratriptan	Amerge Naramig	1998	PO	Amerge: 1, 2.5 mg Naramig: 2.5 mg	2 hrs	5 mg
Rizatriptan	Maxalt Maxalt MLT	1998	PO ODT	5, 10 mg 5, 10 mg	2 hrs	30 mg
Almotriptan	Axert Almogran	2001	PO	6.25, 12.5 mg	2 hrs	25 mg
Frovatriptan	Frova Forvey	2001	PO	2.5 mg	2 hrs	7.5 mg
Eletriptan	Relplax	2002	PO	20, 40, 80 mg	2 hrs	80 mg

Data from Refs. [26, 170]

Abbreviations: *PO* by mouth or orally, *ODT* orally disintegrating tablet, *mL* milliliters, *SC* subcutaneous injection, *hr.(s)* hour(s), *mg* milligram studies for the treatment of acute migraine [43–48]. Differences in pharmacokinetics across the triptan class largely underlie differences in efficacy and adverse effect profiles with medications demonstrating greater efficaciousness (improved 2 hour headache relief and/or higher rates of 2 hour pain free response) also demonstrating higher rates of adverse events (Table 3.3). Comparative studies have shown zolmitriptan and almotriptan perform similarly to sumatriptan with respect to efficacy [46, 49]. Interestingly, despite similar reported rates of efficacy for sumatriptan and almotriptan, one study found that in a group of patients with history of poor response to sumatriptan, a single dose of almotriptan demonstrated statistically significant benefit in these sumatriptan non-responsive patients [50]. Poor or unsatisfactory response to one triptan, therefore, does not exclude therapeutic benefit with other drugs in the class. Across triptans, meta-analyses of multiple clinical trials evaluating the relative efficacy of all triptans found eletriptan to consistently result in the highest treatment effect estimates followed by rizatriptan and zomitriptan [26]. Although efficacy estimates for frovatriptan are only slightly superior to those reported for sumatriptan [47], frovatriptan has a significantly longer plasma half-life compared to other triptans at 26 hours. As a result, treatment with frovatriptan has been shown to result in the lowest headache recurrence rate of all triptans and is likely best suited for patients with long-lasting attacks [51]. Conversely, the rapid onset of rizatriptan makes it a better option for severe, but short-lasting attacks [52].

Table 3.3 Pharmacokinetics, efficacy, and rates of adverse events across triptans

Triptan	Onset to efficacy	Bio-availability	% Improved at 2 hrs	% Pain free at 2 hrs	Half-Life	% reporting adverse effects
Sumatriptan	PO: 30–60 min SC: 10 min Nasal: 10–15 min	14%	PO: 56–61% SC: 70–79% Nasal: 48–61%	PO, mild: 46–58% PO, mod-sev: 25–32% SC: 49–59% Nasal: 4–32%	2 hrs	PO, mild: 16–19% PO, mod-sev: 32–43% SC: 44–71% Nasal: 38%
Zolmitriptan	PO: 30–60 min Nasal: 10–15 min	40–48%	PO: 27–71% Nasal: 60–65%	9–39%	2–3 hrs	15–75%
Naratriptan	1–3 hrs	63–73%	52–69%	19–33%	6 hrs	18–37%
Rizatriptan	30–60 min	45%	48–77%	26–67%	2–3 hrs	29%
Almotriptan	30–60 min	80%	50–80%	20–50% 28–39%	3–4 hrs	23%
Frovatriptan	2–4 hrs	24–30%	36–46%	9–15%	25 hrs	38–41%
Eletriptan	30–60 min	50%	54–77%	25–37%	4 hrs	35–60%

Data from Refs. [26, 44, 171–177]

Abbreviations: *PO* by mouth or orally, *SC* subcutaneous injection; min, minutes, *hr.(s)* hour(s), *mild* patients with mild migraine symptoms, *mod-sev* patients with moderate to severe migraine symptoms

Additional Indications for Triptans

Triptans have demonstrated efficacy for multiple headache types, including migranous and episodic tension-type headaches [53]. Furthermore, despite manufacturer packaging warnings against triptan use for the treatment of hemiplegic migraine, limited studies have reported that potential triptan-related cerebral vasoconstriction not only does not worsen symptoms but actually demonstrates efficacy for amelioration of symptoms for these uncommon forms of migraine with aura [54, 55]. Similarly, triptans also demonstrate benefit in the treatment of basilar-type migraines with minimal adverse effects [56]. Finally, a short course of frovatriptan and zolmitriptan have proven indications in the prophylactic treatment of perimenstrual migraines [57, 58].

Of note, although triptan therapy has demonstrated excellent efficacy in the treatment of migraine with and without aura, the literature remains unclear on the benefit of timing triptan therapy during the aura phase [59]. At minimum, triptan therapy regardless of timing with respect to aura has not been shown to prolong aura, but studies evaluating triptan therapy during aura for preemptive development of headache report mixed results [60, 61].

Adverse Events and Risks of Triptan Therapy

Overall, triptans demonstrate excellent tolerability. Multiple studies report similar rates of adverse events between naratriptan, eletriptan, and placebo [48, 62, 63]. Almotriptan and frovatriptan also demonstrate lower rates of adverse events compared to sumatriptan [64], while rates of adverse events are slightly higher with rizatriptan and zolmitriptan [65, 66]. In general, all triptans demonstrate a dose-responsive relationship with higher relative medication doses demonstrating higher rates of adverse events [67]. CNS effects, including dizziness, somnolence, sedation, and drowsiness, are the most commonly cited adverse events and have been reported in up to 15% of patients [37]. Notably, a weak correlation is noted between lipophilicity and rates of CNS adverse events, with more lipophilic agents, like eletriptan and naratriptan, demonstrating slightly higher rates of CNS adverse events compared to less lipophilic triptans [68]. Across the group, oral formulations are more likely to be associated with transient gastrointestinal distress [49, 69], while intranasal formulations have been associated with dysgeusia [41, 70] and subcutaneous administration with injection site reaction [30].

Coronary and thoracic symptoms are among the most serious adverse events associated with triptan therapy. Although generally uncommon [66, 71–73], the most frequent manifestation of coronary and thoracic symptoms reported by patients include chest tightness, heaviness, pain, or pressure. Patients typically report these symptoms as mild and transient, and accordingly, chest symptoms due to triptan therapy have not been associated with electrocardiographic changes [74]. A consensus statement by the American Headache Society found chest symptoms related to triptan therapy were unlikely due to a cardiovascular or ischemic etiology in patients without concurrent coronary artery disease [75]. However, in patients with coronary artery disease, there have been cases of serious cardiovascular events, some resulting in death, associated with triptan therapy [76]. Cardiovascular events are likely the result of coronary vasospasm as triptans have been shown to cause contraction in isolated human coronary arteries in in vitro studies [77]. While in vitro studies demonstrate that these effects occur only at high plasma concentrations that are unlikely to occur at typical dosing regimens, pretreatment cardiac evaluation is recommended prior to initiating triptan therapy in patients with known coronary risk factors [75]. Furthermore, practitioners should consider the selection of triptans, such as frovatriptan, with known greater cerebrovascular selectivity and concordant lower reported rates of coronary complication, for patients with significant coronary risk factors that are contemplating triptan use [78].

Serotonin syndrome resulting from triptan use in combination with selective serotonin reuptake inhibitor (SSRI) or serotonin-norepinephrine reuptake inhibitor (SNRI) treatment is another potentially life-threatening adverse event associated with triptan treatment [79]. Following multiple case reports reporting serotonin syndrome in patients treated simultaneously with both a triptan and either an SSRI or SNRI, the FDA issued an alert in 2006 recommending patients to be informed of a potential risk for serotonin syndrome with cotreatment [80]. Subsequent reviews of the alert and the associated case studies, however, found insufficient evidence to demonstrate a relationship between cotreatment and increased risk of serotonin syndrome [81]. As a result, the American Headache Society released a position paper in 2010 reporting inadequate evidence to support limiting triptan use in combination with SSRI/SNRI monotherapy [82].

Triptan Therapy in Pregnancy

There are limited studies evaluating the risk of birth defects associated with triptan therapy during pregnancy. Large scale database studies in pregnant women and their resultant children have largely ruled out a significant increase in overall birth defects associated with triptan therapy, particularly during the first trimester [83, 84]. However, triptan use during the second and third trimester has been associated with a statistically significant increase in associated atonic uterus with significant blood loss during labor [85]. Overall, for women in whom migraine is not responsive to other treatments, the benefits of triptan use may outweigh the risks with adequate counseling and appropriate prenatal care.

Ergot Alkaloids

Ergot-containing fungi have been described in the medical literature for headache treatment since the late nineteenth century [86]. Subsequent advancements in modern pharmacology led to isolation of pure ergot compounds in the 1910s and the introduction of ergot alkaloids, including ergotamine and dihydroergotamine. In acute migraine treatment, ergots demonstrate affinity for a variety of noradrenergic, dopaminergic, and serotonergic receptors. Given this breadth of activity, they often have global effects that are hard to isolate, but which have been shown to inhibit the neurogenic inflammatory cascade involved in migraine pathophysiology [87].

Ergot alkaloids were the mainstay of treatment for moderate-to-severe acute migraine since their use was first documented in the 1920s [88], but have largely been replaced by triptans since the 1990s [30, 31]. Both oral and inhaled ergot alkaloids have demonstrated variable efficacy in randomized controlled trials with some studies demonstrating superiority against placebo [89, 90], while other studies reported non-superiority versus placebo [91]. Some comparative studies found oral ergotamine to demonstrate equivalency or even superiority compared to aspirin and other NSAIDs [92–95]. Crossover studies have repeatedly demonstrated various triptans to outperform ergots with respect to short-term headache relief and long-term headache recurrence prevention [89, 96, 97]. Like triptans, ergots can also produce coronary vasoconstriction leading to cardiac ischemia in patients with coronary artery disease [98, 99]. Ergots are also contraindicated in pregnancy as they have been shown to cause fetal growth retardation in animal studies, possibly due to vasoconstriction of uterine vessels [100]. Furthermore, due to a low degree of receptor selectivity, ergot alkaloids have a narrow therapeutic range with relatively poor tolerability compared to triptans. As a result, current recommended practices include the limitation of ergot alkaloids to select patients who suffer from infrequent and long-duration headaches, who are either already established on ergot therapy or are non-responsive to triptan therapy, and are able to comply with dosing restrictions [91, 101].

Selective Serotonin 5-HT$_{1F}$ Receptor Agonists

Recent studies on migraine pathophysiology highlight trigeminovascular dysfunction as a novel target for acute migraine pharmacotherapy [102]. In response, the selective 5-HT$_{1F}$ receptor agonists, which preferentially inhibit trigeminal pathways without concurrent vasoconstrictor activity, were developed [103–105]. The first clinical studies of selective 5-HT$_{1F}$ agonists were on LY334370 with demonstration of superiority versus placebo for treatment of moderate-to-severe acute migraine in a dose-dependent fashion [103]. Unfortunately, due to compound-specific concern for long-term toxicity in animal models, clinical development of LY334370 was halted [106]. Subsequent early studies of LY573144 (now known as lasmiditan), also a selective 5-HT1F agonist, have reported promising efficacy data and good tolerability profiles when administered intravenously or orally [104, 105]. These initial findings have since been confirmed in the first Phase III clinical trials, in which lasmiditan was noted to be more effective than placebo and generally well tolerated [107, 108]. The most common treatment-related adverse reactions included dizziness, paresthesia, somnolence, and nausea, with symptoms generally reported to be mild in severity and self-limiting. Notably, these initial studies reported no triptan-like coronary events (e.g., myocardial infarction, ischemic stroke, or angina) despite enrolling patients with known cardiovascular disease [108, 109]. To date, further studies are still needed to determine the comparative efficacy of 5-HT$_{1F}$ agonists like lasmiditan against triptans, which remain the gold standard of acute migraine treatment. Regardless, these early studies on lasmiditan, particularly given the absence of vasoconstrictive side effects, represent a promising alternative for migraine patients who have contraindications or are nonresponders to triptan therapy. Lasmiditan was granted FDA approval for acute migraine treatment in adults in October 2019 [110].

Sodium Valproate

While sodium valproate is an established agent for migraine prophylaxis [111], some investigational studies also suggest intravenous sodium valproate may have applications for abortive therapy in acute migraine treatment [112, 113]. Open-label studies found sodium valproate infusion to result in especially rapid response times, with mean time to relief of 12 minutes and 75% of patients reporting maximum relief within 60 minutes of treatment [112]. However, outpatient applications of sodium valproate for acute migraine treatment are limited, given the need for intravenous infusion. Furthermore, urine pregnancy test is recommended prior to medication use in women of child-bearing age, as valproate is known to be teratogenic. Intravenous sodium valproate is ideally reserved for known triptan nonresponders who present to the emergency department with severe migraine headache, who seek rapid headache pain relief, and who do not have contraindications to sodium valproate (including liver disease [114] or urea cycle defects [115]).

Adjuvant Therapy

Caffeine

Like many medicinally significant alkaloids, caffeine is believed to function as a naturally occurring pesticide. It is toxic to many insects and grazing animals, and is produced by approximately 60 different plant species [116]. Humans have purposefully ingested caffeine-containing plants (or their extracts) since at least the eleventh century, and caffeinated beverages, including coffee and tea, are the most consumed beverages worldwide, second to water. Given this context, it is perhaps unsurprising that so many differing (and often conflicting) health effects are ascribed to caffeine. Caffeine exerts its effects through multiple mechanisms of action, including adenosine receptor antagonism, intracellular calcium mobilization, and nonselective competitive inhibition of phosphodiesterases [117]. It is also shown to inhibit the synthesis of leukotrienes and prostaglandins which leads to induction of an antinociceptive state [118].

Despite only modest general analgesic effects, caffeine is well-documented in its function as an analgesic adjuvant for acute pain treatment [119]. The mechanism of this effect seems to be in the increased gastric absorption that caffeine promotes by increasing cyclic AMP [118]. In acute migraine treatment, several large-scale studies have found caffeine to demonstrate a significant adjuvant analgesic effect when combined with acetaminophen, paracetamol, or NSAIDs for headache pain reduction [18, 120]. Specifically, combination therapy in which caffeine is co-administered with an NSAID resulted in faster pain reduction compared to an NSAID alone [16]. Furthermore, triple combination therapy – in which aspirin, paracetamol, and caffeine are taken together – provides even greater pain relief than dual therapy using caffeine with aspirin or paracetamol alone [18]. Although caffeine alone is not recommended as abortive monotherapy for migraine relief, caffeine is demonstrated to be an effective NSAID-adjuvant for treatment of mild-moderate migraine headache.

One important caveat to consider in the use of caffeine is that chronic high dose intake can exacerbate analgesic-overuse headache. Furthermore, abrupt discontinuation in individuals who partake in daily caffeine consumption may also precipitate caffeine-withdrawal headaches [118].

Antiemetics

Migraine-associated nausea is reported in at least 60% of migraine sufferers [121] with at least 30% of patients also reporting at least one episode of vomiting during a migraine attack [122]. Accompanying nausea and vomiting can be more functionally disabling than migraine headache pain as these symptoms significantly impede oral intake of food, liquids, and medications. In one study, more than 30% of patients reported nausea had interfered with their ability to take an oral migraine medication [123]. In addition to delaying treatment, there is evidence that gastric stasis underlies migraine-associated nausea, resulting in impairment of gastrointestinal absorption of orally administered medications [124].

Dopamine antagonist antiemetics such as metoclopramide have demonstrated some utility as a primary treatment of migraine headache pain and nausea [125]. Similarly, other dopamine antagonists like domperidone and the phenothiazines have also demonstrated benefit in acute migraine for improvement of pain intensity, reduction of headache length, and amelioration of nausea [126, 127]. Furthermore, comparison studies have found intravenous antiemetics, including metoclopramide and prochlorperazine, to outperform intravenous ketorolac as a single-agent migraine abortive therapy [126, 127]. While there are studies suggesting that metoclopramide in combination with NSAIDs may be similar in efficacy to triptans [128, 129], comparison studies show triptans generally outperform antiemetics as abortive migraine monotherapy, particularly in preventing headache recurrence [130]. However, in patients with significant, severe, and disabling nausea and vomiting associated with migraine attacks, concurrent therapy using a combination triptan and dopaminergic antiemetic has been shown to provide more meaningful headache relief than triptan monotherapy [131].

Butyrophenones, including droperidol and haloperidol, which act as dopamine D2 receptor antagonists, have also been evaluated as abortive therapy for acute migraine [132, 133]. However, concerns for QT prolongation and potentially fatal arrhythmia have generally abandoned further investigation into the butyrophenone class for acute migraine treatment [134]. Furthermore, intravenous or intramuscular droperidol administration has limited studies in acute migraine treatment to emergency department settings with outpatient applications restricted to monitored clinic settings [135, 136].

Intravenous Corticosteroids

Prior to the introduction of triptans, intravenous corticosteroids were commonly used as abortive therapy in acute migraine treatment. Randomized, placebo-controlled trials have since demonstrated intravenous corticosteroids to be ineffective for acute migraine treatment [137, 138]. There are some reports suggesting intravenous corticosteroids may be useful as an adjuvant treatment to reduce headache recurrence when combined with more effective abortive therapy [138, 139].

Opioids

Given their role in the alleviation of so many other varieties of pain, it is not surprising that opioids were once considered a reasonable treatment for headaches. Research has not supported this practice however, as opioids carry significant side effects and risks, including the generation of chronic headache syndromes [140]. Opioids are generally not recommended as first line therapy in acute migraine treatment given the risk of addiction and medication overuse [140], even though placebo-controlled studies have found opioid medications to provide some acute relief of migraine headache [141]. Specifically, only intranasal-administered butorphanol has demonstrated consistent benefit in trials [10, 142]. Comparative studies have demonstrated that non-opioid agents, including ergot alkaloids, NSAIDs, and phenothiazines, provide greater pain reduction with reduced need for rescue medications when compared to opioids [143, 144]. Use of opioids in acute migraine treatment has been associated with potentiation of chronic migraine [145], induction of medication-overuse headache [146], higher rates of headache recurrence [140], and increased disability [147]. Furthermore, concurrent opioid treatment has been demonstrated to decrease triptan efficacy in migraine prevention [148].

Guidelines on Acute Migraine Treatment

Since sumatriptan was approved for acute migraine treatment in 1992, multiple national and international groups have published clinical practice guidelines on acute migraine treatment [149]. Expectedly, guidelines are most frequently developed by groups representing primary care [150], emergency medicine [151], and neurology [10] specialties. Although practice guidelines demonstrate broad-stroke similarities, specific differences are largely due to philosophical differences when applying a stepwise [150] versus a stratified [10] approach.

In general, acute migraine guidelines universally recommend NSAIDs or acetaminophen for mild headache symptoms, with appropriate provisions for cardiovascular, hematologic, renal, and hepatic comorbidities [149, 152]. Some groups recommend multimodal anti-inflammatory therapy with a combination of NSAIDs, ASA, and acetaminophen [24] or combination therapy with an antiemetic [153]. Guidelines showed greater variability on second-line therapy for patients who were unresponsive to first-line treatment, with some recommending repeat NSAID dosing [154], while others recommended progression to migraine-specific therapies such as triptans or ergotamines [10, 150].

While guidelines that recommend a stepwise approach emphasize starting with the safest and least expensive therapies regardless of migraine severity, guidelines recommending a stratified approach recommend earlier intervention with migraine-specific therapies: particularly for moderate or severe symptoms [155]. Although nearly all guidelines consider ergotamine to be effective and generally favorable given low rates of headache recurrence, most guidelines recommend limiting ergotamine use to patients with infrequent and long attacks who are unresponsive to triptan treatment; some reserve ergotamine use for second- or third-line therapy [153, 156]. In addition, acute migraine management using opioids is nearly always discouraged or recommended only as third-line therapy [140, 156].

Practice guidelines are not intended to dictate individual patient care, but rather to provide guidance to improve the quality of care [157]. Indeed, publication of guidelines on accurate migraine diagnosis and appropriate treatment appears concordant with decreased opioid use and increased migraine-prevention medications in the last 20 years [158]. As research efforts clarify migraine pathophysiology, updated clinical practice guidelines are needed to improve granularity in patient stratification, to identify indications for targeted triptan therapy, and to incorporate novel therapies, such as lasmiditan, into regular clinical practice.

References

1. Rose FC. The history of migraine from Mesopotamian to Medieval times. Cephalalgia. 1995;15(Suppl 15):1–3.
2. Becker WJ. Acute migraine treatment in adults. Headache. 2015;55(6):778–93.
3. Marmura MJ, Silberstein SD, Schwedt TJ. The acute treatment of migraine in adults: the American Headache Society evidence assessment of migraine pharmacotherapies. Headache. 2015;55(1):3–20.
4. Yu Y, Ricciotti E, Scalia R, Tang SY, Grant G, Yu Z, et al. Vascular COX-2 modulates blood pressure and thrombosis in mice. Sci Transl Med. 2012;4(132):132ra54.
5. Zhang X, Donnan PT, Bell S, Guthrie B. Non-steroidal anti-inflammatory drug induced acute kidney injury in the community dwelling general population and people with chronic kidney disease: systematic review and meta-analysis. BMC Nephrol. 2017;18(1):256.
6. Kelley BG, Thayer SA. Anandamide transport inhibitor AM404 and structurally related compounds inhibit synaptic transmission between rat hippocampal neurons in culture independent of cannabinoid CB1 receptors. Eur J Pharmacol. 2004;496(1–3):33–9.
7. World Health Organization Model List of Essential Medicines, 21st List. Geneva: World Health Organization; 2019.

8. Hinson JA, Roberts DW, James LP. Mechanisms of acetaminophen-induced liver necrosis. Handb Exp Pharmacol. 2010;196:369–405.
9. Dugan F. Prescription drug products containing acetaminophen: actions to reduce liver injury from unintentional overdose. In: Research CfDEa, editor. https://www.regulations.gov/document?D=FDA-2011-N-0021-0001. Food and Drug Administration; 2011.
10. Silberstein SD. Practice parameter: evidence-based guidelines for migraine headache (an evidence-based review): report of the quality standards Subcommittee of the American Academy of Neurology. Neurology. 2000;55(6):754–62.
11. Suthisisang C, Poolsup N, Kittikulsuth W, Pudchakan P, Wiwatpanich P. Efficacy of low-dose ibuprofen in acute migraine treatment: systematic review and meta-analysis. Ann Pharmacother. 2007;41(11):1782–91.
12. Lange R, Schwarz JA, Hohn M. Acetylsalicylic acid effervescent 1000 mg (Aspirin) in acute migraine attacks; a multicentre, randomized, double-blind, single-dose, placebo-controlled parallel group study. Cephalalgia. 2000;20(7):663–7.
13. Suthisisang CC, Poolsup N, Suksomboon N, Lertpipopmetha V, Tepwitukgid B. Meta-analysis of the efficacy and safety of naproxen sodium in the acute treatment of migraine. Headache. 2010;50(5):808–18.
14. Derry S, Rabbie R, Moore RA. Diclofenac with or without an antiemetic for acute migraine headaches in adults. Cochrane Database Syst Rev. 2013;4:CD008783.
15. Lipton RB, Baggish JS, Stewart WF, Codispoti JR, Fu M. Efficacy and safety of acetaminophen in the treatment of migraine: results of a randomized, double-blind, placebo-controlled, population-based study. Arch Intern Med. 2000;160(22):3486–92.
16. Goldstein J, Silberstein SD, Saper JR, Ryan RE Jr, Lipton RB. Acetaminophen, aspirin, and caffeine in combination versus ibuprofen for acute migraine: results from a multicenter, double-blind, randomized, parallel-group, single-dose, placebo-controlled study. Headache. 2006;46(3):444–53.
17. Kellstein DE, Lipton RB, Geetha R, Koronkiewicz K, Evans FT, Stewart WF, et al. Evaluation of a novel solubilized formulation of ibuprofen in the treatment of migraine headache: a randomized, double-blind, placebo-controlled, dose-ranging study. Cephalalgia. 2000;20(4):233–43.
18. Diener HC, Pfaffenrath V, Pageler L, Peil H, Aicher B. The fixed combination of acetylsalicylic acid, paracetamol and caffeine is more effective than single substances and dual combination for the treatment of headache: a multicentre, randomized, double-blind, single-dose, placebo-controlled parallel group study. Cephalalgia. 2005;25(10):776–87.
19. Diener HC, Montagna P, Gacs G, Lyczak P, Schumann G, Zoller B, et al. Efficacy and tolerability of diclofenac potassium sachets in migraine: a randomized, double-blind, cross-over study in comparison with diclofenac potassium tablets and placebo. Cephalalgia. 2006;26(5):537–47.
20. Gatti G, Barzaghi N, Attardo Parrinello G, Vitiello B, Perucca E. Pharmacokinetics of salicylic acid following administration of aspirin tablets and three different forms of soluble aspirin in normal subjects. Int J Clin Pharmacol Res. 1989;9(6):385–9.
21. Diener HC. Efficacy and safety of intravenous acetylsalicylic acid lysinate compared to subcutaneous sumatriptan and parenteral placebo in the acute treatment of migraine. A double-blind, double-dummy, randomized, multicenter, parallel group study. The ASASUMAMIG Study Group. Cephalalgia. 1999;19(6):581–8. discussion 42
22. Shrestha M, Singh R, Moreden J, Hayes JE. Ketorolac vs chlorpromazine in the treatment of acute migraine without aura. A prospective, randomized, double-blind trial. Arch Intern Med. 1996;156(15):1725–8.
23. Taggart E, Doran S, Kokotillo A, Campbell S, Villa-Roel C, Rowe BH. Ketorolac in the treatment of acute migraine: a systematic review. Headache. 2013;53(2):277–87.
24. Snow V, Weiss K, Wall EM, Mottur-Pilson C, American Academy of Family P, American College of Physicians-American Society of Internal Medicine. Pharmacologic management of acute attacks of migraine and prevention of migraine headache. Ann Intern Med. 2002;137(10):840–9.

25. Risser A, Donovan D, Heintzman J, Page T. NSAID prescribing precautions. Am Fam Physician. 2009;80(12):1371–8.
26. Cameron C, Kelly S, Hsieh SC, Murphy M, Chen L, Kotb A, et al. Triptans in the acute treatment of migraine: a systematic review and network meta-analysis. Headache. 2015;55(Suppl 4):221–35.
27. Classey JD, Bartsch T, Goadsby PJ. Distribution of 5-HT(1B), 5-HT(1D) and 5-HT(1F) receptor expression in rat trigeminal and dorsal root ganglia neurons: relevance to the selective anti-migraine effect of triptans. Brain Res. 2010;1361:76–85.
28. Negro A, Koverech A, Martelletti P. Serotonin receptor agonists in the acute treatment of migraine: a review on their therapeutic potential. J Pain Res. 2018;11:515–26.
29. Pilgrim AJ. Methodology of clinical trials of sumatriptan in migraine and cluster headache. Eur Neurol. 1991;31(5):295–9.
30. The Subcutaneous Sumatriptan International Study Group. Treatment of migraine attacks with sumatriptan. N Engl J Med. 1991;325(5):316–21.
31. Cady RK, Wendt JK, Kirchner JR, Sargent JD, Rothrock JF, Skaggs H Jr. Treatment of acute migraine with subcutaneous sumatriptan. JAMA. 1991;265(21):2831–5.
32. Goadsby PJ, Zagami AS, Donnan GA, Symington G, Anthony M, Bladin PF, et al. Oral sumatriptan in acute migraine. Lancet. 1991;338(8770):782–3.
33. Mathew NT, Dexter J, Couch J, Flamenbaum W, Goldstein J, Rapoport A, et al. Dose ranging efficacy and safety of subcutaneous sumatriptan in the acute treatment of migraine. US Sumatriptan Research Group. Arch Neurol. 1992;49(12):1271–6.
34. Patten JP. Clinical experience with oral sumatriptan: a placebo-controlled, dose-ranging study. Oral Sumatriptan Dose-defining Study Group. J Neurol. 1991;238(Suppl 1):S62–5.
35. Fowler PA, Lacey LF, Thomas M, Keene ON, Tanner RJ, Baber NS. The clinical pharmacology, pharmacokinetics and metabolism of sumatriptan. Eur Neurol. 1991;31(5):291–4.
36. Carpay HA, Matthijsse P, Steinbuch M, Mulder PG. Oral and subcutaneous sumatriptan in the acute treatment of migraine: an open randomized cross-over study. Cephalalgia. 1997;17(5):591–5.
37. Ferrari MD, James MH, Bates D, Pilgrim A, Ashford E, Anderson BA, et al. Oral sumatriptan: effect of a second dose, and incidence and treatment of headache recurrences. Cephalalgia. 1994;14(5):330–8.
38. The Oral Sumatriptan International Multiple-Dose Study Group. Evaluation of a multiple-dose regimen of oral sumatriptan for the acute treatment of migraine. Eur Neurol. 1991;31(5):306–13.
39. Smith TR, Sunshine A, Stark SR, Littlefield DE, Spruill SE, Alexander WJ. Sumatriptan and naproxen sodium for the acute treatment of migraine. Headache. 2005;45(8):983–91.
40. Brandes JL, Kudrow D, Stark SR, O'Carroll CP, Adelman JU, O'Donnell FJ, et al. Sumatriptan-naproxen for acute treatment of migraine: a randomized trial. JAMA. 2007;297(13):1443–54.
41. Tfelt-Hansen P. Efficacy and adverse events of subcutaneous, oral, and intranasal sumatriptan used for migraine treatment: a systematic review based on number needed to treat. Cephalalgia. 1998;18(8):532–8.
42. Goldstein J, Smith TR, Pugach N, Griesser J, Sebree T, Pierce M. A sumatriptan iontophoretic transdermal system for the acute treatment of migraine. Headache. 2012;52(9):1402–10.
43. Tepper SJ, Donnan GA, Dowson AJ, Bomhof MA, Elkind A, Meloche J, et al. A long-term study to maximise migraine relief with zolmitriptan. Curr Med Res Opin. 1999;15(4):254–71.
44. Ashcroft DM, Millson D. Naratriptan for the treatment of acute migraine: meta-analysis of randomised controlled trials. Pharmacoepidemiol Drug Saf. 2004;13(2):73–82.
45. Mathew NT, Kailasam J, Meadors L. Early treatment of migraine with rizatriptan: a placebo-controlled study. Headache. 2004;44(7):669–73.
46. Chen LC, Ashcroft DM. Meta-analysis examining the efficacy and safety of almotriptan in the acute treatment of migraine. Headache. 2007;47(8):1169–77.
47. Poolsup N, Leelasangaluk V, Jittangtrong J, Rithlamlert C, Ratanapantamanee N, Khanthong M. Efficacy and tolerability of frovatriptan in acute migraine treatment: systematic review of randomized controlled trials. J Clin Pharm Ther. 2005;30(6):521–32.

48. Brandes JL, Kudrow D, Cady R, Tiseo PJ, Sun W, Sikes CR. Eletriptan in the early treatment of acute migraine: influence of pain intensity and time of dosing. Cephalalgia. 2005;25(9):735–42.
49. Goadsby PJ, Massiou H, Pascual J, Diener HC, Dahlof CG, Mateos V, et al. Almotriptan and zolmitriptan in the acute treatment of migraine. Acta Neurol Scand. 2007;115(1):34–40.
50. Diener HC, Gendolla A, Gebert I, Beneke M. Almotriptan in migraine patients who respond poorly to oral sumatriptan: a double-blind, randomized trial. Eur Neurol. 2005;53(Suppl 1):41–8.
51. Markus F, Mikko K. Frovatriptan review. Expert Opin Pharmacother. 2007;8(17):3029–33.
52. Belvis R, Pagonabarraga J, Kulisevsky J. Individual triptan selection in migraine attack therapy. Recent Pat CNS Drug Discov. 2009;4(1):70–81.
53. Lipton RB, Stewart WF, Cady R, Hall C, O'Quinn S, Kuhn T, et al. Sumatriptan for the range of headaches in migraine sufferers: results of the Spectrum Study. Headache. 2000;40(10):783–91.
54. Russell MB, Ducros A. Sporadic and familial hemiplegic migraine: pathophysiological mechanisms, clinical characteristics, diagnosis, and management. Lancet Neurol. 2011;10(5):457–70.
55. Artto V, Nissila M, Wessman M, Palotie A, Farkkila M, Kallela M. Treatment of hemiplegic migraine with triptans. Eur J Neurol. 2007;14(9):1053–6.
56. Klapper J, Mathew N, Nett R. Triptans in the treatment of basilar migraine and migraine with prolonged aura. Headache. 2001;41(10):981–4.
57. Silberstein SD, Elkind AH, Schreiber C, Keywood C. A randomized trial of frovatriptan for the intermittent prevention of menstrual migraine. Neurology. 2004;63(2):261–9.
58. Tuchman M, Hee A, Emeribe U, Silberstein S. Efficacy and tolerability of zolmitriptan oral tablet in the acute treatment of menstrual migraine. CNS Drugs. 2006;20(12):1019–26.
59. Loder E. Triptan therapy in migraine. N Engl J Med. 2010;363(1):63–70.
60. Aurora SK, Barrodale PM, McDonald SA, Jakubowski M, Burstein R. Revisiting the efficacy of sumatriptan therapy during the aura phase of migraine. Headache. 2009;49(7):1001–4.
61. Olesen J, Diener HC, Schoenen J, Hettiarachchi J. No effect of eletriptan administration during the aura phase of migraine. Eur J Neurol. 2004;11(10):671–7.
62. Steiner TJ, Diener HC, MacGregor EA, Schoenen J, Muirheads N, Sikes CR. Comparative efficacy of eletriptan and zolmitriptan in the acute treatment of migraine. Cephalalgia. 2003;23(10):942–52.
63. Bomhof M, Paz J, Legg N, Allen C, Vandormael K, Patel K. Comparison of rizatriptan 10 mg vs. naratriptan 2.5 mg in migraine. Eur Neurol. 1999;42(3):173–9.
64. Geraud G, Spierings EL, Keywood C. Tolerability and safety of frovatriptan with short- and long-term use for treatment of migraine and in comparison with sumatriptan. Headache. 2002;42(Suppl 2):S93–9.
65. Gruffyd-Jones K, Kies B, Middleton A, Mulder LJ, Rosjo O, Millson DS. Zolmitriptan versus sumatriptan for the acute oral treatment of migraine: a randomized, double-blind, international study. Eur J Neurol. 2001;8(3):237–45.
66. Visser WH, Terwindt GM, Reines SA, Jiang K, Lines CR, Ferrari MD. Rizatriptan vs sumatriptan in the acute treatment of migraine. A placebo-controlled, dose-ranging study. Dutch/US Rizatriptan Study Group. Arch Neurol. 1996;53(11):1132–7.
67. Fox AW. Comparative tolerability of oral 5-HT1B/1D agonists. Headache. 2000;40(7):521–7.
68. Pascual J, Munoz P. Correlation between lipophilicity and triptan outcomes. Headache. 2005;45(1):3–6.
69. Diamond ML, Hettiarachchi J, Hilliard B, Sands G, Nett R. Effectiveness of eletriptan in acute migraine: primary care for Excedrin nonresponders. Headache. 2004;44(3):209–16.
70. Goadsby PJ, Yates R. Zolmitriptan intranasal: a review of the pharmacokinetics and clinical efficacy. Headache. 2006;46(1):138–49.
71. Klassen A, Elkind A, Asgharnejad M, Webster C, Laurenza A. Naratriptan is effective and well tolerated in the acute treatment of migraine. Results of a double-blind, placebo-controlled, parallel-group study. Naratriptan S2WA3001 Study Group. Headache. 1997;37(10):640–5.

72. Dodick DW. Oral almotriptan in the treatment of migraine: safety and tolerability. Headache. 2001;41(5):449–55.
73. Edmeads JG, Millson DS. Tolerability profile of zolmitriptan (Zomig; 311C90), a novel dual central and peripherally acting 5HT1B/1D agonist. International clinical experience based on > 3000 subjects treated with zolmitriptan. Cephalalgia. 1997;17(Suppl 18):41–52.
74. Welch KM, Mathew NT, Stone P, Rosamond W, Saiers J, Gutterman D. Tolerability of sumatriptan: clinical trials and post-marketing experience. Cephalalgia. 2000;20(8):687–95.
75. Dodick D, Lipton RB, Martin V, Papademetriou V, Rosamond W, MaassenVanDenBrink A, et al. Consensus statement: cardiovascular safety profile of triptans (5-HT agonists) in the acute treatment of migraine. Headache. 2004;44(5):414–25.
76. Dodick DW, Martin VT, Smith T, Silberstein S. Cardiovascular tolerability and safety of triptans: a review of clinical data. Headache. 2004;44(Suppl 1):S20–30.
77. Maassen Van Den Brink A, Saxena PR. Coronary vasoconstrictor potential of triptans: a review of in vitro pharmacologic data. Headache. 2004;44(Suppl 1):S13–9.
78. Buchan P, Wade A, Ward C, Oliver SD, Stewart AJ, Freestone S. Frovatriptan: a review of drug-drug interactions. Headache. 2002;42(Suppl 2):S63–73.
79. Shapiro RE, Tepper SJ. The serotonin syndrome, triptans, and the potential for drug-drug interactions. Headache. 2007;47(2):266–9.
80. Evans RW. The FDA alert on serotonin syndrome with combined use of SSRIs or SNRIs and Triptans: an analysis of the 29 case reports. MedGenMed. 2007;9(3):48.
81. Gillman PK. Triptans, serotonin agonists, and serotonin syndrome (serotonin toxicity): a review. Headache. 2010;50(2):264–72.
82. Evans RW, Tepper SJ, Shapiro RE, Sun-Edelstein C, Tietjen GE. The FDA alert on serotonin syndrome with use of triptans combined with selective serotonin reuptake inhibitors or selective serotonin-norepinephrine reuptake inhibitors: American Headache Society position paper. Headache. 2010;50(6):1089–99.
83. Cunnington M, Ephross S, Churchill P. The safety of sumatriptan and naratriptan in pregnancy: what have we learned? Headache. 2009;49(10):1414–22.
84. Kallen B, Lygner PE. Delivery outcome in women who used drugs for migraine during pregnancy with special reference to sumatriptan. Headache. 2001;41(4):351–6.
85. Nezvalova-Henriksen K, Spigset O, Nordeng H. Triptan exposure during pregnancy and the risk of major congenital malformations and adverse pregnancy outcomes: results from the Norwegian Mother and Child Cohort Study. Headache. 2010;50(4):563–75.
86. Thomson W. Ergot in the treatment of periodic neuralgias. J Nerv Ment Dis. 1894;21:124.
87. Buzzi MG, Moskowitz MA. Evidence for 5-HT1B/1D receptors mediating the antimigraine effect of sumatriptan and dihydroergotamine. Cephalalgia. 1991;11(4):165–8.
88. Maier H. L'ergotamine, inhibiteur du sympathique etudie en clinque, comme moyen d'exploration et comme agent therapeutique. Rev Neurol. 1926;33:1104–8.
89. Diener HC, Jansen JP, Reches A, Pascual J, Pitei D, Steiner TJ, et al. Efficacy, tolerability and safety of oral eletriptan and ergotamine plus caffeine (Cafergot) in the acute treatment of migraine: a multicentre, randomised, double-blind, placebo-controlled comparison. Eur Neurol. 2002;47(2):99–107.
90. Gallagher RM. Acute treatment of migraine with dihydroergotamine nasal spray. Dihydroergotamine Working Group. Arch Neurol. 1996;53(12):1285–91.
91. Tfelt-Hansen P, Saxena PR, Dahlof C, Pascual J, Lainez M, Henry P, et al. Ergotamine in the acute treatment of migraine: a review and European consensus. Brain. 2000;123(Pt 1):9–18.
92. Hakkarainen H, Gustafsson B, Stockman O. A comparative trial of ergotamine tartrate, acetyl salicylic acid and a dextropropoxyphene compound in acute migraine attacks. Headache. 1978;18(1):35–9.
93. Hakkarainen H, Quiding H, Stockman O. Mild analgesics as an alternative to ergotamine in migraine. A comparative trial with acetylsalicylic acid, ergotamine tartrate, and a dextropropoxyphene compound. J Clin Pharmacol. 1980;20(10):590–5.
94. Hakkarainen H, Vapaatalo H, Gothoni G, Parantainen J. Tolfenamic acid is as effective as ergotamine during migraine attacks. Lancet. 1979;2(8138):326–8.

95. Treves TA, Streiffler M, Korczyn AD. Naproxen sodium versus ergotamine tartrate in the treatment of acute migraine attacks. Headache. 1992;32(6):280–2.
96. Winner P, Ricalde O, Le Force B, Saper J, Margul B. A double-blind study of subcutaneous dihydroergotamine vs subcutaneous sumatriptan in the treatment of acute migraine. Arch Neurol. 1996;53(2):180–4.
97. Lainez MJ, Galvan J, Heras J, Vila C. Crossover, double-blind clinical trial comparing almotriptan and ergotamine plus caffeine for acute migraine therapy. Eur J Neurol. 2007;14(3):269–75.
98. Galer BS, Lipton RB, Solomon S, Newman LC, Spierings EL. Myocardial ischemia related to ergot alkaloids: a case report and literature review. Headache. 1991;31(7):446–50.
99. Goldfischer J. Acute myocardial infarction secondary to ergot therapy – report of a case and review of the literature. N Engl J Med. 1960;262:860–3.
100. Banhidy F, Acs N, Puho E, Czeizel AE. Ergotamine treatment during pregnancy and a higher rate of low birthweight and preterm birth. Br J Clin Pharmacol. 2007;64(4):510–6.
101. Neurology QSSotAAo. Practice parameter: appropriate use of ergotamine tartrate and dihydroergotamine in the treatment of migraine and status migrainosus. Neurology. 1995;45:585–7.
102. Goadsby PJ, Lipton RB, Ferrari MD. Migraine – current understanding and treatment. N Engl J Med. 2002;346(4):257–70.
103. Goldstein DJ, Roon KI, Offen WW, Ramadan NM, Phebus LA, Johnson KW, et al. Selective seratonin 1F (5-HT(1F)) receptor agonist LY334370 for acute migraine: a randomised controlled trial. Lancet. 2001;358(9289):1230–4.
104. Ferrari MD, Farkkila M, Reuter U, Pilgrim A, Davis C, Krauss M, et al. Acute treatment of migraine with the selective 5-HT1F receptor agonist lasmiditan–a randomised proof-of-concept trial. Cephalalgia. 2010;30(10):1170–8.
105. Nelson DL, Phebus LA, Johnson KW, Wainscott DB, Cohen ML, Calligaro DO, et al. Preclinical pharmacological profile of the selective 5-HT1F receptor agonist lasmiditan. Cephalalgia. 2010;30(10):1159–69.
106. Buchanan TM, Ramadan NM, Aurora S. Future pharmacologic targets for acute and preventive treatments of migraine. Expert Rev Neurother. 2004;4(3):391–430.
107. Loo LS, Ailani J, Schim J, Baygani S, Hundemer HP, Port M, et al. Efficacy and safety of lasmiditan in patients using concomitant migraine preventive medications: findings from SAMURAI and SPARTAN, two randomized phase 3 trials. J Headache Pain. 2019;20(1):84.
108. Krege JH, Rizzoli PB, Liffick E, Doty EG, Dowsett SA, Wang J, et al. Safety findings from phase 3 lasmiditan studies for acute treatment of migraine: results from SAMURAI and SPARTAN. Cephalalgia. 2019;39(8):957–66.
109. Farkkila M, Diener HC, Geraud G, Lainez M, Schoenen J, Harner N, et al. Efficacy and tolerability of lasmiditan, an oral 5-HT(1F) receptor agonist, for the acute treatment of migraine: a phase 2 randomised, placebo-controlled, parallel-group, dose-ranging study. Lancet Neurol. 2012;11(5):405–13.
110. Administration UFaD. FDA approves new treatment for patients with migraine https://www.fda.gov/news-events/press-announcements/fda-approves-new-treatment-patients-migraine2019. Updated 10/11/2019.
111. Rothrock JF. Clinical studies of valproate for migraine prophylaxis. Cephalalgia. 1997;17(2):81–3.
112. Shahien R, Saleh SA, Bowirrat A. Intravenous sodium valproate aborts migraine headaches rapidly. Acta Neurol Scand. 2011;123(4):257–65.
113. Mathew NT, Kailasam J, Meadors L, Chernyschev O, Gentry P. Intravenous valproate sodium (depacon) aborts migraine rapidly: a preliminary report. Headache. 2000;40(9):720–3.
114. Itoh S, Yamaba Y, Matsuo S, Saka M, Ichinoe A. Sodium valproate-induced liver injury. Am J Gastroenterol. 1982;77(11):875–9.
115. Hjelm M, de Silva LV, Seakins JW, Oberholzer VG, Rolles CJ. Evidence of inherited urea cycle defect in a case of fatal valproate toxicity. Br Med J (Clin Res Ed). 1986;292(6512):23–4.

116. Caballero B, Finglas PM, Toldra F, Fernandez ML, Andersen CJ. Caffeine: characterization and properties. In: The Encyclopedia of Food and Health (1st Ed). Academic Press 2015. p. 556–7.
117. Cappelletti S, Piacentino D, Sani G, Aromatario M. Caffeine: cognitive and physical performance enhancer or psychoactive drug? Curr Neuropharmacol. 2015;13(1):71–88.
118. Espinosa Jovel CA, Sobrino Mejia FE. Caffeine and headache: specific remarks. Neurologia. 2017;32(6):394–8.
119. Derry CJ, Derry S, Moore RA. Caffeine as an analgesic adjuvant for acute pain in adults. Cochrane Database Syst Rev. 2014;12:CD009281.
120. Laska EM, Sunshine A, Mueller F, Elvers WB, Siegel C, Rubin A. Caffeine as an analgesic adjuvant. JAMA. 1984;251(13):1711–8.
121. Lainez MJ, Garcia-Casado A, Gascon F. Optimal management of severe nausea and vomiting in migraine: improving patient outcomes. Patient Relat Outcome Meas. 2013;4:61–73.
122. Lipton RB, Stewart WF, Diamond S, Diamond ML, Reed M. Prevalence and burden of migraine in the United States: data from the American Migraine Study II. Headache. 2001;41(7):646–57.
123. Silberstein SD. Migraine symptoms: results of a survey of self-reported migraineurs. Headache. 1995;35(7):387–96.
124. Aurora SK, Kori SH, Barrodale P, McDonald SA, Haseley D. Gastric stasis in migraine: more than just a paroxysmal abnormality during a migraine attack. Headache. 2006;46(1):57–63.
125. Tfelt-Hansen P, Olesen J, Aebelholt-Krabbe A, Melgaard B, Veilis B. A double blind study of metoclopramide in the treatment of migraine attacks. J Neurol Neurosurg Psychiatry. 1980;43(4):369–71.
126. MacGregor EA, Wilkinson M, Bancroft K. Domperidone plus paracetamol in the treatment of migraine. Cephalalgia. 1993;13(2):124–7.
127. Kelly AM, Walcynski T, Gunn B. The relative efficacy of phenothiazines for the treatment of acute migraine: a meta-analysis. Headache. 2009;49(9):1324–32.
128. Friedman BW, Garber L, Yoon A, Solorzano C, Wollowitz A, Esses D, et al. Randomized trial of IV valproate vs metoclopramide vs ketorolac for acute migraine. Neurology. 2014;82(11):976–83.
129. Seim MB, March JA, Dunn KA. Intravenous ketorolac vs intravenous prochlorperazine for the treatment of migraine headaches. Acad Emerg Med. 1998;5(6):573–6.
130. Tfelt-Hansen P, Henry P, Mulder LJ, Scheldewaert RG, Schoenen J, Chazot G. The effectiveness of combined oral lysine acetylsalicylate and metoclopramide compared with oral sumatriptan for migraine. Lancet. 1995;346(8980):923–6.
131. Schulman EA, Dermott KF. Sumatriptan plus metoclopramide in triptan-nonresponsive migraineurs. Headache. 2003;43(7):729–33.
132. Honkaniemi J, Liimatainen S, Rainesalo S, Sulavuori S. Haloperidol in the acute treatment of migraine: a randomized, double-blind, placebo-controlled study. Headache. 2006;46(5):781–7.
133. Wang SJ, Silberstein SD, Young WB. Droperidol treatment of status migrainosus and refractory migraine. Headache. 1997;37(6):377–82.
134. Kelley NE, Tepper DE. Rescue therapy for acute migraine, part 2: neuroleptics, antihistamines, and others. Headache. 2012;52(2):292–306.
135. Richman PB, Reischel U, Ostrow A, Irving C, Ritter A, Allegra J, et al. Droperidol for acute migraine headache. Am J Emerg Med. 1999;17(4):398–400.
136. Thomas MC, Musselman ME, Shewmaker J. Droperidol for the treatment of acute migraine headaches. Ann Pharmacother. 2015;49(2):233–40.
137. Friedman BW, Greenwald P, Bania TC, Esses D, Hochberg M, Solorzano C, et al. Randomized trial of IV dexamethasone for acute migraine in the emergency department. Neurology. 2007;69(22):2038–44.
138. Colman I, Friedman BW, Brown MD, Innes GD, Grafstein E, Roberts TE, et al. Parenteral dexamethasone for acute severe migraine headache: meta-analysis of randomised controlled trials for preventing recurrence. BMJ. 2008;336(7657):1359–61.

139. Innes GD, Macphail I, Dillon EC, Metcalfe C, Gao M. Dexamethasone prevents relapse after emergency department treatment of acute migraine: a randomized clinical trial. CJEM. 1999;1(1):26–33.
140. Tepper SJ. Opioids should not be used in migraine. Headache. 2012;52(Suppl 1):30–4.
141. Levin M. Opioids in headache. Headache. 2014;54(1):12–21.
142. Hoffert MJ, Couch JR, Diamond S, Elkind AH, Goldstein J, Kohlerman NJ 3rd, et al. Transnasal butorphanol in the treatment of acute migraine. Headache. 1995;35(2):65–9.
143. Friedman BW, Kapoor A, Friedman MS, Hochberg ML, Rowe BH. The relative efficacy of meperidine for the treatment of acute migraine: a meta-analysis of randomized controlled trials. Ann Emerg Med. 2008;52(6):705–13.
144. Lane PL, McLellan BA, Baggoley CJ. Comparative efficacy of chlorpromazine and meperidine with dimenhydrinate in migraine headache. Ann Emerg Med. 1989;18(4):360–5.
145. Bigal ME, Lipton RB. Excessive opioid use and the development of chronic migraine. Pain. 2009;142(3):179–82.
146. Dodick D, Freitag F. Evidence-based understanding of medication-overuse headache: clinical implications. Headache. 2006;46(Suppl 4):S202–11.
147. Buse D, Manack A, Serrano D, Reed M, Varon S, Turkel C, et al. Headache impact of chronic and episodic migraine: results from the American Migraine Prevalence and Prevention study. Headache. 2012;52(1):3–17.
148. Ho TW, Rodgers A, Bigal ME. Impact of recent prior opioid use on rizatriptan efficacy. A post hoc pooled analysis. Headache. 2009;49(3):395–403.
149. Schuurmans A, van Weel C. Pharmacologic treatment of migraine. Comparison of guidelines. Can Fam Physician. 2005;51:838–43.
150. Becker WJ, Findlay T, Moga C, Scott NA, Harstall C, Taenzer P. Guideline for primary care management of headache in adults. Can Fam Physician. 2015;61(8):670–9.
151. Ducharme J. Canadian Association of Emergency Physicians Guidelines for the acute management of migraine headache. J Emerg Med. 1999;17(1):137–44.
152. Antonaci F, Dumitrache C, De Cillis I, Allena M. A review of current European treatment guidelines for migraine. J Headache Pain. 2010;11(1):13–9.
153. Diener HC, Brune K, Gerber WD, Gobel H, Pfaffenrath V. Treatment of migraine attacks and migraine prophylaxis: recommendations of the German Migraine and Headache Society. Med Monatsschr Pharm. 1998;21(2):30–9.
154. Pryse-Phillips WE, Dodick DW, Edmeads JG, Gawel MJ, Nelson RF, Purdy RA, et al. Guidelines for the diagnosis and management of migraine in clinical practice. Canadian Headache Society. CMAJ. 1997;156(9):1273–87.
155. Worthington I, Pringsheim T, Gawel MJ, Gladstone J, Cooper P, Dilli E, et al. Canadian Headache Society Guideline: acute drug therapy for migraine headache. Can J Neurol Sci. 2013;40(5 Suppl 3):S1–S80.
156. Silberstein SD, Holland S, Freitag F, Dodick DW, Argoff C, Ashman E, et al. Evidence-based guideline update: pharmacologic treatment for episodic migraine prevention in adults: report of the quality standards Subcommittee of the American Academy of Neurology and the American Headache Society. Neurology. 2012;78(17):1337–45.
157. Natsch S, van der Meer JW. The role of clinical guidelines, policies and stewardship. J Hosp Infect. 2003;53(3):172–6.
158. Altalib HH, Fenton BT, Sico J, Goulet JL, Bathulapalli H, Mohammad A, et al. Increase in migraine diagnoses and guideline-concordant treatment in veterans, 2004-2012. Cephalalgia. 2017;37(1):3–10.
159. Amar PJ, Schiff ER. Acetaminophen safety and hepatotoxicity–where do we go from here? Expert Opin Drug Saf. 2007;6(4):341–55.
160. American Headache S. The American Headache Society position statement on integrating new migraine treatments into clinical practice. Headache. 2019;59(1):1–18.
161. Andersson PG, Hinge HH, Johansen O, Andersen CU, Lademann A, Gotzsche PC. Double-blind study of naproxen vs placebo in the treatment of acute migraine attacks. Cephalalgia. 1989;9(1):29–32.

162. Blondell RD, Azadfard M, Wisniewski AM. Pharmacologic therapy for acute pain. Am Fam Physician. 2013;87(11):766–72.
163. Evers S, Afra J, Frese A, Goadsby PJ, Linde M, May A, et al. EFNS guideline on the drug treatment of migraine – revised report of an EFNS task force. Eur J Neurol. 2009;16(9):968–81.
164. Lipton RB, Goldstein J, Baggish JS, Yataco AR, Sorrentino JV, Quiring JN. Aspirin is efficacious for the treatment of acute migraine. Headache. 2005;45(4):283–92.
165. McAleer SD, Majid O, Venables E, Polack T, Sheikh MS. Pharmacokinetics and safety of ketorolac following single intranasal and intramuscular administration in healthy volunteers. J Clin Pharmacol. 2007;47(1):13–8.
166. Nestvold K, Kloster R, Partinen M, Sulkava R. Treatment of acute migraine attack: naproxen and placebo compared. Cephalalgia. 1985;5(2):115–9.
167. Rao AS, Gelaye B, Kurth T, Dash PD, Nitchie H, Peterlin BL. A randomized trial of ketorolac vs. Sumatripan vs. placebo nasal spray (KSPN) for acute migraine. Headache. 2016;56(2):331–40.
168. Smolinske SC, Hall AH, Vandenberg SA, Spoerke DG, McBride PV. Toxic effects of nonsteroidal anti-inflammatory drugs in overdose. An overview of recent evidence on clinical effects and dose-response relationships. Drug Saf. 1990;5(4):252–74.
169. Society AP. Principles of analgesic use in the treatment of acute pain and cancer pain. American Pain Society; Glenview, IL 2009.
170. Rapoport AM, Tepper SJ, Bigal ME, Sheftell FD. The triptan formulations: how to match patients and products. CNS Drugs. 2003;17(6):431–47.
171. Bird S, Derry S, Moore RA. Zolmitriptan for acute migraine attacks in adults. Cochrane Database Syst Rev. 2014;5:CD008616.
172. Dahlof CG, Dodick D, Dowson AJ, Pascual J. How does almotriptan compare with other triptans? A review of data from placebo-controlled clinical trials. Headache. 2002;42(2):99–113.
173. Derry CJ, Derry S, Moore RA. Sumatriptan (all routes of administration) for acute migraine attacks in adults - overview of Cochrane reviews. Cochrane Database Syst Rev. 2014;5:CD009108.
174. Havanka H, Dahlof C, Pop PH, Diener HC, Winter P, Whitehouse H, et al. Efficacy of naratriptan tablets in the acute treatment of migraine: a dose-ranging study. Naratriptan S2WB2004 Study Group. Clin Ther. 2000;22(8):970–80.
175. Oldman AD, Smith LA, McQuay HJ, Moore RA. Rizatriptan for acute migraine. Cochrane Database Syst Rev. 2001;3:CD003221.
176. Ryan R, Geraud G, Goldstein J, Cady R, Keywood C. Clinical efficacy of frovatriptan: placebo-controlled studies. Headache. 2002;42(Suppl 2):S84–92.
177. Smith LA, Oldman AD, McQuay HJ, Moore RA. Eletriptan for acute migraine. Cochrane Database Syst Rev. 2001;3:CD003224.

4 Prophylaxis of Migraine Protocols and Options

Rakhi Dayal and Adrian Darryll Sulindro

Migraine headaches are among the top reasons for patients to visit emergency departments as well as outpatient visit and are prevalent in almost 16% of the population, with it being more common in women [1]. The prevalence estimates have remained remarkably stable over many years [2]. Migraine commonly affects people in the 18–44 age group with a higher prevalence in people with low socioeconomic status, unemployed, or working part-time. Several of these patients may have reduced access to healthcare and treatment. Hence, a sizable proportion of migraine headaches are under-recognized and undertreated. When present, migraine headaches can be significantly burdensome. Most migraineurs have from one to four headache attacks per month [3]. The attack frequency and associated impairment consequently leads to reduced functionality and quality of life. This also attributes significantly to the public health burden associated with the disease.

Episodic and chronic migraine headaches are essential to recognize and differentiate. Most migraineurs present with episodic migraine which are defined as headaches less than 15 days a month. Episodic migraine are further classified as low-frequency migraine if they have less than ten migraines a month, and high-frequency migraines are between 10 and 14 migraines a month. Chronic migraines are less common than episodic migraines and are defined as having headaches 15 times a month for at least 3 months, and at least 8 days per month meet the diagnostic criteria of migraine [4], and have shown to lead to poorer quality of life. Influenced by various migraine triggers, episodic migraine commonly evolves to chronic migraine, thereby leading to overuse of acute migraine medications [5]. Drug overuse itself also contributes to the progression of episodic migraine to chronic migraine [6]. Hence, the importance of migraine prophylaxis to stop this

R. Dayal
Department of Anesthesiology, University of California Irvine Health, Orange, CA, USA

A. D. Sulindro (✉)
Biohealth Pain Management, Lawndale, CA, USA

© Springer Nature Switzerland AG 2021

S. Shah (ed.), *Migraine*, https://doi.org/10.1007/978-3-030-75239-2_4

self-perpetuating cycle should be established. Though several patients may meet the criteria for migraine prevention treatment, many may not be receiving it. Lipton et al. suggested that approximately 38% of patients with migraine headaches would benefit from migraine prophylaxis; however, only 3–13% of people seek treatment for migraine prophylaxis [3].

Treatment of migraine attacks may reduce frequency, burden of care, and prevent the development of chronic migraine [7]. This chapter outlines the indications and principal practice guidelines for initiating and managing migraine prophylaxis. We delve into various modalities used for prophylaxis such as pharmacological agents, nonpharmacological options, psychological therapies, interventional procedures, and neuromodulation. Also, we include the most recent scientific breakthrough in developing new medications targeting CGRP neurochemical. In addition, this chapter comprises an overview of key clinical evidence for the recommended modalities.

Indications for Migraine Prophylaxis

We summarize the indications here based on review of several guidelines. As of this writing, the most recent position statement update in 2018, by the American Headache Society for preventative treatment guidelines is included [8]. International guidelines published as recently as 2019 by Diener et al. is included as well [9]. They recommend initiation of migraine prevention treatment in the following patients:

- Attacks significantly interfere with patients' daily routines despite acute treatment
- Frequent attacks (≥4 monthly headache days)
- Three or more migraine attacks per month with a negative impact on the quality of life
- Migraine attacks which regularly last longer than 72 h
- Attacks which are unresponsive to acute therapy (including triptans)
- Patients who cannot tolerate the side effects of acute therapy
- Contraindication to, failure, or overuse of acute treatments, with overuse defined as:
  - Ten or more days per month for ergot derivatives, triptans, opioids, combination analgesics, and a combination of drugs from different classes that are not individually overused
  - Fifteen or more days per month for nonopioid analgesics, acetaminophen, and nonsteroidal anti-inflammatory drugs (NSAIDs [including aspirin])
- Complicated migraine attacks with debilitating (e.g. hemiplegic) and/or long-lasting auras
- Following migrainous brain infarction when other causes of stroke can be excluded

Basic Outline and Practical Tips for Implementing Migraine Prophylaxis

Starting migraine prophylaxis may be considered when patients' frequency and severity of headaches increase and they have difficulty managing or tolerating them. Prophylactic treatment targets to reduce frequency by 50%, reduce the intensity, and improve response to acute migraine treatment. Furthermore, high-frequency use of acute headache medications such as nonsteroidal anti-inflammatories may cause medication-overuse headaches. Adherence to prophylactic treatment can reduce the incidence of medication overuse headaches. The overall goal is to improve functionality and reduce disability associated with migraine headaches.

Starting medications greatly depend on patient preference, but following standards of care may improve the success of preventative therapy [10].

1. Start medications with highest level of evidence.
2. Consider co-morbid conditions and side effects which may cause contraindications to certain medications.
3. Start with the lowest effective dose, and titrate every 2–4 weeks until therapeutic effect develops and patient is unable to tolerate side effects.
4. Give the selected preventative medication an adequate trial of 2–6 months.
5. Goal setting and constant monitoring of frequency and severity of headaches.
6. Re-evaluation every couple month and titrate dose or change therapy.
7. Consider discontinuing or decreasing therapy if migraines are controlled for over six months.

Counsel the patients well about possible adverse effects with pharmacological agents. Encourage the patient to adhere to the titration regimen. Maintaining a migraine diary is a useful tool in assessing response to treatment. In general, monotherapy is preferred. However, it may not suffice due to unfavorable tolerance or inadequate response, in which case implement combination treatment.

It is established practice to continue prophylactic treatment for at least 6–9 months, longer if needed. Stopping the medication is indicated in the following conditions:

- If there is no improvement with an adequate trial of 2–6 months
- If the patient develops significant adverse effect at any time
- If the patient is migraine free for over 6 months, wean as tolerated to stop medications. Intermittent re-evaluations are recommended for recurrence of symptoms

Pharmacological Interventions

When considering what pharmacological agents to start the patient on, it is important to consider patient preference, comorbidities, and the pharmacological profile of the medication. We reviewed the FDA indications and the guidelines put forth by

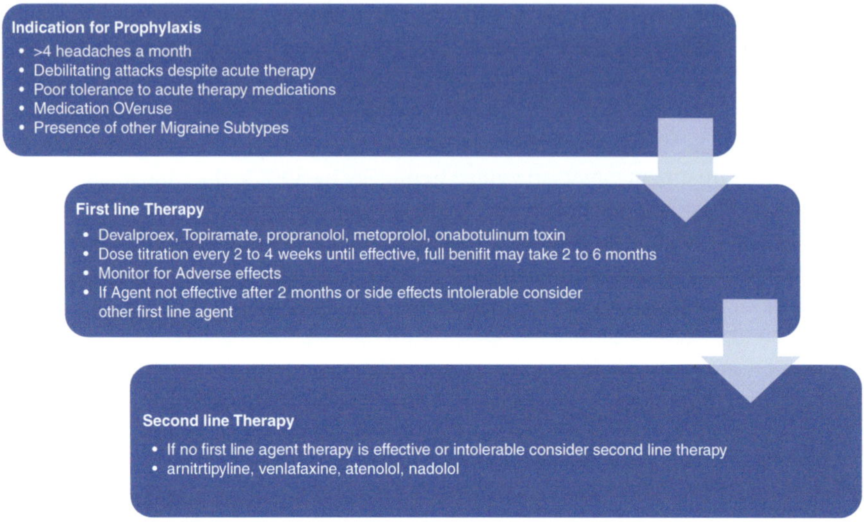

Fig. 4.1 Initiation of Medical Management of migraine (Data from Migraine Prophylaxis Am Fam Physician 2019 [12] and American Headache Society [13])

the American Academy of Neurology and the American Headache Society [11–13] for first-line and second-line medication for medications detailed below. These recommendations do not include the considerations for CGRP antibodies as the FDA approved them in 2018–2019, while the recommendations by AAN/AHS are from 2012. In the future, we may expect inclusion of these medications in the migraine prophylaxis guidelines depending on how these medications perform in the phase 4 clinical trials. An outline for indications of preventative treatment, medications, and management is detailed in Fig. 4.1.

Traditional Pharmacological Agents

Here we discuss commonly used migraine prophylaxis medications. We have discussed the newer CGRP antibodies in a separate section below titled new pharmacological advancements. Interestingly, the traditional migraine prophylaxis medications are not specifically targeted to migraine pathophysiological pathways. They were developed for different medical conditions and demonstrated significant clinical improvement in patients with migraine.

Anticonvulsants

Topiramate and divalproex sodium are FDA approved for migraine prophylaxis. Of the various anticonvulsants only topiramate and valproic acid have the most significant literature support for >50% reduction in migraine headaches. Interestingly, with continued pharmacological developments, medications such as topiramate, though classified as an anticonvulsant, may rarely be considered for that indication.

It has a more predominant role in migraine prophylaxis than seizure prophylaxis. Of the anticonvulsants, gabapentin, pregabalin, carbamazepine, oxcarbazepine, and lamotrigine were considered for treatment of migraine prophylaxis; however, subsequent studies did not demonstrate significant improvement [14, 15]. Interestingly, with continued pharmacological developments, medications such as topiramate, though classified as an anticonvulsant, may rarely be considered for that indication. It has a more predominant role in migraine prophylaxis than seizure prophylaxis.

Topiramate Topiramate is FDA approved for migraine prophylaxis. It has level-A evidence for use per the AAN/AHS guidelines. Topiramate reduces the frequency of headaches by 50% or more when compared to placebo. It blocks multiple channels such as voltage-dependent sodium and calcium channels [16]. It has also shown to inhibit glutamate-mediated excitatory neurotransmission and carbonic anhydrase activity [17], as well as reduce CGRP secretion from trigeminal neurons during stimulus [18]. The multiple molecular targets may account for why topiramate is effective in migraine while most other, more specific, anticonvulsants are not [19]. A favorable weight loss profile, in addition to its neuronal stabilizing mechanism, makes it an attractive migraine prophylaxis medication. Other adverse effects include kidney stones, and closed-angle glaucoma [20]. Migraine patients at baseline have a higher risk of kidney stones independent of the use of topamax, and adequate hydration should be encouraged in all migraine patients [19]. Acute angle closure glaucoma is a rare idiosyncratic effect that may be reversible with discontinuation of the medication. Mental slowing and difficulty with word-finding may occur; start at a low dose, go slow. Tachyphylaxis on long term is not evident. Doses range from 100 to 200 mg/day, although studies have suggested that a dose of 200 mg/day is no more effective and has more adverse effects than 100 mg/day in patients [21]. In a placebo-controlled, randomized, double-blinded study, topamax 100 mg/d demonstrated similar efficacy as propranolol 160 mg/d [22].

Valproic acid (Sodium Valproate/Divalproex) Divalproex sodium is approved by FDA for migraine prophylaxis. It is a good option for patients with concurrent seizure disorder and bipolar disorder and has shown to be effective in multiple trials compared to placebo. Common side effects include gastrointestinal distress, nausea, somnolence, and vomiting. Risks of thrombocytopenia, liver failure, and pancreatitis warrant periodic laboratory monitoring. It should be avoided in pregnancy as it increases risk for neural tube defects [23]. Similar to topiramate, there are multiple mechanisms at play and they include enhancing GABAergic inhibition and blocking excitatory ion channels [16]. It can also suppress protein kinase C which is a regulator in the glutamatergic neurotransmission [24] and in recent studies, the inhibition of the NF-kB pathway as a potential mechanism of action in migraine [25].

Zonisamide In a comparative study with topiramate, zonisamide demonstrated similar efficacy for migraine prophylaxis [26]. Most concerning adverse effects are Stevens-Johnson syndrome and toxic epidermal lysis. Initiate at low doses, and subsequet slow titration is recommended to prevent adverse effects. Recommended dose is 50–200 mg per day.

Lamotrigine Lamotrigine has a suppressive effect on cortical spreading depression. Some studies have suggested improved outcomes in migraine with aura, though not in migraine without aura [21]. Silberstein et al. demonstrated lamotrigine to be ineffective for migraine prophylaxis, (Level A evidence) [11].

Beta-Blockers

Beta-blockers are well established in their role for migraine prophylaxis. Interestingly, their role in migraine started with the accidental discovery of propranolol for migraine prophylaxis when studied for angina [27]. Mechanisms for beta-blockers in migraine prophylaxis are not completely understood, but inhibition of **β**1-mediated effects is the proposed mechanism of action. Further studies support beta-blocker's effects on noradrenaline synthesis, reduced neuronal firing rate in the locus coeruleus, regulation of firing rate of the periaqueductal gray matter via GABA-mediated actions, interfering with chronic sensitization, counteracting facilitation of trigeminovascular transmission, interaction with the serotonergic system, inhibition of nitric oxide production, and membrane stabilizing properties. These mechanisms may all contribute to antimigraine actions of beta-blockers.

Propranolol, metoprolol, nadolol, and timolol are the commonly studied beta-blockers for migraine prophylaxis. Based on clinical trials, propranolol and metoprolol have the highest ratings for migraine prophylaxis amongst the beta-blockers. Differences in the methodology of review of data have led to a disparity in the recommendation from several significant organizations regarding which specific beta-blocker is for first-line use for migraine prophylaxis. Danesh et al. consolidated the recommendations from the American Headache Society/American Association of Neurology (AAN/AHS), the Canadian Headache Society (CHS), and the European Federation of Neurological Societies (EFNS). Consistently, metoprolol and propranolol were cited as first-line use by all the organizations. Timolol and nadolol were cited by one organization, each as first-line use. There are only two FDA-approved beta-blockers, propranolol and timolol.

Beta-blockers have variability in their ability to cross the blood brain barrier, possibly attributing to their varying efficacy for migraine prophylaxis [28]. Beta-blockers with intrinsic sympathomimetic activity such as acebutolol, alprenolol, oxprenolol, and pindolol are not effective for migraine prevention [29]. Beta-blockers would be a preferred choice for migraine prophylaxis in patients with hypertension. It would be contraindicated in patients with asthma or hypertension.

Propranolol There are numerous trials showing the effectiveness of propranolol in migraine prophylaxis as a first-line treatment for medications. Usually they are a good option for patients with concurrent hypertension, but adverse effects, including hypotension, triggers of asthma, should be monitored [11]. Clinical studies support the efficacy of propranolol, timolol, bisoprolol, and metoprolol in migraine preventive treatment [30].

Metoprolol Similar to propranolol, metoprolol has the highest level of evidence across the three guidelines by AAN/AHS, CHS, and EFNS. Unlike propranolol, it does not have an affinity for serotonin receptors. However, metoprolol is not approved by FDA for migraine prophylaxis. Efficacy is dose dependent, 100 mg twice daily is more effective than 50 mg twice daily [31].

Timolol Level A evidence for use per the AAN/AHS guidelines. Other guidelines did not demonstrate similar support.

Atenolol and Nadolol Level B evidence for use per the AAN/AHS.

Antidepressants

Tricyclic antidepressants, serotonin norepinephrine reuptake inhibitors [SNRIs], and selective serotonin reuptake inhibitors [SSRIs] have all been studied for migraine prophylaxis. Amitriptyline and venlafaxine have level B evidence for migraine prophylaxis per the AAN/AHS recommendations.

Tricyclic Antidepressants Tricyclic Antidepressants (TCAs) were the first agents shown to be effective in the prophylaxis of headaches in 1964 [32]. TCAs have a broad mechanism of action as antihistamine, anticholinergic, serotonin, and norepinephrine reuptake inhibition. They have been used extensively for migraine prophylaxis with numerous studies demonstrating >50% improvement in migraine headaches. Tertiary tricyclics (amitriptyline or doxepin) and secondary tricyclics (nortriptyline) may be used. An adverse effect of all of the TCAs is sedation – tertiary TCAs are more associated with adverse effects compared to secondary TCAs. Other adverse effects are predominantly anticholinergic and include urinary retention, constipation, epigastric distress, hypertension, tachycardia, palpitations, and prolonged Qtc, to name a few. Antidepressants would be a preferred preventative migraine medication with concurrent depression. Its use would be relatively contraindicated in patients with mania.

Amitriptyline While multiple other antidepressants are used clinically in migraine prevention, amitriptyline has the most data to support its effectiveness. However, given its high incidence of adverse effects, many patients are unable to tolerate continuation of amitriptyline. It is a good medication for patients with depression or insomnia, but runs the risk of anticholinergic effects, orthostatic hypotension, and prolonged QT [33]. Given its effects of being a mixed serotonin-norepinephrine reuptake pump inhibitor, it is thought to facilitate descending noxious inhibition as well as have some mediation by a-2 agonists as well [34]. Dodick et al. demonstrated similar efficacy in reducing the monthly rate of migraine episodes with amitriptyline 100 mg/d and topiramate 100 mg/d in a multicenter, randomized, double-blinded, noninferiority study [35].

Nortriptyline Nortriptyline is a metabolite of amitriptyline and hence expected to be of similar efficacy with lesser adverse effects [36].

Serotonin Norepinephrine Reuptake Inhibitors (SNRIs): Venlafaxine, Duloxetine Serotonin norepinephrine reuptake inhibitors (SNRIs) have also demonstrated a positive role in migraine prevention. At times, there is reduced tolerability to tricyclic antidepressants because of their adverse effects, the patient's age, or the patient's comorbidities. SNRIs can be an alternative in such clinical scenarios. SNRIs increase neurotransmitter serotonin in the extracellular space by inhibiting its presynaptic reuptake. Potential adverse effects are sexual dysfunction, anxiety, nervousness, insomnia, drowsiness, fatigue, tremor, sweating, anorexia, nausea, vomiting, and dizziness or lightheadedness. Randomized controlled studies have demonstrated good efficacy of venlafaxine for migraine and tension type headaches [36]. Similar positive results have not been demonstrated with duloxetine. Hence, venlafaxine is the preferred choice among the two.

Selective serotonin reuptake inhibitors (SSRIs) SSRIs have been evaluated for prevention of migraine headaches. However, based on reviews, SSRIs are no more efficacious than placebo in patients with migraine; however, they may show benefit in tension-type headaches [37].

Recent comparative analysis between amitriptyline, SNRI, and SSRI demonstrates similar efficacy for migraine prophylaxis [33]. TCAs, SSRIs, and SNRIs can all cause weight gain. Overall, SSRIs and SNRIs have a better tolerance profile vs. TCAs.

Triptans

Triptans are commonly used as abortive treatment for acute migraine episodes. Interestingly, they also play a role in short-term prevention of menstruation-related migraine. The patient only uses the medication for 5–6 days of the month when the period is expected. Frovatriptan, naratriptan, and zomitriptan have been used. Frovatriptan uniquely has a long half-life of 26 hrs versus the other triptans. In addition, it has favorable tolerability and significantly lower rate of relapse over 48 hours versus the other triptans [38]. Triptans exert their effect via serotonin receptors. They are strong vasoconstrictors hence contraindicated in patients with significant cardiovascular or cerebrovascular event risk.

The first-line and second-line agents summarize various pharmacological agents that have been used in the prophylaxis of migraine (Tables 4.1 and 4.2) [39]. Further below we discuss the agents that have lesser but some efficacy in migraine prevention. Medications that have conflicting data or are established as ineffective therapies are listed below for completion.

Clinical Considerations for Selection of Pharmacological Agents

- Avoid prophylactic migraine treatment, especially topiramate and valproate in pregnant women, women planning to conceive, and lactating women.

Table 4.1 Summary of pharmacological agents adapted from AAN and AHS guidelines

First-line agents	Second-line agents	Possible effective agents	Conflicting data and/or inadequate support	Medications that are established as likely not effective
Anticonvulsants	*Antidepressants*	*Anticonvulsants*	*Anticonvulsants*	*Anticonvulsants*
Divalproex	Amitriptyline	Carbamazepine	Gabapentin	Lamotrigine
Topiramate	Venlafaxine	*ACE inhibitors*	*Antidepressants*	Oxcarbazepine
B-blockers	*B-blockers*	Lisinopril	Fluoxetine	Clomipramine
Propranolol	Atenolol	*ARBs*	Fluvoxamine	Acebutalol
Metoprolol	Nadolol	Candesartan	Protriptyline	*Benzodiazepines*
Triptans	*Triptans*	*α-Agonists*	*Anti-thrombotics*	Clonazepam
Frovatriptan	Naratriptan	Clonidine	Coumadin	*ARBs*
Onabotulinumtoxin A	Zolmitriptan	*Antihistamines*	*Beta-blockers*	Telmisartan
		Cyproheptadine	Bisoprolol	*NSAIDS*
		Guafacine	*Calcium Channel blockers*	Nabumetone
		B-blockers	Nicardipine	
		Nebivolol	Nifedipine	
		Pindolol	Nimodipine	
			Verapamil	
			Carbonic anhydrase inhibitors	
			Acetazolamide	

From Silberstein et al. [11], with permission

- Propranolol, sodium valproate, amitriptyline, and nortriptyline are cleared by hepatic metabolism which may be a limiting factor in a patient with liver pathology.

New Pharmacological Agents: CGRP Antagonists and Monoclonal Antibodies

FDA recently approved three CGRP inhibitors for migraine prophylaxis:

1. Erenumab (Aimovig)
2. Galacanezumab (Emgality)
3. Fremanezumab (Ajovy)

CGRP is produced in the central and peripheral neurons, and acts as a potent vasodilator. There is good evidence that CGRP is released during severe migraine attacks [40]. CGRP monoclonal antibodies are the first example of immunopharmacology in which antibodies target a molecular pathway instead of modifying immune pathways [41].Clinical trials involving anti-CGRP medications have positively shown effectiveness in treatment of acute attacks, prevention of attack onset, or reduction in attacks [42]. CGRP antagonists "gepants," such as ubrogepant, have

Table 4.2 Common First and Second-Line Agents

First-/second-line agents	Starting dose	Daily dose	Adverse effects	Contraindications
Anticonvulsants				
Divalproex	250 mg	250 mg to 500 mg twice a day	Nausea, dizziness, pancreatitis, hepatic failure, thrombocytopenia, tremors	Liver disease, pregnancy
Topiramate	25 mg	25 to 200 mg daily	Paresthesia (common), decreased appetite, difficulty in concentration, fatigue, kidney stones, fatigue, nausea	Pregnancy
Beta-blockers				
Metoprolol	50 mg twice a day	37.5 to 200 mg daily	Bradycardia, depression, fatigue, hypotension impotence, lethargy	Asthma, bradycardia, COPD
Propranolol	40 mg divided in two or three times a day	120 to 240 mg two to three times daily	Bradycardia, depression, fatigue, hypotension impotence, lethargy	Asthma, bradycardia, COPD
Timolol		20–30 mg daily or 10–15 mg twice daily	Bradycardia, depression, fatigue, hypotension impotence, lethargy	Asthma, bradycardia, COPD
Atenolol	50 mg	100 mg daily	Bradycardia, depression, fatigue, hypotension impotence, lethargy	Asthma, bradycardia, COPD
Nadolol	40 to 80 mg	20 to 160 mg daily	Bradycardia, depression, fatigue, hypotension impotence, lethargy	Asthma, bradycardia, COPD
Antidepressants				
Amitriptyline	10 mg	25 t0 150 mg daily	Blurry vision, constipation, decreased seizure threshold, dry mouth, QT prolongation, hypotension, sedation, urinary retention	Avoid with MAO-inhibitors, avoid in acute MI, seizure disorder, prolonged QT syndrome
Venlafaxine	37.5 mg	150 mg daily	Dry mouth, hypertension, insomnia, mydriasis, nausea, seizures	Avoid with MAO-inhibitors
Triptans				
Frovatriptan	2.5 mg	Not to exceed 7.5 mg daily, or > 2x a week	Dizziness, headache, nausea, paresthesias, flushing, abdominal pain, dry mouth	Avoid in vascular disease, severe renal or hepatic disease

From Loder et al. [39], with permission

demonstrated a robust role in the management of acute migraine. Monoclonal antibodies against CGRP (eptinezumab, fremanezumab, and galcanezumab) or the CGRP receptor (erenumab) effectively prevent migraine attacks [43, 44]. For chronic migraine, CGRP agents appear to have similar efficacy in reduction of monthly migraine days as well as a slightly higher responder rate than topiramate, with less adverse side effects [45]. The unique advantage versus currently prevalent prophylactic therapies is that they specifically target the trigeminal pain system and have a broad safety margin. All four CGRP monoclonal antibodies have shown good tolerability, with few adverse events, mostly with respect to injection site reactions, no serious side effects, and high retention rates of subjects in the studies [43]. Early trials of some cGRP receptor antagonists caused liver toxicity with transient increases of transaminases; however, none of the current drugs on the market showed liver toxicity [46]. Interestingly, CGRP receptor agonists have no effect on cerebral or systemic hemodynamics [47] so they could be safe in patients with triptan contraindications, such as previous myocardial infarction, angina, or previous stroke [48].

Monoclonal Antibodies to cGRP Receptor or Ligand

These medications bind or affect the calcitonin gene-related peptide receptor that mediates migraine pain pathways. Usage of this therapy has demonstrated efficacy in decreasing monthly migraine days, and these monoclonal antibodies are usually well tolerated, with the biggest side effect being constipation and injection site pain. However, long-term studies on its effectiveness and adverse effect profile still need to be completed [49].

Role of Newer Pharmacological Agents

Most medications available for acute and preventative drugs for migraine act on several neurotransmitters and may be ineffective or have a litany of side effects which lead to poor compliance and responder rates (40–50%) in most studies [43]. In addition, for the numerous migraine prophylaxis medications, most recommendations for pharmacological interventions are studied in only a few randomized controlled trials and or open-label studies [50, 51]. All the approved CGRP inhibitors have a unique rapid onset and favorable adverse effect profile; therefore, optimistic clinical results can be expected from these emerging treatments. With time and further study, their long-term adverse effects and clinical outcomes will be established.

Recommendations on When to Use Anti-CGRP

These treatments come at a high cost. Cost-effective care requires recognition of appropriate indications while ensuring access to treatment. The American headache society has published a position statement on the use of CGRP inhibitors [8, 50, 51].

Indications include the following:

1. Episodic migraine, high frequency (8 to 14 monthly headache days), patients must have demonstrated inability to tolerate (due to adverse effects) or inadequate response to a 6-week trial of at least two previous therapies. Episodic migraine, low frequency (4 to 7 monthly headache days), patients must also have had at least moderate disability, as defined by a Migraine Disability Assessment Scale (MIDAS) score of >11 or a Headache Impact Text-6 (HIT-6) score of >50.
2. Chronic migraine (>15 monthly headache days), patients must have either inability to tolerate (due to adverse effects) or inadequate response to a 6-week trial of at least two previous therapies and inability to tolerate or inadequate response to a minimum of two quarterly injection (six months) of onabotulinumtoxin A.

Medication Administration

The three prophylactic CGRP inhibitors are administered as injections and not orally. They vary from the oral prophylactic medications as the dose does not need to be initiated low and titrated slow. The dose recommendations are detailed in Table 4.3 [52, 53].

Criteria of Continuation of Treatment

Response to treatment should be evaluated at 4 weeks, 3 months and 6 months. Criteria for continuation of treatment, as recommended by the American Headache Society is as follows [8, 50]:

1. A reduction in mean monthly headache days of 50% or more relative to the pretreatment baseline (Diary documentation is recommended but not required).
2. A clinically meaningful improvement in a validated migraine-specific patient-reported outcome measure, including but not limited to:
   - A reduction of at least 5 points or more in Migraine Disability Assessment (MIDAS) score for those whose baseline score was between 11 and 20
   - A 30% reduction in MIDAS score for those with baseline scores above 20.
   - Reduction of 5 or more points on the Migraine Physical Function Impact Diary (MPFID)
   - Reduction in scores on the 6-item Headache Impact Test (HIT-6) of at least 5 points 58
   - Other documented benefits reported by clinician and patient

Table 4.3 Dose Recommendations for CGRP Inhibitors

Medication	Dose	Comments
Erenumab	2 doses, 70 mg and 140 mg	Either of which can be used as a starting dose
Fremanezumab [52]	2 doses, 225 mg and 675 mg	225 mg, monthly regimen 675 mg, quarterly regimen
Galcanezumab [53]	2 doses, 120 mg and 240	Initial loading, 240 mg Monthly, 120 mg dose

Of note, in the above cases, the AHS recommends either to continue treatment with CGRP inhibitors or consider neuromodulation.

Nonpharmacological Therapies

Nonpharmacological therapies are increasingly used over the last few decades. These include nutraceuticals, acupuncture, psychotherapy, behavior therapy, and neuromodulation.

The US Headache Consortium [54] suggested that nonpharmacologic treatments might be particularly useful for patients who

- prefer nonpharmacologic interventions.
- have inadequate response, poor tolerance, or medical contraindications to specific pharmacologic treatments.
- are pregnant, lactating, or planning to become pregnant.
- have a history of acute medication overuse.
- exhibit significant stress or deficient stress-coping skills.

Nutraceutical Approach for the Treatment of Migraine [55]

Most established evidence supports the use of butterbur, magnesium, and riboflavin for migraine headaches. Less established nutraceutical supplement such as feverfew and CoQ10 are also listed below for completion.

Butterbur

The AAN/AHS guidelines reported level A evidence of the use of butterbur for migraine prophylaxis. Two randomized controlled studies demonstrated good efficacy [56]. Underlying mechanism is antispasmodic and anti- inflammatory. The recommended dosage is 50–75 mg twice daily. Common side effects include gastrointestinal distress; however, serious hepato-toxicity may occur [57, 58].

Magnesium Dicitrate

It is well established that migraine deficiency is associated with migraine headaches. Mody et al. demonstrated increased NMDA sensitivity leading to glutamate-induced cortical-spreading depression [59]. There have been conflicting results in demonstrating improvement in migraine outcomes with replacement with migraine. Intravenous magnesium demonstrated improvement with acute migraine management [60]. Oral magnesium supplementation for prophylaxis may reduce the frequency and intensity of the migraine headache. Variations in response to magnesium replacement for patients with migraine associated with aura and without aura have been noted, with the former responding better [61]. The dose is not well established (add commonly used dose). Diarrhea may present as an adverse effect.

Riboflavin

Migraine attacks are associated with oxidative stress and mitochondrial dysfunction. Vitamin B2, riboflavin, can replenish mitochondrial energy production [62]. Studies have suggested that it may have a role in migraine prophylaxis. Daily recommended dose 400 mg.

Coenzyme Q10

CoQ10, a key cofactor of mitochondrial electron transport chain, has unique antioxidant and anti-inflammatory properties. Several studies have demonstrated the efficacy of CoQ10 as adjunctive therapy in cardiovascular, neurodegenerative diseases, and mitochondrial myopathies [63]. Mitochondrial dysfunction, subsequent oxidative stress contributes to the pathogenesis of migraine. Both CoQ10 and riboflavin demonstrate antioxidant properties useful for migraine prophylaxis. The recommended dose for CoQ10 is 100 mg three times a day.

Feverfew (*Tanacetum parthenium*)

A herbal remedy for migraine. Feverfew, belonging to the family Asteraceae (daisies), is a daisy-like perennial plant found commonly in gardens and along roadsides. The name originates from a Latin word *febrifugia, meaning "fever reducer."* [64]. Historically, the medication was used for ancient Greek and European medicine. Reports suggest anti- inflammatory and antinociceptive effects as the contributory mechanisms of action. The medication was used over the ages for several different conditions such as fever, arthritis, psoriasis, asthma, constipation, and nausea to name a few. In the 1980s, the medication gained recognition for use in migraine prophylaxis [65]. No serious adverse effects have been reported, nausea and bloating may occur. The recommended dose is 125 mg daily. The product should contain at least 0.2% parthenolide.

Acupuncture

Acupuncture is a therapy in which thin needles are inserted into the skin at certain points. Acupuncture has level A evidence, supported by consistent, good-quality patient-oriented evidence for efficacy in migraine prophylaxis [12]. In multiple trials, usage of acupuncture halved the frequency of headaches compared to patients with usual care only. Furthermore, sham or "fake" acupuncture was less effective than real acupuncture. Acupuncture has also been compared to pharmacologic treatment and shown to be just as effective, with less side effects from people receiving drug prophylaxis treatment. Consensus of a recent Cochrane report stated that acupuncture, consisting at least six treatment sessions, can be a valuable option for people with migraine [66].

Psychological Therapies

Psychological therapies are a useful tool for the prevention of migraine headaches. The conversion from episodic to chronic migraine may rely on conditions of increased cortical excitability, which is favored by stress through an adrenergic overflow [67]. Behavior therapy reduces the frequency of migraine attacks by reducing adrenergic flow, improving sleep patterns, reducing migraine stressors, improving quality of life, and adherence to migraine treatment. Different types of behavior therapy are: cognitive behavior therapy, biofeedback, and relaxation.

- Cognitive Behavior Therapy is improving the way the patient feels by influencing the way they think. This addresses maladaptive thinking and behaviors, consequentially encouraging risk avoidance for migraine triggers.
- Biofeedback utilizes special instruments that provide objective physiological information to patients as they practice biofeedback-guided relaxation.
- Relaxation is a strategy to relax muscle tension. Video programs, audio programs, guided imagery, deep breathing, and meditation are different techniques utilized.

Behavior Modification

Migraine triggers are specific to various individuals and avoidance of these triggers can help in migraine prophylaxis (Table 4.4). Utilizing a headache diary to identify these triggers is a simple helpful tool that can assist patients monitor the number of headache days and assess for therapeutic response. Common triggers include certain smells, menstruation, stress, cold weather, humidity, lack of meals, caffeine, red wine, chocolate, soft cheeses, and artificial additives and sweeteners [68, 69].

Table 4.4 Common migraine triggers

Migraine triggers
Modifiable
Additives
Alcohol
Artificial sweeteners
Caffeine (over consumption or acute withdrawal from regular use
Erratically scheduled meals
Exercise
Certain foods (chocolates, soft cheeses)
Bright lights
Odors
Oral contraceptives
Red wine
Sleep disturbances (e.g. insomnia, obstructive sleep apnea)
Smoking
Stress
Nonmodifiable
Psychiatric comorbidities
Weather changes
Menses

From Kelman [68], with permission

Interventional Procedures

OnabotulinumtoxinA (BoNT-A)

OnabotulinumtoxinA (BoNT-A) is FDA approved for prevention of chronic migraine. OnaBoNT-A is established as effective and should be offered to increase headache-free days (Level A) and is probably effective and should be considered to improve health-related quality of life (Level B) in chronic migraine. OnaBoNT-A is established as ineffective and should not be offered for episodic migraine (Level A) and is probably ineffective for chronic tension-type headaches (Level B) [70].

Usage of botox in several placebo-controlled studies showed reduction in frequency of total headache days as well as improvement in quality of life, with minor side effects, most commonly, injection site pain. However, while reduction of headache days is statistically superior, the magnitude of the difference is small (reduction of headache days: 1.7 for placebo and 2.3 for Botox). Botox should be used as a treatment after failure of oral medications [71].

A series of studies called the Placebo-controlled phase III Research Evaluating Migraine Prophylaxis Therapy (PREEMPT) treated patients with chronic migraine with BoNT-A at fixed sites (procerus, corrugator, frontalis, temporalis, occipitalis, cervical paraspinals, trapezius) in fixed doses (5 units per site for 155 units total). These studies showed significance in reducing headache and migraine days, headache hours, and improvement in patients' quality of life and is now the standard protocol for BoNT-A in Migraine prophylaxis [72–74].

There are several fixed sites for the injection of botox. The injection locations are easy to learn as most of the injection sites are around the head in a circular pattern starting from the forehead frontalis muscle, then the temporalis, the occipitalis, and the cervical paraspinal muscles. There are additional injection sites on the face and over the back. In the front, the sites are by the eyebrows in the corrugator and procerus muscles. In the back, they are located in the trapezius muscle. Total recommended injection sites are 31. Since 5 units of botox are injected at each site, it totals 155 units for the complete treatment. Variation in injection sites has been documented with improved success. The symptoms of the patients usually guide the location of the additional injections. After the injection, the patients should be counseled not to rub or massage the sites of injection for concerns of spreading the botox. Adverse effects commonly seen are soreness; other possibilities are bruising and swelling, more so in the more vascular regions of the face such as the eyebrows. Patients could develop flu-like symptoms if they have a mild allergic reaction. The most concerning adverse effects, though extremely rare, are neck weakness and dysphagia. The former has been reported with cervical paraspinal muscle injections. The latter is more so when the injection is done in the neck muscles for torticollis and not a typical location for the treatment of migraine headaches.

While it was initially thought that BoNT-A had its effects on headaches by relaxation of muscles in the headache and neck, it turned out it is ineffective in disorders of muscle tension such as in tension type headaches. It is believed that BoNT-A acts by inhibiting peripheral sensitization by attenuating neuropeptide and neurotransmitter exocytosis from peripheral sensory neurons, thereby reducing central sensitization which is why it plays a more important role in chronic versus episodic migraine [75]. The most remarkable improvement with Onabotulinum A is demonstrated within the first year of treatment and sustained for a long time [76]. Increasing the dosage improves efficacy without any change in the safety profile [77].

Neuromodulation

In neuromodulation, stimulation, either electric or magnetic, is applied either centrally or peripherally to modulate the pain pathways. While the bulk of migraine prophylaxis relies on the usage of medications, pharmacologic treatments are not efficacious in almost 50% of cases and a large majority of drugs are poorly tolerated due to their adverse effects [78], leading to a need for research into nonpharmacologic treatment options. Non-invasive Brain stimulation (NIBS) represents a treatment to act on neural plasticity by modifying brain excitability which may help improve migraine symptoms and lead to possible future treatment modalities. Transcranial magnetic stimulation for acute treatment of migraines has shown effectiveness [79] but recent guidelines suggest that patients who prefer non-drug therapies or those who have failed to respond or have contraindications to pharmacotherapy may be candidates for neuromodulation [8]. Based on results demonstrating efficacy and safety in clinical trials, the US Food and Drug Administration has approved the following [80, 81]:

1. Single-pulse transcranial magnetic stimulation for the acute and preventive treatment of migraine
2. Electrical trigeminal nerve stimulation for the acute and preventive treatment of migraine
3. Noninvasive vagus nerve stimulation for the acute treatment of migraine

Transcranial Magnetic Stimulation (TMS)

The magnetic field creates an electrical stimulus in the underlying cerebral cortex. Studies have demonstrated its ability to block cortical spreading depression which plays a significant role in migraine pathophysiology.

(a) Usage of a hand-held single pulse TMS device has shown to help in a reduction in the number of headache days compared to baseline [80, 82].
(b) Repetitive TMS has also been studied and shown to reduce headache frequency over placebo [83].

Trigeminal Nerve Stimulation

Many headaches and migraines involve the trigeminal nerve with the superior branch ending at the eye socket, underneath the forehead. External trigeminal nerve stimulation generates impulses to stimulate the nerve endings of the trigeminal nerve and repetitive impulses help reduce the number of migraine attacks [84].

(a) Usage shows statistically significant decrease in mean number of migraine days.
(b) There was significant decrease in monthly intake of migraine drugs for acute attacks.
(c) No change in mean headache severity per migraine day.

Transcutaneous Vagus Nerve Stimulator

Similar to stimulation by devices at the trigeminal nerve, transcutaneous vagus nerve stimulators stimulate the vagus nerve which has purported roles in pain regulation

(a) Usage shows that it significantly treats acute migraine attacks more effectively than sham stimulation, with significant pain improvement [85].
(b) There was no significant difference in frequency of headache days a month compared to placebo [86].

Conclusion

Migraine is the most common neurological condition affecting both women and men. Impaired function, missed work or school days, and reduced quality of life increase the burden associated with the disease. Despite this, it is a remarkably underdiagnosed and undertreated disease. Of those diagnosed, about a third of the patients would benefit from migraine prophylaxis. There are numerous pharmacological and nonpharmacological treatment options for migraine prophylaxis. Of the pharmacological agents, topiramate, divalproex, propranolol, metoprolol, amovig, emgality, ajovy, and Onabotulinum are FDA approved for migraine prophylaxis. We recommend the use of FDA approved medications for migraine prophylaxis prior to considering the other medications for off-label use. Besides the above, several antidepressants, triptans, anticonvulsants, and beta blockers have also demonstrated high levels of efficacy in migraine prophylaxis.

Though remarkably efficacious, the commonly used medications for migraine prophylaxis, listed as traditional medications for migraine prophylaxis in this chapter, have several shortcomings. These include adverse effects, poor tolerance, poor adherence to treatment, and increased pharmacological interactions. Adherence and persistence, when compared between anticonvulsants, antidepressants, and beta blockers, were shown to be below the acceptable threshold (<80%) after six months among both observational and RCT data. Common reason cited is adverse effects [87]. These are opportunities for improvement in therapeutic management. The newer agents have demonstrated high efficacy with an improved safety profile. Further studies will guide their continued role in migraine prophylaxis. Of the non-pharmacological agents, nutraceuticals, acupuncture, behavior therapy, neuromodulation have great potential. Several studies support their use for migraine prevention, larger randomized controlled studies are needed to guide their appropriate use going forward.

References

1. Smitherman TA, Burch R, Sheikh H, Loder E. The prevalence, impact, and treatment of migraine and severe headaches in the United States: a review of statistics from national surveillance studies. Headache. 2013;53:427–36.
2. Burch R, Rizzoli P, Loder E. The prevalence and impact of migraine and severe headache in the United States: figures and trends from government health studies. Headache. 2018;58:496–505.
3. Lipton RB, Bigal ME, Diamond M, Freitag F, Reed ML, Stewart WF, AMPP Advisory Group. Migraine prevalence, disease burden, and the need for preventive therapy. Neurology. 2007;68:343–9.
4. Schwedt TJ. Chronic migraine. BMJ. 2014;348:g1416.
5. Negro A, Martelletti P. Chronic migraine plus medication overuse headache: two entities or not? J Headache Pain. 2011;12:593–601.
6. Negro A, Rocchietti-March M, Fiorillo M, Martelletti P. Chronic migraine: current concepts and ongoing treatments. Eur Rev Med Pharmacol Sci. 2011;15:1401–20.
7. Katsarava Z, Buse DC, Manack AN, Lipton RB. Defining the differences between episodic migraine and chronic migraine. Curr Pain Headache Rep. 2012;16:86–92.
8. Society AH. The American Headache Society position statement on integrating new migraine treatments into clinical practice. Headache. 2019;59:1–18.
9. Diener H-C, Holle-Lee D, Nägel S, et al. Treatment of migraine attacks and prevention of migraine: guidelines by the German Migraine and Headache Society and the German Society of Neurology. Clinical and translational. Neuroscience. 2019;3:2514183X1882337.
10. Silberstein SD. Preventive migraine treatment. Continuum. 2015;21:973–89.
11. Silberstein SD, Holland S, Freitag F, Dodick DW, Argoff C, Ashman E, Quality Standards Subcommittee of the American Academy of Neurology and the American Headache Society. Evidence-based guideline update: pharmacologic treatment for episodic migraine prevention in adults: report of the Quality Standards Subcommittee of the American Academy of Neurology and the American Headache Society. Neurology. 2012;78:1337–45.
12. Ha H, Gonzalez A. Migraine headache prophylaxis. Am Fam Physician. 2019;99:17–24.
13. Society AH, American Headache Society. The American Headache Society position statement on integrating new migraine treatments into clinical practice. Headache. 2018; https://doi.org/10.1111/head.13456.
14. Linde M, Mulleners WM, Chronicle EP, McCrory DC. Antiepileptics other than gabapentin, pregabalin, topiramate, and valproate for the prophylaxis of episodic migraine in adults. Cochrane Database Syst Rev. 2013;6:CD010608.
15. Linde M, Mulleners WM, Chronicle EP, McCrory DC. Gabapentin or pregabalin for the prophylaxis of episodic migraine in adults. Cochrane Database Syst Rev. 2013;6:CD010609.
16. Cutrer FM. Antiepileptic drugs: how they work in headache. Headache. 2001;41(Suppl 1):S3–10.
17. Shank RP, Doose DR, Streeter AJ, Bialer M. Plasma and whole blood pharmacokinetics of topiramate: the role of carbonic anhydrase. Epilepsy Res. 2005;63:103–12.

18. Durham PL, Niemann C, Cady R. Repression of stimulated calcitonin gene-related peptide secretion by topiramate. J Headache Pain. 2006;46(8):1291–5.
19. Silberstein SD. Topiramate in migraine prevention: a 2016 perspective. Headache. 2017;57:165–78.
20. Linde M, Mulleners WM, Chronicle EP, McCrory DC. Topiramate for the prophylaxis of episodic migraine in adults. Cochrane Database Syst Rev. 2013;6:CD010610.
21. Parikh SK, Silberstein SD. Current status of antiepileptic drugs as preventive migraine therapy. Curr Treat Options Neurol. 2019;21:16.
22. Diener H-C, Tfelt-Hansen P, Dahlof C, Lainez J, Sandrini G, Wang S-J, Neto W, Jacobs D, et al. Topiramate in migraine prophylaxis: results from a placebo-controlled trial including an active comparator-propranolol. Cephalalgia. 2003;251(8):943–50.
23. Freitag FG, Collins SD, Carlson HA, et al. A randomized trial of divalproex sodium extended-release tablets in migraine prophylaxis. Neurology. 2002;58:1652–9.
24. Chen G, Manji HK, Hawver DB, Wright CB, Potter WZ. Chronic sodium valproate selectively decreases protein kinase C α and ε in vitro. J Neurochem. 1994;63:2361–4.
25. Li Y, Zhang Q, Qi D, Zhang L, Yi L, Li Q, Zhang Z. Valproate ameliorates nitroglycerin-induced migraine in trigeminal nucleus caudalis in rats through inhibition of NF-κB. J Headache Pain. 2016;17:49.
26. Mohammadianinejad SE, Abbasi V, Sajedi SA, Majdinasab N, Abdollahi F, Hajmanouchehri R, Faraji A. Zonisamide versus Topiramate in migraine prophylaxis. Clin Neuropharmacol. 2011;34:174–7.
27. Rabkin R, Stables DP, Levin NW, Suzman MM. The prophylactic value of propranolol in angina pectoris. Am J Cardiol. 1966;18:370–83.
28. Danesh A, Gottschalk PCH. Beta-blockers for migraine prevention: a review article. Curr Treat Options Neurol. 2019;21:20.
29. Limmroth V, Michel MC. The prevention of migraine: a critical review with special emphasis on β-adrenoceptor blockers. Br J Clin Pharmacol. 2001;52:237–43.
30. Sprenger T, Viana M, Tassorelli C. Current prophylactic medications for migraine and their potential mechanisms of action. Neurotherapeutics. 2018;15:313–23.
31. Steiner TJ, Joseph R, Hedman C, Rose FC. Metoprolol in the prophylaxis of migraine: parallel-groups comparison with Placebo and dose-ranging follow-up. Headache. 1988;28:15–23.
32. Lance JW, Curran DA. Treatment of chronic tension headache. Lancet. 1964;1:1236–9.
33. Xu X-M, Liu Y, Dong M-X, Zou D-Z, Wei Y-D. Tricyclic antidepressants for preventing migraine in adults. Medicine. 2017;96:e6989.
34. Gray AM, Pache DM, Sewell RD. Do alpha2-adrenoceptors play an integral role in the antinociceptive mechanism of action of antidepressant compounds? Eur J Pharmacol. 1999;378:161–8.
35. Dodick DW, Freitag F, Banks J, Saper J, Xiang J, Rupnow M, Biondi D, Greenberg SJ, Hulihan J. Topiramate versus amitriptyline in migraine prevention: a 26-week, multicenter, randomized, double-blind, double-dummy, parallel-group noninferiority trial in adult migraineurs. Clin Ther. 2009;31:542–59.
36. Smitherman TA, Brooke Walters A, Maizels M, Penzien DB. The use of antidepressants for headache prophylaxis. CNS Neurosci Ther. 2011;17:462–9.
37. Moja L, Cusi C, Sterzi R, Canepari C. Selective serotonin re-uptake inhibitors (SSRIs) for preventing migraine and tension-type headaches. Cochrane Database Syst Rev. 2005;3:CD002919.
38. Allais G, Benedetto C. Spotlight on frovatriptan: a review of its efficacy in the treatment of migraine. Drug Des Devel Ther. 2016;10:3225.
39. Loder E, Burch R, Rizzoli P. The 2012 AHS/AAN guidelines for prevention of episodic migraine: a summary and comparison with other recent clinical practice guidelines. Headache. 2012;52:930–45.
40. Diener H-C, Charles A, Goadsby PJ, Holle D. New therapeutic approaches for the prevention and treatment of migraine. Lancet Neurol. 2015;14:1010–22.
41. Goadsby PJ. Incredible progress for an era of better migraine care. Nat Rev Neurol. 2015;11:621–2.

42. Edvinsson L. The Trigeminovascular pathway: role of CGRP and CGRP receptors in migraine. Headache. 2017;57:47–55.
43. Grimsrud KW, Halker Singh RB. Emerging treatments in episodic migraine. Curr Pain Headache Rep. 2018;22:1–6.
44. Edvinsson L, Haanes KA, Warfvinge K, Krause DN. CGRP as the target of new migraine therapies — successful translation from bench to clinic. Nat Rev Neurol. 2018;14:338–50.
45. Deen M, Correnti E, Kamm K, Kelderman T, Papetti L, Rubio-Beltrán E, Vigneri S, Edvinsson L, Van Den Brink AM. Blocking CGRP in migraine patients--a review of pros and cons. J Headache Pain. 2017;18:96.
46. Deen M, On behalf of the European Headache Federation School of Advanced Studies (EHF-SAS), Correnti E, Kamm K, Kelderman T, Papetti L, Rubio-Beltrán E, Vigneri S, Edvinsson L, Van Den Brink AM. Blocking CGRP in migraine patients – a review of pros and cons. J Headache Pain. 2017; https://doi.org/10.1186/s10194-017-0807-1.
47. Petersen KA, Birk S, Lassen LH, Kruuse C, Jonassen O, Lesko L, Olesen J. The CGRP-antagonist, BIBN4096BS does not affect cerebral or systemic haemodynamics in healthy volunteers. Cephalalgia. 2005;25:139–47.
48. Dodick D, Lipton RB, Martin V, et al. Consensus statement: cardiovascular safety profile of triptans (5-HT agonists) in the acute treatment of migraine. Headache. 2004;44:414–25.
49. Goadsby PJ, Reuter U, Hallström Y, Broessner G, Bonner JH, Zhang F, Sapra S, Picard H, Mikol DD, Lenz RA. A controlled trial of Erenumab for episodic migraine. N Engl J Med. 2017;377:2123–32.
50. Cho S-J, Song T-J, Chu MK. Treatment update of chronic migraine. Curr Pain Headache Rep. 2017; https://doi.org/10.1007/s11916-017-0628-6.
51. Negro A, Martelletti P. Patient selection for migraine preventive treatment with anti-CGRP(r) monoclonal antibodies. Expert Rev Neurother. 2019;19:769–76.
52. Silberstein SD, Dodick DW, Bigal ME, Yeung PP, Goadsby PJ, Blankenbiller T, Grozinski-Wolff M, Yang R, Ma Y, Aycardi E. Fremanezumab for the preventive treatment of chronic migraine. N Engl J Med. 2017;377:2113–22.
53. Stauffer VL, Dodick DW, Zhang Q, Carter JN, Ailani J, Conley RR. Evaluation of Galcanezumab for the prevention of episodic migraine: the EVOLVE-1 randomized clinical trial. JAMA Neurol. 2018;75:1080–8.
54. Silberstein SD. Practice parameter: evidence-based guidelines for migraine headache (an evidence-based review): report of the quality standards Subcommittee of the American Academy of neurology. Neurology. 2000;55:754–62.
55. D'Onofrio F, Raimo S, Spitaleri D, Casucci G, Bussone G. Usefulness of nutraceuticals in migraine prophylaxis. Neurol Sci. 2017;38:117–20.
56. Lipton RB, Gobel H, Einhaupl KM, Wilks K, Mauskop A. Petasites hybridus root (butterbur) is an effective preventive treatment for migraine. Neurology. 2004;63:2240–4.
57. Rajapakse T, Pringsheim T. Nutraceuticals in migraine: a summary of existing guidelines for use. Headache. 2016;56:808–16.
58. Von Luckner A, Riederer F. Magnesium in migraine prophylaxis—is there an evidence-based rationale? A systematic review. Headache. 2018;58:199–209.
59. Mody I, Lambert JD, Heinemann U. Low extracellular magnesium induces epileptiform activity and spreading depression in rat hippocampal slices. J Neurophysiol. 1987;57:869–88.
60. Xu F, Arakelyan A, Spitzberg A, Green L, Cesar P-H, Csere A, Nworie O, Sahai-Srivastava S. Experiences of an outpatient infusion center with intravenous magnesium therapy for status migrainosus. Clin Neurol Neurosurg. 2019;178:31–5.
61. Hansen JM, Charles A. Differences in treatment response between migraine with aura and migraine without aura: lessons from clinical practice and RCTs. J Headache Pain. 2019;20:96.
62. Colombo B, Saraceno L, Comi G. Riboflavin and migraine: the bridge over troubled mitochondria. Neurol Sci. 2014;35(Suppl 1):141–4.
63. Littarru GP, Tiano L. Clinical aspects of coenzyme Q10: an update. Nutrition. 2010;26:250–4.
64. Pareek A, Suthar M, Rathore GS, Bansal V. Feverfew (Tanacetum parthenium L.): a systematic review. Pharmacogn Rev. 2011;5:103.

65. Feverfew–a new drug or an old wives' remedy? Lancet. 1985; 1:1084.
66. Linde K, Allais G, Brinkhaus B, Fei Y, Mehring M, Vertosick EA, Vickers A, White AR. Acupuncture for the prevention of episodic migraine. Cochrane Database Syst Rev. 2016;6:CD001218.
67. Pistoia F, Sacco S, Carolei A. Behavioral Therapy for Chronic Migraine. Curr Pain Headache Rep. 2013; https://doi.org/10.1007/s11916-012-0304-9.
68. Kelman L. The triggers or precipitants of the acute migraine attack. Cephalalgia. 2007;27:394–402.
69. Starling AJ, Dodick DW. Best practices for patients with chronic migraine: burden, diagnosis, and management in primary care. Mayo Clin Proc. 2015;90:408–14.
70. Simpson DM, Hallett M, Ashman EJ, et al. Practice guideline update summary: botulinum neurotoxin for the treatment of blepharospasm, cervical dystonia, adult spasticity, and headache. Neurology. 2016;86:1818–26.
71. Simpson DM, Hallett M, Ashman EJ, et al. Practice guideline update summary: botulinum neurotoxin for the treatment of blepharospasm, cervical dystonia, adult spasticity, and headache: report of the guideline development Subcommittee of the American Academy of Neurology. Neurology. 2016;86:1818–26.
72. Aurora SK, Dodick DW, Turkel CC, DeGryse RE, Silberstein SD, Lipton RB, Diener HC, Brin MF. OnabotulinumtoxinA for treatment of chronic migraine: results from the double-blind, randomized, placebo-controlled phase of the PREEMPT 1 trial. Cephalalgia. 2010;30:793–803.
73. Dodick DW, Turkel CC, DeGryse RE, Aurora SK, Silberstein SD, Lipton RB, Diener H-C, Brin MF. OnabotulinumtoxinA for treatment of chronic migraine: pooled results from the double-blind, randomized, placebo-controlled phases of the PREEMPT clinical program. Headache. 2010;50:921–36.
74. Diener HC, Dodick DW, Aurora SK, Turkel CC, DeGryse RE, Lipton RB, Silberstein SD, Brin MF, PREEMPT 2 Chronic Migraine Study Group. OnabotulinumtoxinA for treatment of chronic migraine: results from the double-blind, randomized, placebo-controlled phase of the PREEMPT 2 trial. Cephalalgia. 2010;30:804–14.
75. Aoki KR. Review of a proposed mechanism for the antinociceptive action of botulinum toxin type A. Neurotoxicology. 2005;26:785–93.
76. Guerzoni S, Pellesi L, Baraldi C, Cainazzo MM, Negro A, Martelletti P, Pini LA. Long-term treatment benefits and prolonged efficacy of OnabotulinumtoxinA in patients affected by chronic migraine and medication overuse headache over 3 years of therapy. Front Neurol. 2017; https://doi.org/10.3389/fneur.2017.00586.
77. Negro A, Curto M, Lionetto L, Martelletti P. A two years open-label prospective study of OnabotulinumtoxinA 195 U in medication overuse headache: a real-world experience. J Headache Pain. 2015;17:1.
78. Blumenfeld AM, Bloudek LM, Becker WJ, Buse DC, Varon SF, Maglinte GA, Wilcox TK, Kawata AK, Lipton RB. Patterns of use and reasons for discontinuation of prophylactic medications for episodic migraine and chronic migraine: results from the second international burden of migraine study (IBMS-II). Headache. 2013;53:644–55.
79. Lefaucheur J-P, André-Obadia N, Antal A, et al. Evidence-based guidelines on the therapeutic use of repetitive transcranial magnetic stimulation (rTMS). Clin Neurophysiol. 2014;125:2150–206.
80. Starling AJ, Tepper SJ, Marmura MJ, et al. A multicenter, prospective, single arm, open label, observational study of sTMS for migraine prevention (ESPOUSE Study). Cephalalgia. 2018;38:1038–48.
81. Chou DE, Gross GJ, Casadei CH, Yugrakh MS. External trigeminal nerve stimulation for the acute treatment of migraine: open-label trial on safety and efficacy. Neuromodulation. 2017;20:678–83.
82. Bhola R, Kinsella E, Giffin N, Lipscombe S, Ahmed F, Weatherall M, Goadsby PJ. Single-pulse transcranial magnetic stimulation (sTMS) for the acute treatment of migraine: evaluation of outcome data for the UK post market pilot program. J Headache Pain. 2015; https://doi.org/10.1186/s10194-015-0535-3.

83. Misra UK, Kalita J, Bhoi SK. High-rate repetitive transcranial magnetic stimulation in migraine prophylaxis: a randomized, placebo-controlled study. J Neurol. 2013;260:2793–801.
84. Riederer F, Penning S, Schoenen J. Transcutaneous supraorbital nerve stimulation (t-SNS) with the Cefaly® device for migraine prevention: a review of the available data. Pain Ther. 2015;4:135–47.
85. Martelletti P, on Behalf of the PRESTO Study Group, Barbanti P, et al. Consistent effects of non-invasive vagus nerve stimulation (nVNS) for the acute treatment of migraine: additional findings from the randomized, sham-controlled, double-blind PRESTO trial. J Headache Pain. 2018; https://doi.org/10.1186/s10194-018-0929-0.
86. Silberstein SD, Calhoun AH, Lipton RB, et al. Chronic migraine headache prevention with noninvasive vagus nerve stimulation: the EVENT study. Neurology. 2016;87:529–38.
87. Hepp Z, Bloudek LM, Varon SF. Systematic review of migraine prophylaxis adherence and persistence. J Manag Care Pharm. 2014;20:22–33.

CGRP and Immune Modulation: Evidence-Based Therapy

5

Hsiangkuo Yuan and Stephen D. Silberstein

Tremendous progress has been made in the field of migraine pathophysiology and pharmacotherapy in the past decade. Calcitonin gene-related peptide (CGRP), a 37-amino acid neuropeptide discovered 30 years ago [1], plays a significant role in migraine pathogenesis. Such an understanding has led to the development of multiple new migraine therapeutics for acute and preventive use. At the time of writing, the United States Food and Drug Administration (FDA) has approved two CGRP small molecules for acute treatment of migraine and four CGRP biologics for preventive treatment of migraine. The American Headache Society (AHS) guidelines recommend starting preventive treatment if: the patient has ≥3 headache days per month with severe disability, ≥4 headache days per month with mild disability, or ≥6 headache days per month with no disability. If the patient demonstrates an inability to tolerate (due to side effects) or an inadequate response to a 6-week trial of at least two classes of preventive medications or a 6-month trial of onabotulinumtoxinA, a CGRP functional blocking monoclonal antibody (MAb) injection may be used [2]. In this chapter, we will focus on the discussion of CGRP and its functional blockage through immunoglobulins.

CGRP Ligand, Receptor, and Its Role in Migraine

CGRP belongs to the calcitonin family of peptides, including calcitonin, amylin, adrenomedullin, and adrenomedullin-2. There are two isoforms of CGRP, α-CGRP, and β-CGRP, encoded by two different genes; they are structurally similar with overlapping functions but differ in regional potency and regulation. CGRP is found

H. Yuan (✉) · S. D. Silberstein
Jefferson Headache Center, Thomas Jefferson University, Philadelphia, PA, USA

© Springer Nature Switzerland AG 2021

S. Shah (ed.), *Migraine*, https://doi.org/10.1007/978-3-030-75239-2_5

throughout the body serving multiple functions (e.g., sensory, digestive, vascular, vestibular, hemopoietic, immunomodulatory, nociceptive, energy homeostasis, and tissue healing) [3]. CGRP is the most abundant neuropeptide in the trigeminal system, where it is found mainly in trigeminal ganglion (TG) and unmyelinated capsaicin-sensitive trigeminal nociceptive C fibers (less in A- or B-fibers). These peptidergic C-fibers are pseudounipolar nerves, which run along arteries and then spread into non-vascular tissue peripherally or project into the trigeminal cervical complex centrally. Activation of trigeminal nociceptive fibers releases CGRP that binds to the canonical CGRP receptor and the amylin1 (AMY_1) receptor, activating adenylyl cyclase to generate cyclic AMP (cAMP) and subsequent intracellular messengers depending on the cell type. In the TG, 70% of these CGRP neurons express vanilloid-sensitive transient receptor potential (TRPV1) channel, which triggers the release of CGRP in response to capsaicin, noxious heat, acidity, hydrogen sulfide, or injury. Other factors, such as nerve growth factor, angiotensin II, norepinephrine, cholecystokinin, and cannabinoids, are also involved. Once released, CGRP acts on nearby receptive cells, diffuses beyond the release site via volume transmission or gets metabolized by proteases without reuptake. Unmetabolized CGRP may leak into circulation. CGRP has a serum half-life of ~7 min (fast phase) and 26 min (slow phase). The tissue half-life is thought to be longer [4].

The CGRP receptor is a G-protein coupled receptor (GPCR) widely expressed throughout the body. It belongs to the secretin family that reacts to a variety of peptides. The CGRP receptor is formed by the heterodimerization of two components (calcitonin receptor-like receptor [CLR] and a single transmembrane-spanning protein called receptor activity-modifying protein 1 [$RAMP_1$]) then coupled with receptor component protein (RCP) for effective intracellular signaling (Table 5.1; Fig. 5.1). CGRP binds strongly to both the CGRP receptor and AMY_1 receptor (formed by calcitonin receptor with RAMP1), with lower affinity to adrenomedullin receptors (formed by CLR and $RAMP_2$ [AM_1] or RAMP3 [AM_2]), with minimal affinity to AMY_3 receptors (formed by calcitonin receptor (CTR) and RAMP3). Amylin, in contrast, binds weakly to the CGRP receptor [7]. CGRP receptors can signal not only via surface plasma membrane but also from intracellular endosomes [8]. Transient stimulation induces brief internalization of the receptor to endosomes; chronic exposure to CGRP leads to receptor degradation in lysosomes.

Table 5.1 Calcitonin family of ligands and receptors with rank of ligand potency

Ligand	Receptor component	Relative potency
CGRP	CLR + $RAMP_1$	CGRP >AM ≥ AMY ≥ CT
Adrenomedullin1 (AM_1)	CLR + $RAMP_2$	AM > AM_2 > CGRP > AMY > CT
Adrenomedullin2 (AM_2)	CLR + $RAMP_3$	AM = AM_2 > CGRP > AMY > CT
Calcitonin (CT)	CTR	CT > AMY, CGRP > AM
Amylin1 (AMY_1)	CTR + $RAMP_1$	AMY ≥ CGRP > CT > AM
Amylin3 (AMY_3)	CTR + $RAMP_3$	AMY > CGRP > AM

Data from Hay et al. [5] and Edvinsson et al. [6]

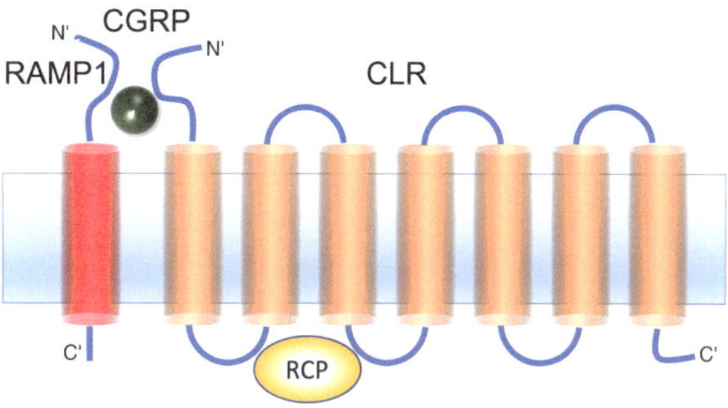

Fig. 5.1 CGRP receptor. A heterodimer of calcitonin receptor-like receptor (CLR) and receptor activity modifying protein (RAMP) coupled with receptor component protein (RCP) to facilitate adenylyl cyclase activation to form cAMP

The function of CGRP receptors varies. In the central nervous system, CGRP receptors are found almost exclusively in the neuronal process throughout the brain with complex functions [9]. Since central antagonism of CGRP is not required for therapeutic efficacy, the role of the central CGRP receptors in migraine is still to be determined. CGRP receptors can be found on the endothelial and smooth muscle cells of major cerebral arteries [10]. The intracranial and dural vascular smooth muscle layers receive CGRP from axonal varicosities interspersed the nerve fiber causing vasodilation; CGRP is one of the most potent vasodilators [11]. CGRP receptors are also found on ganglionic satellite glial cells (SGCs), perivascular mast cells (in rodents but not in humans), and immune cells modulating regional immune functions [11]. CGRP stimulates ganglionic SGCs to release cytokines; [12, 13] glial inhibition reverses CGRP-induced thermal nociception [12]. Within the dura mater and TG, CGRP receptors are found on Aδ-fibers but not C-fibers [11]. Axon-axon interactions occur near varicosities where CGRP is released to CGRP receptors located within the Ranvier's nodes of Aδ-sensory nerves; such an interaction occurs along the entire trigeminal pathway [14]. Interestingly, neither IV nor topical dural application of CGRP sensitizes meningeal nociceptors [15]. Instead of directly stimulating the nociceptors, CGRP's interaction with multiple cell types likely facilitates cross-talks within the trigeminal nervous system leading to neurogenic neuroinflammation and pain sensitization [16, 17].

CGRP was first demonstrated to play a role in migraines in 1990, when its levels were found to be increased in the jugular vein during acute migraine attacks [18]. Although the serum CGRP measurement's reliability is still a debatable issue, elevated CGRP levels have been frequently reported during spontaneous migraine attacks [18–22]. Treatment with triptans, topiramate, and onabotulinumtoxinA normalized CGRP levels [18–20, 23, 24]. In human migraine models using nitroglycerin (NTG), CGRP concentration correlated with the timing of headache and was reversed by triptan administration [25]. NTG-provoked migraine-like attacks were observed mostly in those with migraines but much less in healthy controls. Similarly, CGRP intravenous (IV) infusion triggered delayed migraine-like attacks (no other somatic pain) in roughly 68% of migraine subjects but not in healthy controls, individuals with tension-type headaches, or familial hemiplegic migraine [26–29]. This selective therapeutic response may reflect an underlying genetic predisposition and heightened sensitivity of the trigeminal nociceptive network in patients with migraine [30]. Two-hour CGRP infusion also caused gastrointestinal (GI) hypermotility symptoms (pain, nausea, diarrhea, urge to defecate), while pre-treatment with sumatriptan had no effect on CGRP-provoked headache or GI symptoms [31]. Since CGRP is impermeable to the blood-brain barrier (BBB), it likely acts somewhere with leaky or no BBB. Lack of central adverse events (AEs) from CGRP provocation also suggests a peripheral mechanism. It is reasonable to assume that, via a peripheral mechanism, CGRP mediates neurogenic neuroinflammation, modulates nociceptive inputs, and promotes pain sensitization that contributes to migraines [17, 32]. Blocking CGRP signaling is, therefore, a rational strategy to treat migraines.

Rationale for CGRP Monoclonal Antibody as Migraine Therapeutics

Animal studies of CGRP neutralization started in the late 1980s. In the early 2000s, migraine trials of CGRP functional-blocking MAbs began concurrently with the development of CGRP antagonizing small molecules (also known as gepants). Gepant binds competitively and preferentially to CGRP receptor and less to AMY_1 receptor [33, 34]. It blocks cAMP production and cAMP response element-binding protein (CREB) phosphorylation, inhibits trigeminovascular nociceptive activation, and subsequently reverses CGRP-induced vasodilation and neurogenic inflammation that leads to migraines [35, 36]. A peripheral site of action has been suggested, as earlier gepants of limited BBB permeability still achieved clinical efficacy, and a clinically efficacious dose of telcagepant (140 mg PO) showed only low receptor occupancy in the brain in a human PET study [37, 38].

Gepant is a new class of acute migraine medication successfully developed since the first triptan (sumatriptan) approval in 1991. Olcegepant (BIBN-4096; Boehringer Ingelheim GmbH, Germany), telcagepant (MK-0974; Merck, Kenilworth, NJ), MK-3207 (Merck, Kenilworth, NJ) are early gepants (Table 5.2)

Table 5.2 CGRP antagonizing small molecules (gepants)

Name	Company	Route	$T_{1/2}$	T_{max}
Olcegepant	Boehringer Ingelheim	IV	2.5 h	10 min
Telcagepant	Merck	PO	6 h	1.5 h
MK-3207	Merck	PO	3–6 h	1–2 h
Ubrogepant	Abbvie	PO	5–7 h	0.7–1.5 h
Atogepant	Abbvie	PO	10 h	~2 h
Rimegepant	Biohaven	PO	11–12 h	1.5–2 h
Zavegepant[a]	Biohaven	IN, PO	–	15–20 min

IV intravenous, *PO* oral, *IN* intranasal, $T_{1/2}$ circulatory half-life, T_{max} time to maximal serum concentration

[a]Zavegepant used to call vazegepant. Its half-life data is unobtainable at the time of writing

whose developments were halted by their potential hepatotoxic effects when dosed regularly [39]. The four new gepants, ubrogepant (MK-1602; Ubrelvy®, Abbvie, North Chicago, IL), atogepant (MK-8031, AGN-241689; Abbvie, North Chicago, IL), rimegepant (BMS-927711, BHV-3000; Nurtec ODT®, Biohaven, New Haven, CT), and zavegepant (BMS-742413, BHV-3500; Biohaven, New Haven, CT), in contrast, showed no significant hepatotoxicity so far. At the time of writing, both ubrogepant and rimegepant have received the FDA approval for acute migraine use. With a different mechanism of action and no vasoconstrictive effect, gepant is an attractive alternative to patients who are unresponsive, intolerant, or contraindicated to triptan. In preclinical models, gepant displayed a lower risk than triptan for medication overuse headaches [40, 41]. Preventive use of rimegepant (every other day) and atogepant (daily) has been demonstrated in clinical trials, but it is currently under FDA review [42, 43]. A detailed discussion of gepant's efficacy in clinical trials is reviewed elsewhere [44].

To date, there are four FDA-approved CGRP biologics (Table 5.3) for use in migraine prevention, namely eptinezumab (ALD-403; Vyepti®, H. Lundbeck A/S, Denmark), erenumab (AMG-334; Aimovig®, Amgen, Thousand Oaks, CA), fremanezumab (Rinat RN-307, Labrys LBR-101, TEV-48125; Ajovy®; TEVA, Petah Tikva, Israel), and galcanezumab (LY2951742; Emgality®; Eli Lilly, Indianopolis, IN). While eptinezumab is administered through IV infusion, all others are administered via autoinjectors for subcutaneous (SC) injection. Erenumab targets the CGRP receptors, while all others bind to CGRP ligands (both α and β forms). Compared to oral gepants, these biologics have distinct advantages such as long half-lives, insignificant antibody-drug interaction, negligible off-target effect, and minimal influence from hepatic/renal dysfunction. Due to their unique macromolecular structure, they display a pharmacokinetic (PK) and pharmacodynamic (PD) profile different from small molecule medications.

Table 5.3 CGRP functional blocking monoclonal antibodies

Name	Company	IgG	Route	$T_{1/2}$	T_{max}	Dose	Frequency
Eptinezumab-jjmr	Lundbeck	$IgG_{1\kappa}$	IV	27D	0.5–1 h[a]	100 mg	QTLY
						300 mg	QTLY
Erenumab-aooe	Amgen	$IgG_{2\lambda}$	SC	28D	6D	70 mg	QM
						140 mg	QM
Fremanezumab-vfrm	Teva	IgG_{2a}	SC	31D	5–7D	225 mg	QM
						675 mg	QTLY
Galcanezumab-gnlm	Eli Lilly	IgG_4	SC	27D	5D	120 mg[b]	QM

IV intravenous, *SC* subcutaneous, $T_{1/2}$ circulatory half-life, T_{max} time to maximal serum concentration, *QTLY* quarterly, *QM* monthly

[a]Depends on the infusion time

[b]Starts with 240 mg loading

Monoclonal Antibody Structure and Nomenclature

MAbs are immunoglobulins (Igs) engineered with a monovalent affinity to their target. There are five subtypes of Ig, namely, α (IgA), δ (IgD), ε (IgE), γ (IgG), and μ (IgM), where IgG is most commonly used as a therapeutic antibody. It is made up of two light chains and two heavy chains with a mass of 150 kDa (~7–10 nm). It is structurally divided into three parts (2 Fab and 1 Fc regions). The Fab contains complementarity-determining regions (CDRs) that bind to a specific antigen; the Fc plays a major role in effector cell activation (e.g., phagocytosis) and antibody recycling. Glycosylation on the Fc or Fab regions affects the immunoregulatory and functional properties of the IgG. There are four subclasses of IgG named in order of decreasing abundance (IgG_1, IgG_2, IgG_3, IgG_4); they are structurally conserved but different in their constant regions (e.g., hinges, upper CH2 domain) [45]. Since IgG_3 has a relatively shorter half-life, most therapeutic MAbs are made of IgG_1, IgG_2, or IgG_4. At the time of writing, there are more than 90 MAb formulations approved by the FDA, where more than three-quarters are indicated for cancer or autoimmune conditions [46].

For clinical use, therapeutic MAbs ideally should display high target specificity, long circulatory half-life, and low immunogenicity. They are designed with great target specificity through unique selection strategies. Numerous methods were developed to lower the immune-clearance response from the host to increase half-life. Traditionally, MAbs were made by an immortalized hybridoma, a fusion of antibody-producing B cells and immortalized myeloma cells, pioneered by Milstein and Köhler in 1975. Early therapeutic MAbs contained foreign non-human components; their clinical use was limited by high immunogenicity and short half-life. Chimerization and humanization were thus developed to lower the non-human antibody content. Chimeric antibodies (-ximab) are defined by having <85% human sequence on V gene, while humanized antibodies (-zumab) have ≥85% derived from human DNA with only the CDR being foreign (e.g., non-human or synthetic). However, human anti-chimeric antibody responses and CDR grafting difficulties can be problematic. To solve these issues, fully human antibodies (-umab) were developed using technologies such as phage display, yeast display, and transgenic mice [47, 48]. Importantly, estimating immunogenicity based purely on the foreign content ratio is oversimplified. Many other factors (e.g., Fc glycosylation, route of administration, antibody stoichiometry) play specific roles in triggering adverse immune reactions; this explains why new chimeric moieties are still in development for clinical use. Furthermore, modern humanization engineering techniques cause confusion of the term "human" or "humanization". The World Health Organization and the American Medical Association thus proposed in 2017 a new naming system based not on the species but on the target, such as -ne- for neural or -ta- for tumor [49]. It is worth noting that while MAbs can be engineered with low immunogenicity, some MAbs are designed to target the immune system (e.g., for autoimmune disorders) or to induce an immune response (e.g., for neoplastic disorders). For CGRP functional blockade, in contrast, the MAbs are designed to neutralize CGRP ligands or receptors without causing an immune reaction.

Pharmacodynamics and Pharmacokinetics

The PK and PD profiles determine the MAbs mechanism of action. MAbs are glycoproteins with unique properties (e.g., size, surface charge, target/off-target affinity, absorption, distribution, metabolism, and excretion) strikingly distinct from small molecules. MAbs can be created with picomolar affinity, which is usually several-fold potent and more specific than that of small molecules. In an equilibrium PK/PD model, greater affinity, higher dose, and slower clearance of MAb lead to greater and longer suppression of free ligand activity [50]. It has minimal off-site targeting (i.e., low binding to other ligands or receptors) and MAb-drug interaction (i.e., low binding to other drugs). Since MAb binding is governed by thermoequilibrium, its action is a dynamic process that favors association over dissociation. It is not a fixed binding of the antibody to the ligand. The association rate (K_a) and dissociation rate (K_d) determine how fast and stable the MAb binds, respectively. At any given time, there will always be both free MAbs and their ligands. This may explain why despite higher concentration, CGRP's functional blockade is not 100% [51]; basal CGRP function is probably less affected than reactive CGRP function. MAbs have high target specificity; their effects and adverse effects depend on the target's function and distribution. Blocking CGRP's protective function (e.g., decidualization, homeostasis, vasodilation) in certain regions (e.g., placenta, bone marrow, coronary vessel) is not ideal. Blocking a ligand is also not the same as blocking a receptor due to biological redundancy in the GPCR system (i.e., different ligands on a single receptor or the same ligand on different receptors). With modern bioengineering technology, MAbs can certainly be designed with high target specificity and minimal immunogenicity. The major action and AE thus depend on the target's function and the MAb's local concentration at the relevant target sites.

Therapeutic MAbs are typically delivered via IV or SC administration to avoid degradation in the GI tract. Compared to IV injection, SC injection is more convenient but may be more painful and have lower bioavailability. Due to their large size and positive surface charge, as well as local proteolysis and immunophagocytosis, the transportation of MAbs through SC tissue and the lymphatic system into circulation is much slower than IV administration. For IV administration, the T_{max} (time to reach maximal serum concentration [C_{max}]) occurs at the end of infusion with 100% bioavailability. In contrast, it takes 3–8 days after SC injection to reach C_{max} with 40–80% bioavailability. Due to delayed T_{max} and reduced bioavailability, SC injection of MAbs is thus not ideal for acute treatment and may sometimes require higher dosing.

The distribution of MAbs depends on their extravasation and convection through vessels and tissues, respectively. Extravasation is a passive process that depends on the hydrostatic/oncotic pressure and the size of the paracellular pores in the vascular epithelia (e.g., fenestrated capillaries, sinusoids). Receptor-mediated transcytosis, in contrast, is an active process to transport MAb via specific surface receptors. Here, we focus on mechanisms and barriers of passive IgG delivery. Once extravasated, MAbs convect through the extracellular matrix until they bind to the target, get metabolized, or enter the lymphatic system. MAbs are usually distributed in organs with leaky vasculatures such as thyroid, skin, liver, and spleen. In the brain parenchyma, due to the tight BBB, IgG concentration is very low (0.2%) relative to plasma concentration. However, in the central nervous system, the dura mater, pituitary, and circumventricular organs are much leakier than regions inside the BBB or brain-CSF barrier (arachnoid mater). Sensory ganglia (TG, cervical, vagus, sphenopalatine, etc.) are also highly permeable but with interganglionic differences [52]. IgG accumulates much greater in dura mater (11%) and TG (5.2%) than in cortex (0.23%), hypothalamus (0.34%), or CSF (0.12%) [53]. Inside the ganglia, IgGs are found surrounding individual neurons possibly on the satellite glial cells (SGCs) [54]. Since dura and sensory ganglia not only contain leaky vasculature but also play critical roles in migraine pathogenesis, they are the presumed action sites for CGRP MAbs. The effect of CGRP MAbs in other regions remains to be determined. To date, the use of CGRP MAb has yet resulted in any major cardiac, pulmonary or hepatic AE in clinical trials, and the real-world data is becoming available.

MAbs are not typically filtered by the kidney or metabolized by microsomal/mitochondrial oxidation in the liver. IgG catabolism is estimated to be 33%, 24%, 16%, and 12% from skin, muscle, liver, and gut, respectively [55]. This unique distribution explains why body surface area or body weight is often used to guide MAb dosing. IgGs are metabolized inside the cells upon either receptor-mediated endocytosis (minor) or nonspecific pinocytosis (major). The former takes place at the target cell or immune cell surface; the latter is a nonspecific fluid-phase endocytosis utilized by endothelial cells throughout the body. Interestingly, IgG has a much longer circulatory half-life than IgM or IgA due to a salvage pathway mediated by neonatal Fc receptor (FcRN) to escape intracellular breakdown. Without FcRn, IgG catabolism is similar to that of IgM or IgA [56]. In fetuses and neonates, FcRN mediates IgG transport via placenta and intestine, respectively. FcRN is highly expressed in skin, muscle, liver, and spleen, where vascular endothelia and reticuloendothelia are the major sites of IgG homeostasis [57]. FcRN, which is expressed in the brain microvascular endothelium and choroid plexus epithelium, also facilitates IgG transport from the brain parenchyma and cerebrospinal fluid, respectively, back to blood vessels [58]. This salvage pathway is saturable, rendering a non-linear elimination at higher MAb concentration [59]. At lower doses, MAb may exhibit non-linear PK due to receptor-mediated clearance [60]. Anti-drug antibody (ADA), a polyclonal response that can be either neutralizing or non-neutralizing, plays a minor role in IgG elimination. Neutralizing ADAs reduce MAb's specific binding to the target; non-neutralizing ADAs form ADA-mAb immune complexes that are cleared via the reticuloendothelial system. Other time-varying MAb PK profiles are still to be studied [61]. A significant variation exists in PK between individuals with the same MAbs or even the same individual with time. Overall, MAb's unique PK allows for a longer dosing interval with no adjustment need for hepatic/renal dysfunction, but each individual's response may vary.

Possible Mechanisms of CGRP Functional Blocking Monoclonal Antibody

The main questions are: how do CGRP MAbs work, and are there any differences? They likely act similarly to gepants by blocking CGRP's function and CGRP-induced downstream cAMP signaling pathway but have no effect in the absence of CGRP [62]. In 2008, RN-307 (now fremanezumab) first demonstrated long-lasting neurogenic vasodilatation inhibition without affecting heart rate or blood pressure in rat models [63]. Fremanezumab, despite having no effect on baseline tactile thresholds, significantly inhibited both bright light stress- and nitric oxide donor-induced cutaneous allodynia in rats that were previously primed with sumatriptan or morphine [64]. In a cortical spreading depression (CSD) rat model, fremanezumab prevented the sensitization of high-threshold but not wide-dynamic range neurons [65]. It selectively inhibits the responsiveness of Aδ-fibers but not C-fibers of afferent meningeal nociceptors [66]. Fremanezumab IV did not prevent CSD-induced dural arterial dilatation and plasma protein extravasation (PPE) but prevented CGRP-induced dural arterial dilatation [67]. Even when the BBB was compromised, fremanezumab IV still failed to prevent CSD [68]. Eptinezumab (another MAb) alleviated and prevented the cutaneous mechanical hypersensitivity induced by NTG in rats. The onset and duration of action from eptinezumab were longer than that from olcegepant (a gepant) [69]. Both eptinezumab and olcegepant, when administered intracerebroventricularly in mice, failed to change the mechanical sensitivity threshold; this is suggestive for the lack of central action [70]. Eptinezumab also attenuated the peripheral CGRP-induced light aversion behaviors and diarrhea in mice [71, 72]. Although these studies were from different CGRP MAbs preparations, we can probably assume they share a similar mechanism: systemic pretreatment of CGRP functional blocking MAbs likely blocks the pain sensitization primed by medication or CSD via a peripheral mechanism.

Although they bind to CGRP ligand or receptor with similar picomolar affinity, each CGRP MAb exhibits a unique characteristic. In binding analyses, galcanezumab and eptinezumab engage the CGRP ligand quicker (higher K_a) than fremanezumab; [73] quicker binding may be beneficial for acute usage. Eptinezumab and fremanezumab dissociate much slower (smaller K_d) than galcanezumab. Galcanezumab and erenumab are thus usually considered having reversible target binding [73, 74]. Whether these binding features result in a clinical difference remains to be seen. To quantify CGRP's activity clinically, capsaicin-induced dermal blood flow (CIDBF) was used. For erenumab, the maximum possible DBF inhibition estimated by modeling was 89% (95% CI 87.3–91.4). It required less concentration than other CGRP ligand-targeting MAbs to achieve maximum CIDBF inhibition; the magnitude of maximum CIDBF inhibition was also higher. Only the CIDBF, but not the basal DBF, was affected [74]. The dermal response, however, does not predict clinical anti-migraine efficacy.

The major clinical difference is determined by the target type (ligand vs. receptor) and the administration route (IV vs. SC). Although there is no head-to-head comparison, the three CGRP ligand MAbs are probably equally effective in migraine prevention, but that remains to be examined. GPCR redundancy likely renders CGRP ligand MAb less prone to adverse reaction than receptor MAb. This probably explains why constipation ranked second for erenumab but did not make the top ten AEs for fremanezumab or galcanezumab [75]. In addition, due to administration route difference, eptinezumab is associated with shorter T_{max} and greater exposure (as assessed by C_{max} or area under curve) than fremanezumab, galcanezumab, and erenumab administered at single therapeutic doses [76]; IV administration explains why the treatment effect for eptinezumab can be seen from day 1 [77], but its real-world clinical benefit remains to be explored.

Clinical Evidence for CGRP Monoclonal Antibody in Migraine

Eptinezumab is a humanized $IgG_{1\kappa}$ targeting both the α- and β-CGRP ligands. It is produced by yeast as opposed to mammalian cells. It requires quarterly infusion and is the only IV formulation available. In their studies, eptinezumab 100 mg or above consistently showed significant clinical efficacy in reducing migraine frequency (Table 5.4) and improving quality of life. Overall, there were significant mean monthly migraine day reduction (placebo-adjusted) of 0.7–1.1 days in EM and 2.0–2.6 days in CM. ≥50% responder rate was also higher in the treatment than placebo groups: 12.4–18.9% more in EM and 14.6–22.1% more in CM. Eptinezumab has rapid clinical benefit as it was effective from day 1 [77]. A 104-week open-label safety study (NCT02985398) on eptinezumab 300 mg for patients with CM showed improvement in disease burden and quality of life [82]. Overall, the

Table 5.4 Summary of eptinezumab-related clinical trials

Trial information	Drug dose (mg)	Primary endpoint
NCT01772524 [78] Phase 1b, EM, $n = 163$	1000 vs. placebo	Safety profile in 24 weeks. (MMD change from baseline: −1.0)[a]
NCT02275117 [79] Phase 2b, CM, $n = 616$	300, 100, 30, 10 vs. placebo	≥75% responder rates: 33.3%*, 31.4%*, 28.2%, 26.8%, vs. 20.7% (MMD change from baseline: −2.7*, −2.1*, −2.4*, −1.2)[a]
NCT02559895 [80] Phase 3, EM, $n = 888$	300, 100, 30 vs. placebo	MMD change from baseline: −1.1*, −0.7*, −0.8*
NCT02974153 [81] Phase 3, CM, $n = 1072$	300, 100 vs. placebo	MMD change from baseline: −2.6*, −2.0*

All studies were evaluated over 12-week unless otherwise specified

EM episodic migraine, *CM* chronic migraine, *MMD* mean monthly migraine days

[a]Secondary endpoint

*Statistically significant

treatment-emergent AEs were similar between treatment and placebo groups, with the most common AEs being nasopharyngitis, upper respiratory tract infection, sinusitis, and influenza; 2–6% resulted in discontinuation of therapy. The development of neutralizing ADA was 2.2% and 7.8% in the phase 3 trials. At this moment, a trial investigating eptinezumab 100 mg IV for acute migraine use (NCT04152083) has met statistical significance on the co-primary endpoints with no new safety signal identified, but the detail has yet to be released [83].

Erenumab, a fully human $IgG_{2\lambda}$ targeting the CGRP receptor, has been shown to reduce migraine frequency (Table 5.5) and improve quality of life. All trials reached their primary endpoint from monthly erenumab SC injection 70 mg or above. There were significant mean monthly migraine days reduction (placebo-adjusted) of 1.0–1.9 days in EM and 2.5 days in CM. ≥50% responder rate was also higher in the treatment than placebo groups: 10–23% more in EM (including those who failed 2–4 preventives) and 17–18% more in CM. Those achieving ≥50% response achieved twice mean monthly migraine days' reduction than that of the overall study population [89]. In a 52-week open-label study (NCT02174861), 74% stayed in the study where 59% achieved ≥50% reduction in mean monthly migraine days and a reduction of −9.3 days [90]. Subjects with pre-existing medication overuse also responded similarly. Higher dose erenumab showed a greater clinical benefit but no worse AEs. Most frequent AEs were injection pain, viral upper respiratory tract infection, upper respiratory tract infection, sinusitis, and arthralgia. However, serious constipation requiring hospitalizations was reported in post-marketing analysis. "Constipation with serious complications" was then added to the Aimovig® FDA label as a warning. Erenumab was not associated with vasoactive properties per se but specifically inhibited CGRP-induced relaxation [91]. However, a rare vascular complication has been reported possibly from the loss of CGRP's protective vasodilatory response [92]. Since erenumab was found to worsen cardiac

Table 5.5 Summary of erenumab-related clinical trials

Trial information	Drug dose (mg)	Primary endpoint
NCT01952574 [84] Phase 2, EM, $n = 483$	70, 21, 7 vs. placebo	MMD change from baseline: −1.1*, −0.1, 0.1
NCT02483585 [85] Phase 3, EM, $n = 577$	70 vs. placebo	MMD change from baseline: −1.0*
NCT02456740 [86] Phase 3, EM, $n = 955$	140, 70 vs. placebo	MMD change from baseline[a]: −1.9*, −1.4*
NCT03096834 [87] Phase 3b, EM[b], $n = 246$	140 vs. placebo	≥50% response in MMD reduction: 30% vs. 14%, OR 2.7*
NCT02066415 [88] Phase 2, CM, $n = 667$	140, 70 vs. placebo	MMD change from baseline: −2.5*, −2.5*

All studies were evaluated over 12-week unless otherwise specified
EM episodic migraine, *CM* chronic migraine, *MMD* mean monthly migraine days, *OR* odds ratio
[a]24-week trial, averaged from last 3 months
[b]Failed 2–4 migraine preventives
*Statistically significant

dysfunction in chronic hypertensive mice [93], "new-onset or worsening of pre-existing hypertension" was also added to the label as a warning.

Fremanezumab is a humanized IgG_{2a} targeting both the α- and β-CGRP ligands administered SC monthly or quarterly. All studies met their primary endpoints (Table 5.6) and demonstrated improvement in migraine frequency, disease burden, and quality of life. In the 12-week study period, there were significant reduction in mean monthly migraine days (placebo-adjusted) of 1.3–2.8 days in EM and 1.7–2.0 days in CM. ≥50% responder rate was also higher in the treatment than placebo groups: 17–31% more in EM and 20–24% more in CM. In CM subjects with medication overuse at baseline, more than 50% reported no medication overuse during the treatment [99]. Discontinuation due to AEs or SAEs occurred in <1% of patients treated. Efficacy and safety of fremanezumab were maintained over 12 months [100]. After completion of the 1-year extension study, 69% of patients expressed a preference for quarterly dosing [101]. In those who failed 2–4 classes of migraine preventives (EM/CM combined, 52% overuse acute medication, 18% moderate/severe depression), both regimens resulted in mean monthly migraine days reductions of 3.1–3.5 days and acute medication use day reductions of 3.1–3.4 days; the higher therapeutic gains may be due to lower placebo response. The clinical effect continued in the open-label extension at 6 months [102]. In two post hoc analyses, the clinical effect was observed at week 1 with separation from placebo by day 2 [103, 104]. The incidence of AEs was similar to those from placebo; the most common AEs were injection-site erythema, injection-site induration,

Table 5.6 Summary of fremanezumab-related clinical trials

Trial information	Drug dose (mg)[a]	Primary endpoint
NCT02021773 [94] Phase 2b, CM, *n* = 264	900, 675/225[b] vs. placebo	MHH change from baseline: −30.4*, −22.7* (MMD change from baseline: −2.0*, −1.7*)[c]
NCT02025556 [95] Phase 2b, HFEM, *n* = 297	675, 225, vs. placebo	MMD change from baseline: −2.6*, −2.8*
NCT02621931 [96] Phase 3, CM, *n* = 376	675 quarterly, 675/225[b] vs. placebo	MHD change from baseline: −1.8*, −2.1* (MMD change from baseline: −1.7*, −1.8*)[c]
NCT02629861 [97] Phase 3, EM, *n* = 875	675 quarterly, 675/225[b] vs. placebo	MMD change from baseline: −1.3*, −1.5*
NCT03308968 [98] Phase 3b, EM/CM[d], *n* = 838	675 quarterly, 675/225[b] vs. placebo	MMD change from baseline: −3.1 (−3.0/−3.2)*, −3.5 (−3.2/−3.8)[e],*

All studies were evaluated over 12 weeks

EM episodic migraine, *CM* chronic migraine, *MHH* mean headache hours, *MMD* mean monthly migraine day, *MHD* mean monthly headache day (≥4 h & moderate/severe intensity or use acute migraine med)

[a]Administered monthly unless noted otherwise

[b]675 mg loading followed by 275 mg monthly

[c]Secondary endpoint

[d]Failed 2–4 classes of migraine preventives

[e]EM/CM results

*Statistically significant

and nasopharyngitis. There was no cardiovascular safety signal. The most common cardiovascular AEs were hypertension (2%), palpitation (<1%), and hot flush (<1%) [105].

Galcanezumab, a humanized IgG_4 that targets the α- and β-CGRP ligands, also demonstrated its clinical efficacy in reducing migraine frequency and improving quality of life. All studies reached their primary endpoints (Table 5.7). In the 3–6-month study period, there was significant reduction in mean monthly migraine/probable migraine days (placebo-adjusted) in EM (1.2–2.0 days) and in CM (1.9–2.1 days) as well as acute medication use days in EM (1.6–1.8 days) and in CM (2.0–2.5 days). ≥50% responder rate was also higher in the treatment than placebo groups: 20.5–25.0% more in EM and 12.1–12.2% more in CM. Its effect likely started at day 1 after injection [111]. In a long-term open-label extension study (n = 270), 77.8% completed the open-label phase, and 4.8% discontinued due to AEs; the migraine days were reduced (−5.6 for 120 mg, −6.5 for 240 mg) [112]. In those who failed 2–4 categories of migraine preventives, galcanezumab treatment resulted in a mean monthly migraine/probable migraine days reduction of 3.1 days (with low placebo response) and improvement in depressive symptoms [113]. Galcanezumab demonstrated a favorable safety and tolerability profile for up to 1 year of treatment for the prevention of migraine [114]. Overall the most common AEs were injection site pain, nasopharyngitis, upper respiratory tract infection, injection site reaction, back pain, and sinusitis. Although 2–9% developed ADA, there was no discernible effect of ADA on treatment efficacy or tolerability.

Based on the phase 3 studies, CGRP functional blocking MAbs reduced mean monthly migraine days of 2.9–4.7 (placebo-adjusted 0.7–2.0) in EM, 4.3–8.2 (placebo adjusted 1.8–2.6) in CM, and 1.8–4.5 (placebo-adjusted 1.6–3.8) in those who failed more than two preventives. The 50% responder rates ranged between 39.7–62.2% (placebo-adjusted 10.2–23.6%) in EM and 27.6–61.4% (placebo-adjusted 8.2–23.0%) in CM. Acute medication use reduction (placebo-adjusted)

Table 5.7 Summary of galcanezumab-related clinical trials

Trial information	Drug dose (mg)	Primary endpoint
NCT01625988 [106] Phase 2, EM, n = 218	150 vs. placebo	MMD change from baseline (3-month average): −1.2*
NCT02614183 [107] Phase 3, EM, n = 858	240, 120[a] vs. placebo	MMD change from baseline (6-month average): −1.8*; −1.9*
NCT02614196 [108] Phase 3, EM, n = 915	240, 120[a] vs. placebo	MMD change from baseline (6-month average): −1.9*; −2.0*
NCT02614261 [109] Phase 3, CM, n = 1113	240, 120[a] vs. placebo	MMD change from baseline (3-month average): −1.9*; −2.1*
NCT03559257 [110] Phase 3, EM/CM[b], n = 462	120[a] vs. placebo	MMD change from baseline (3-month average): −3.1*

All studies were evaluated over 12-week unless otherwise specified
EM episodic migraine, *CM* chronic migraine, *MMD* mean monthly migraine/probable migraine day
[a]240 mg loading followed by 120 mg monthly
[b]Failed 2–4 migraine preventive category
*Statistically significant

was 0.5–3 days in EM and 1.6–1.9 days in CM. The onset of action is usually less than 1 week, but maybe quicker if administered via infusion. Early non-responders may still respond by later months [115]. The effect may sustain beyond 4–5 years. It has been our personal experience that a second mAb agent may be successful if the first one fails or has significant AEs. ADA may develop, but so far with no discernible clinical effect. With a complementary mechanism and minimal drug interactions, CGRP functional blocking mAbs likely will gain additional clinical benefit when used in combination with current preventive medications. Its utility with gepants remains to be explored. Despite their wonderful AE profile, CGRP functional blocking MAbs have not been studied in certain susceptible populations (BMI >40, age <18 or >75, with cardiovascular disease or other major comorbidities, pregnant or breast-feeding). Migraine patients with above-described conditions should be treated with caution. Discontinuation of these MAbs 3–6 months prior to conception may be needed.

Conclusion

CGRP functional blocking MAbs have recently emerged as a promising treatment option in the migraine therapeutic armamentarium. These MAbs likely block CGRP functions on large neurons, Aδ-fibers, and SGCs within TG, alleviating neurogenic neuroinflammation and pain sensitization in the trigeminal system, but other mechanisms remain to be explored. Clinical evidence suggests that MAbs targeting CGRP ligands and receptors not only reduce migraine days and acute medication use but also improve quality of life and psychosocial burden. Their convenient monthly/quarterly dosing and favorable safety profile improve medication compliance and reduce migraine chronification. However, individual effect varies. Their safety has not been tested in certain patient populations. More well-designed clinical trials are still needed.

References

1. Amara SG, Jonas V, Rosenfeld MG, Ong ES, Evans RM. Alternative RNA processing in calcitonin gene expression generates mRNAs encoding different polypeptide products. Nature. 1982;298(5871):240–4.
2. American Headache Society. The American Headache Society position statement on integrating new migraine treatments into clinical practice. Headache. 2019;59(1):1–18.
3. Russell FA, King R, Smillie SJ, Kodji X, Brain SD. Calcitonin gene-related peptide: physiology and pathophysiology. Physiol Rev. 2014;94(4):1099–142.
4. Kraenzlin ME, Ch'ng JL, Mulderry PK, Ghatei MA, Bloom SR. Infusion of a novel peptide, calcitonin gene-related peptide (CGRP) in man. Pharmacokinetics and effects on gastric acid secretion and on gastrointestinal hormones. Regul Pept. 1985;10(2–3):189–97.
5. Hay DL, Poyner DR, Sexton PM. GPCR modulation by RAMPs. Pharmacol Ther. 2006;109(1–2):173–97.
6. Edvinsson L, Grell AS, Warfvinge K. Expression of the CGRP family of neuropeptides and their receptors in the trigeminal ganglion. J Mol Neurosci. 2020;70(6):930–44.

7. Walker CS, Eftekhari S, Bower RL, Wilderman A, Insel PA, Edvinsson L, et al. A second trigeminal CGRP receptor: function and expression of the AMY1 receptor. Ann Clin Transl Neurol. 2015;2(6):595–608.
8. Yarwood RE, Imlach WL, Lieu T, Veldhuis NA, Jensen DD, Klein Herenbrink C, et al. Endosomal signaling of the receptor for calcitonin gene-related peptide mediates pain transmission. Proc Natl Acad Sci U S A. 2017;114(46):12309–14.
9. Warfvinge K, Edvinsson L. Distribution of CGRP and CGRP receptor components in the rat brain. Cephalalgia. 2019;39(3):342–53.
10. Miller S, Liu H, Warfvinge K, Shi L, Dovlatyan M, Xu C, et al. Immunohistochemical localization of the calcitonin gene-related peptide binding site in the primate trigeminovascular system using functional antagonist antibodies. Neuroscience. 2016;328:165–83.
11. Eftekhari S, Warfvinge K, Blixt FW, Edvinsson L. Differentiation of nerve fibers storing CGRP and CGRP receptors in the peripheral trigeminovascular system. J Pain. 2013;14(11):1289–303.
12. Afroz S, Arakaki R, Iwasa T, Oshima M, Hosoki M, Inoue M, et al. CGRP induces differential regulation of cytokines from satellite glial cells in trigeminal ganglia and orofacial nociception. Int J Mol Sci. 2019;20(3):711.
13. Capuano A, De Corato A, Lisi L, Tringali G, Navarra P, Dello Russo C. Proinflammatory-activated trigeminal satellite cells promote neuronal sensitization: relevance for migraine pathology. Mol Pain. 2009;5:43.
14. Edvinsson JCA, Warfvinge K, Krause DN, Blixt FW, Sheykhzade M, Edvinsson L, et al. C-fibers may modulate adjacent Aδ-fibers through axon-axon CGRP signaling at nodes of Ranvier in the trigeminal system. J Headache Pain. 2019;20(1):105.
15. Levy D, Burstein R, Strassman AM. Calcitonin gene-related peptide does not excite or sensitize meningeal nociceptors: implications for the pathophysiology of migraine. Ann Neurol. 2005;58(5):698–705.
16. Messlinger K, Balcziak LK, Russo AF. Cross-talk signaling in the trigeminal ganglion: role of neuropeptides and other mediators. J Neural Transm (Vienna). 2020;127(4):431–44.
17. Edvinsson L, Haanes KA, Warfvinge K. Does inflammation have a role in migraine? Nat Rev Neurol. 2019;15(8):483–90.
18. Goadsby PJ, Edvinsson L, Ekman R. Vasoactive peptide release in the extracerebral circulation of humans during migraine headache. Ann Neurol. 1990;28(2):183–7.
19. Goadsby PJ, Edvinsson L. The trigeminovascular system and migraine: studies characterizing cerebrovascular and neuropeptide changes seen in humans and cats. Ann Neurol. 1993;33(1):48–56.
20. Sarchielli P, Alberti A, Codini M, Floridi A, Gallai V. Nitric oxide metabolites, prostaglandins and trigeminal vasoactive peptides in internal jugular vein blood during spontaneous migraine attacks. Cephalalgia. 2000;20(10):907–18.
21. Gallai V, Sarchielli P, Floridi A, Franceschini M, Codini M, Glioti G, et al. Vasoactive peptide levels in the plasma of young migraine patients with and without aura assessed both interictally and ictally. Cephalalgia. 1995;15(5):384–90.
22. Cernuda-Morollon E, Larrosa D, Ramon C, Vega J, Martinez-Camblor P, Pascual J. Interictal increase of CGRP levels in peripheral blood as a biomarker for chronic migraine. Neurology. 2013;81(14):1191–6.
23. Cernuda-Morollon E, Ramon C, Martinez-Camblor P, Serrano-Pertierra E, Larrosa D, Pascual J. OnabotulinumtoxinA decreases interictal CGRP plasma levels in patients with chronic migraine. Pain. 2015;156(5):820–4.
24. Akerman S, Goadsby PJ. Topiramate inhibits trigeminovascular activation: an intravital microscopy study. Br J Pharmacol. 2005;146(1):7–14.
25. Juhasz G, Zsombok T, Modos EA, Olajos S, Jakab B, Nemeth J, et al. NO-induced migraine attack: strong increase in plasma calcitonin gene-related peptide (CGRP) concentration and negative correlation with platelet serotonin release. Pain. 2003;106(3):461–70.
26. Lassen LH, Haderslev PA, Jacobsen VB, Iversen HK, Sperling B, Olesen J. CGRP may play a causative role in migraine. Cephalalgia. 2002;22(1):54–61.

27. Hansen JM, Hauge AW, Olesen J, Ashina M. Calcitonin gene-related peptide triggers migraine-like attacks in patients with migraine with aura. Cephalalgia. 2010;30(10):1179–86.
28. Hansen JM, Thomsen LL, Olesen J, Ashina M. Calcitonin gene-related peptide does not cause migraine attacks in patients with familial hemiplegic migraine. Headache. 2011;51(4):544–53.
29. Ashina M, Bendtsen L, Jensen R, Schifter S, Olesen J. Calcitonin gene-related peptide levels during nitric oxide-induced headache in patients with chronic tension-type headache. Eur J Neurol. 2001;8(2):173–8.
30. De Felice M, Ossipov MH, Wang R, Lai J, Chichorro J, Meng I, et al. Triptan-induced latent sensitization: a possible basis for medication overuse headache. Ann Neurol. 2010;67(3):325–37.
31. Falkenberg K, Bjerg HR, Olesen J. Two-hour CGRP infusion causes gastrointestinal hyperactivity: possible relevance for CGRP antibody treatment. Headache. 2020;60(5):929–37.
32. Russo AF. Calcitonin gene-related peptide (CGRP): a new target for migraine. Annu Rev Pharmacol Toxicol. 2015;55(1):533–52.
33. Pan KS, Siow A, Hay DL, Walker CS. Antagonism of CGRP signaling by rimegepant at two receptors. Front Pharmacol. 2020;11:1240.
34. Moore E, Fraley ME, Bell IM, Burgey CS, White RB, Li CC, et al. Characterization of ubrogepant: a potent and selective antagonist of the human calcitonin gene-related peptide receptor. J Pharmacol Exp Ther. 2020;373:160–66.
35. Filiz A, Tepe N, Eftekhari S, Boran HE, Dilekoz E, Edvinsson L, et al. CGRP receptor antagonist MK-8825 attenuates cortical spreading depression induced pain behavior. Cephalalgia. 2019;39(3):354–65.
36. Walker CS, Raddant AC, Woolley MJ, Russo AF, Hay DL. CGRP receptor antagonist activity of olcegepant depends on the signalling pathway measured. Cephalalgia. 2018;38(3):437–51.
37. Tfelt-Hansen P, Olesen J. Possible site of action of CGRP antagonists in migraine. Cephalalgia. 2011;31(6):748–50.
38. Hostetler ED, Joshi AD, Sanabria-Bohorquez S, Fan H, Zeng Z, Purcell M, et al. In vivo quantification of calcitonin gene-related peptide receptor occupancy by telcagepant in rhesus monkey and human brain using the positron emission tomography tracer [11C]MK-4232. J Pharmacol Exp Ther. 2013;347(2):478–86.
39. Ho TW, Connor KM, Zhang Y, Pearlman E, Koppenhaver J, Fan X, et al. Randomized controlled trial of the CGRP receptor antagonist telcagepant for migraine prevention. Neurology. 2014;83(11):958–66.
40. Navratilova E, Behravesh S, Oyarzo J, Dodick DW, Banerjee P, Porreca F. Ubrogepant does not induce latent sensitization in a preclinical model of medication overuse headache. Cephalalgia. 2020;40(9):892–902.
41. Saengjaroentham C, Strother LC, Dripps I, Sultan Jabir MR, Pradhan A, Goadsby PJ, et al. Differential medication overuse risk of novel anti-migraine therapeutics. Brain. 2020;143(9):2681–8.
42. Goadsby PJ, Dodick DW, Ailani J, Trugman JM, Finnegan M, Lu K, et al. Safety, tolerability, and efficacy of orally administered atogepant for the prevention of episodic migraine in adults: a double-blind, randomised phase 2b/3 trial. Lancet Neurol. 2020;19(9):727–37.
43. Biohaven Pharmaceuticals. Biohaven achieves positive results in pivotal trial of oral NURTEC™, dosed every other day, for the preventive treatment of migraine. 2020. Available from: https://www.biohavenpharma.com/investors/news-events/press-releases/03-30-2020.
44. Yuan H, Chen A, Silberstein SD. CGRP therapeutics for the treatment of migraine – a narrative review. Ann Head Med. 2020;(01.03):1–22.
45. Vidarsson G, Dekkers G, Rispens T. IgG subclasses and allotypes: from structure to effector functions. Front Immunol. 2014;5:520.
46. Antibody Society. Antibody therapeutics approved or in regulatory review in the EU or US. Available from: https://www.antibodysociety.org/resources/approved-antibodies/.
47. Kim SJ, Park Y, Hong HJ. Antibody engineering for the development of therapeutic antibodies. Mol Cells. 2005;20(1):17–29.

48. Saeed AF, Wang R, Ling S, Wang S. Antibody engineering for pursuing a healthier future. Front Microbiol. 2017;8:495.
49. Mayrhofer P, Kunert R. Nomenclature of humanized mAbs: early concepts, current challenges and future perspectives. Hum Antibodies. 2019;27(1):37–51.
50. Davda JP, Hansen RJ. Properties of a general PK/PD model of antibody-ligand interactions for therapeutic antibodies that bind to soluble endogenous targets. MAbs. 2010;2(5):576–88.
51. Kielbasa W, Helton DL. A new era for migraine: pharmacokinetic and pharmacodynamic insights into monoclonal antibodies with a focus on galcanezumab, an anti-CGRP antibody. Cephalalgia. 2019;39(10):1284–97.
52. Anzil AP, Blinzinger K, Herrlinger H. Fenestrated blood capillaries in rat cranio-spinal sensory ganglia. Cell Tissue Res. 1976;167(4):563–7.
53. Johnson KW, Morin SM, Wroblewski VJ, Johnson MP. Peripheral and central nervous system distribution of the CGRP neutralizing antibody [(125)I] galcanezumab in male rats. Cephalalgia. 2019;39(10):1241–8.
54. Noseda R, Schain AJ, Melo-Carrillo A, Tien J, Stratton J, Mai F, et al. Fluorescently-labeled fremanezumab is distributed to sensory and autonomic ganglia and the dura but not to the brain of rats with uncompromised blood brain barrier. Cephalalgia. 2020;40(3):229–40.
55. Garg A, Balthasar JP. Physiologically-based pharmacokinetic (PBPK) model to predict IgG tissue kinetics in wild-type and FcRn-knockout mice. J Pharmacokinet Pharmacodyn. 2007;34(5):687–709.
56. Junghans RP, Anderson CL. The protection receptor for IgG catabolism is the beta2-microglobulin-containing neonatal intestinal transport receptor. Proc Natl Acad Sci U S A. 1996;93(11):5512–6.
57. Pyzik M, Sand KMK, Hubbard JJ, Andersen JT, Sandlie I, Blumberg RS. The neonatal Fc receptor (FcRn): a misnomer? Front Immunol. 2019;10:1540.
58. Schlachetzki F, Zhu C, Pardridge WM. Expression of the neonatal Fc receptor (FcRn) at the blood-brain barrier. J Neurochem. 2002;81(1):203–6.
59. Xiao JJ. Pharmacokinetic models for FcRn-mediated IgG disposition. J Biomed Biotechnol. 2012;2012:282989.
60. de Hoon J, Van Hecken A, Vandermeulen C, Yan L, Smith B, Chen JS, et al. Phase I, randomized, double-blind, placebo-controlled, single-dose, and multiple-dose studies of erenumab in healthy subjects and patients with migraine. Clin Pharmacol Ther. 2018;103(5):815–25.
61. Petitcollin A, Bensalem A, Verdier MC, Tron C, Lemaitre F, Paintaud G, et al. Modelling of the time-varying pharmacokinetics of therapeutic monoclonal antibodies: a literature review. Clin Pharmacokinet. 2020;59(1):37–49.
62. Manoukian R, Sun H, Miller S, Shi D, Chan B, Xu C. Effects of monoclonal antagonist antibodies on calcitonin gene-related peptide receptor function and trafficking. J Headache Pain. 2019;20(1):44.
63. Zeller J, Poulsen KT, Sutton JE, Abdiche YN, Collier S, Chopra R, et al. CGRP function-blocking antibodies inhibit neurogenic vasodilatation without affecting heart rate or arterial blood pressure in the rat. Br J Pharmacol. 2008;155(7):1093–103.
64. Kopruszinski CM, Xie JY, Eyde NM, Remeniuk B, Walter S, Stratton J, et al. Prevention of stress- or nitric oxide donor-induced medication overuse headache by a calcitonin gene-related peptide antibody in rodents. Cephalalgia. 2017;37(6):560–70.
65. Melo-Carrillo A, Noseda R, Nir RR, Schain AJ, Stratton J, Strassman AM, et al. Selective inhibition of trigeminovascular neurons by fremanezumab: a humanized monoclonal anti-CGRP antibody. J Neurosci. 2017;37(30):7149–63.
66. Melo-Carrillo A, Strassman AM, Nir RR, Schain AJ, Noseda R, Stratton J, et al. Fremanezumab – a humanized monoclonal anti-CGRP antibody-inhibits thinly myelinated (Aδ) but not unmyelinated (C) meningeal nociceptors. J Neurosci. 2017;37(44):10587–96.
67. Schain AJ, Melo-Carrillo A, Stratton J, Strassman AM, Burstein R. CSD-induced arterial dilatation and plasma protein extravasation are unaffected by fremanezumab: implications for CGRP's role in migraine with aura. J Neurosci. 2019;39(30):6001–11.

68. Melo-Carrillo A, Schain AJ, Stratton J, Strassman AM, Burstein R. Fremanezumab and its isotype slow propagation rate and shorten cortical recovery period but do not prevent occurrence of cortical spreading depression in rats with compromised blood-brain barrier. Pain. 2020;161(5):1037–43.
69. Christensen SL, Petersen S, Kristensen DM, Olesen J, Munro G. Targeting CGRP via receptor antagonism and antibody neutralisation in two distinct rodent models of migraine-like pain. Cephalalgia. 2019;39(14):1827–37.
70. Christensen SL, Ernstsen C, Olesen J, Kristensen DM. No central action of CGRP antagonising drugs in the GTN mouse model of migraine. Cephalalgia. 2020;40(9):924–34.
71. Kaiser EA, Rea BJ, Kuburas A, Kovacevich BR, Garcia-Martinez LF, Recober A, et al. Anti-CGRP antibodies block CGRP-induced diarrhea in mice. Neuropeptides. 2017;64:95–9.
72. Mason BN, Kaiser EA, Kuburas A, Loomis MM, Latham JA, Garcia-Martinez LF, et al. Induction of migraine-like photophobic behavior in mice by both peripheral and central CGRP mechanisms. J Neurosci. 2017;37(1):204–16.
73. Karasek C, Ojala E, Allison D, Latham J. Characterization of the intrinsic binding features of three anti-CGRP therapeutic antibodies effective in preventing migraine: a comparative preclinical case study of ALD403, LY-2951742, TEV-48125, 2016 November 9, 2019. Available from: http://www.alderbio.com/wp-content/uploads/2016/09/EU-Glasgow-2016-ALD403-Comparative-Poster-Latham-v2a-2016-09-08-FINAL2.pdf.
74. Vu T, Ma P, Chen JS, de Hoon J, Van Hecken A, Yan L, et al. Pharmacokinetic-pharmacodynamic relationship of erenumab (AMG 334) and capsaicin-induced dermal blood flow in healthy and migraine subjects. Pharm Res. 2017;34(9):1784–95.
75. Silberstein SD, Reshef S, Cohen JM, Gandhi S, Seminerio M, Campos VR, et al. Adverse event profiles of therapies that target the calcitonin gene-related peptide (CGRP) pathway, during the first six months after launch: a real-world data analysis using the FDA adverse events reporting system (FAERS) (4315). Neurology. 2020;94(15 Supplement):4315.
76. Baker B, Beliveau M, Pederson S, Schaeffler B. Differences in exposure between intravenously (IV) administered eptinezumab and subcutaneously (SC) administered CGRP inhibitor monoclonal antibodies after single therapeutic doses (708). Neurology. 2020;94(15 Supplement):708.
77. Dodick DW, Gottschalk C, Cady R, Hirman J, Smith J, Snapinn S. Eptinezumab demonstrated efficacy in sustained prevention of episodic and chronic migraine beginning on day 1 after dosing. Headache. 2020;60(12):2220–31.
78. Dodick DW, Goadsby PJ, Silberstein SD, Lipton RB, Olesen J, Ashina M, et al. Safety and efficacy of ALD403, an antibody to calcitonin gene-related peptide, for the prevention of frequent episodic migraine: a randomised, double-blind, placebo-controlled, exploratory phase 2 trial. Lancet Neurol. 2014;13(11):1100–7.
79. Dodick DW, Lipton RB, Silberstein S, Goadsby PJ, Biondi D, Hirman J, et al. Eptinezumab for prevention of chronic migraine: a randomized phase 2b clinical trial. Cephalalgia. 2019;39(9):1075–85.
80. Ashina M, Saper J, Cady R, Schaeffler BA, Biondi DM, Hirman J, et al. Eptinezumab in episodic migraine: a randomized, double-blind, placebo-controlled study (PROMISE-1). Cephalalgia. 2020;40(3):241–54.
81. Lipton RB, Goadsby PJ, Smith J, Schaeffler BA, Biondi DM, Hirman J, et al. Efficacy and safety of eptinezumab in patients with chronic migraine: PROMISE-2. Neurology. 2020;94(13):e1365–e77.
82. Dhillon S. Eptinezumab: first approval. Drugs. 2020;80(7):733–9.
83. Lundbeck. Initiating VYEPTI™ (eptinezumab-jjmr) migraine prevention during a migraine attack demonstrated positive results in the RELIEF study. 2020. Available from: https://www.newsroom.lundbeckus.com/news-release/2020/positive-headline-results-from-the-vyepti-eptinezumab-jjmr-relief-study.
84. Sun H, Dodick DW, Silberstein S, Goadsby PJ, Reuter U, Ashina M, et al. Safety and efficacy of AMG 334 for prevention of episodic migraine: a randomised, double-blind, placebo-controlled, phase 2 trial. Lancet Neurol. 2016;15(4):382–90.

85. Dodick DW, Ashina M, Brandes JL, Kudrow D, Lanteri-Minet M, Osipova V, et al. ARISE: a phase 3 randomized trial of erenumab for episodic migraine. Cephalalgia. 2018;38(6):1026–37.
86. Goadsby PJ, Reuter U, Hallstrom Y, Broessner G, Bonner JH, Zhang F, et al. A controlled trial of erenumab for episodic migraine. N Engl J Med. 2017;377(22):2123–32.
87. Reuter U, Goadsby PJ, Lanteri-Minet M, Wen S, Hours-Zesiger P, Ferrari MD, et al. Efficacy and tolerability of erenumab in patients with episodic migraine in whom two-to-four previous preventive treatments were unsuccessful: a randomised, double-blind, placebo-controlled, phase 3b study. Lancet. 2018;392(10161):2280–7.
88. Tepper S, Ashina M, Reuter U, Brandes JL, Dolezil D, Silberstein S, et al. Safety and efficacy of erenumab for preventive treatment of chronic migraine: a randomised, double-blind, placebo-controlled phase 2 trial. Lancet Neurol. 2017;16(6):425–34.
89. Brandes JL, Diener H-C, Dolezil D, Freeman MC, McAllister PJ, Winner P, et al. The spectrum of response to erenumab in patients with chronic migraine and subgroup analysis of patients achieving ≥50%, ≥75%, and 100% response. Cephalalgia. 2019;40(1):28–38.
90. Tepper SJ, Ashina M, Reuter U, Brandes JL, Dolezil D, Silberstein SD, et al. Long-term safety and efficacy of erenumab in patients with chronic migraine: results from a 52-week, open-label extension study. Cephalalgia. 2020;40(6):543–53.
91. Ohlsson L, Haanes KA, Kronvall E, Xu C, Snellman J, Edvinsson L. Erenumab (AMG 334), a monoclonal antagonist antibody against the canonical CGRP receptor, does not impair vasodilatory or contractile responses to other vasoactive agents in human isolated cranial arteries. Cephalalgia. 2019;39(14):1745–52.
92. Yuan H, Nahas SJ, Berk MA. Acute reversible cerebral vasoconstriction syndrome with low-dose dihydroergotamine possibly potentiated by valproic acid and erenumab: a case report. J Neurol Res. 2020;10(1):20–4.
93. Skaria T, Mitchell KJ, Vogel O, Walchli T, Gassmann M, Vogel J. Blood pressure normalization-independent cardioprotective effects of endogenous, physical activity-induced alphaCGRP (alpha calcitonin gene-related peptide) in chronically hypertensive mice. Circ Res. 2019;125(12):1124–40.
94. Bigal ME, Edvinsson L, Rapoport AM, Lipton RB, Spierings EL, Diener HC, et al. Safety, tolerability, and efficacy of TEV-48125 for preventive treatment of chronic migraine: a multicentre, randomised, double-blind, placebo-controlled, phase 2b study. Lancet Neurol. 2015;14(11):1091–100.
95. Bigal ME, Dodick DW, Rapoport AM, Silberstein SD, Ma Y, Yang R, et al. Safety, tolerability, and efficacy of TEV-48125 for preventive treatment of high-frequency episodic migraine: a multicentre, randomised, double-blind, placebo-controlled, phase 2b study. Lancet Neurol. 2015;14(11):1081–90.
96. Silberstein SD, Dodick DW, Bigal ME, Yeung PP, Goadsby PJ, Blankenbiller T, et al. Fremanezumab for the preventive treatment of chronic migraine. N Engl J Med. 2017;377(22):2113–22.
97. Dodick DW, Silberstein SD, Bigal ME, Yeung PP, Goadsby PJ, Blankenbiller T, et al. Effect of fremanezumab compared with placebo for prevention of episodic migraine: a randomized clinical trial. JAMA. 2018;319(19):1999–2008.
98. Ferrari MD, Diener HC, Ning X, Galic M, Cohen JM, Yang R, et al. Fremanezumab versus placebo for migraine prevention in patients with documented failure to up to four migraine preventive medication classes (FOCUS): a randomised, double-blind, placebo-controlled, phase 3b trial. Lancet. 2019;394(10203):1030–40.
99. Silberstein SD, Cohen JM, Seminerio MJ, Yang R, Ashina S, Katsarava Z. The impact of fremanezumab on medication overuse in patients with chronic migraine: subgroup analysis of the HALO CM study. J Headache Pain. 2020;21(1):114.
100. Goadsby PJ, Silberstein SD, Yeung PP, Cohen JM, Ning X, Yang R, Dodick DW. Long-term safety, tolerability, and efficacy of fremanezumab in migraine. Neurology. 2020;95:e2487–e2499.

101. Cowan RP, Gandhi SK, Cloud B, Cohen JM, Buse DC, Ramirez-Campos V, et al. Patient preference for dosing regimen and perception of dosing flexibility with fremanezumab for migraine: results from a patient survey following completion of a 1-year extension study (4219). Neurology. 2020;94(15 Supplement):4219.
102. Gladstone J, Ning X, Cohen JM, Ramirez-Campos V, Yang R, Spierings ELH. Clinically meaningful responses to fremanezumab in patients with migraine and documented inadequate response to 2–4 migraine preventive medication classes in the open–label period of the international, multicenter phase 3b FOCUS study (4398). Neurology. 2020;94(15 Supplement):4398.
103. Winner PK, Spierings ELH, Yeung PP, Aycardi E, Blankenbiller T, Grozinski-Wolff M, et al. Early onset of efficacy with fremanezumab for the preventive treatment of chronic migraine. Headache. 2019;59(10):1743–52.
104. Brandes JL, Ramirez-Campos V, Yang R, Cohen J, Galic M, Ning X, et al. Very early onset of action of fremanezumab in patients with migraine and documented inadequate response to 2–4 classes of migraine preventive medications: results of the international, multicenter, randomized, placebo-controlled FOCUS study (4371). Neurology. 2020;94(15 Supplement):4371.
105. Ning X, Faulhaber N, Lang N, Yeung P, Schiemann J, Cohen J, et al. Fremanezumab cardiovascular and cerebrovascular safety profile: pooled data from placebo-controlled and long-term studies (S17.005). Neurology. 2019;92(15 Supplement):S17.005.
106. Dodick DW, Goadsby PJ, Spierings EL, Scherer JC, Sweeney SP, Grayzel DS. Safety and efficacy of LY2951742, a monoclonal antibody to calcitonin gene-related peptide, for the prevention of migraine: a phase 2, randomised, double-blind, placebo-controlled study. Lancet Neurol. 2014;13(9):885–92.
107. Stauffer VL, Dodick DW, Zhang Q, Carter JN, Ailani J, Conley RR. Evaluation of galcanezumab for the prevention of episodic migraine: the EVOLVE-1 randomized clinical trial. JAMA Neurol. 2018;75(9):1080–8.
108. Skljarevski V, Matharu M, Millen BA, Ossipov MH, Kim BK, Yang JY. Efficacy and safety of galcanezumab for the prevention of episodic migraine: results of the EVOLVE-2 phase 3 randomized controlled clinical trial. Cephalalgia. 2018;38(8):1442–54.
109. Detke HC, Goadsby PJ, Wang S, Friedman DI, Selzler KJ, Aurora SK. Galcanezumab in chronic migraine: the randomized, double-blind, placebo-controlled REGAIN study. Neurology. 2018;91(24):e2211–e21.
110. Mulleners W, Kim B-K, Lainez M, Lanteri-Minet M, Aurora S, Nichols R, et al. A randomized, placebo-controlled study of galcanezumab in patients with treatment-resistant migraine: double-blind results from the CONQUER study (162). Neurology. 2020;94(15 Supplement):162.
111. Andreou AP, Wright P, Detke H, Ruff D, Reuter U. Galcanezumab shows efficacy as early as day 1 after initial treatment vs. placebo for the prevention of episodic and chronic migraine (4014). Neurology. 2020;94(15 Supplement):4014.
112. Camporeale A, Kudrow D, Sides R, Wang S, Van Dycke A, Selzler KJ, et al. A phase 3, long-term, open-label safety study of galcanezumab in patients with migraine. BMC Neurol. 2018;18(1):188.
113. Maizels M, Buse DC, Jedynak J, Hand AL, Ford J, Detke H. Changes in depression and anxiety in a randomized, double-blind, placebo-controlled study of galcanezumab in adults with treatment-resistant migraine: results from the CONQUER study (1383). Neurology. 2020;94(15 Supplement):1383.
114. Bangs ME, Kudrow D, Wang S, Oakes TM, Terwindt GM, Magis D, et al. Safety and tolerability of monthly galcanezumab injections in patients with migraine: integrated results from migraine clinical studies. BMC Neurol. 2020;20(1):25.
115. Goadsby PJ, Dodick DW, Martinez JM, Ferguson MB, Oakes TM, Zhang Q, et al. Onset of efficacy and duration of response of galcanezumab for the prevention of episodic migraine: a post-hoc analysis. J Neurol Neurosurg Psychiatry. 2019;90(8):939–44.

6 OnabotulinumtoxinA (Botox®) Evidence-Based Therapy

Shalini Shah and Michael-David Calderon

Background

In 2016, the Global Burden of Diseases, Injuries, and Risk Factors (GBD) estimated almost 3 billion individuals have a headache disorder – migraine ranked sixth out of 328 diseases and injuries. Migraine also ranked second out of the top 10 most disabling disorders in each of the GBD regions, particularly among young aged 5–15 and middle-aged women aged 20–49 [1]. The most recent version of the International Classification of Headache Disorders (ICHD-3) in 2018 classifies migraines into two major types: (1) migraine without aura and (2) migraine with aura. The common features of migraine include, but are not limited to, headache, fatigue, difficulty concentrating, neck stiffness, sensitivity to light and/or sounds, nausea, blurred vision, yawning, and pallor [2]. Chronic migraine is complex and ideally requires a collaborative multidisciplinary team – neurologist, psychiatrist, and pain specialist [3] – to (1) accurately quantify the clinical nature of the condition, followed by a (2) systematic and proactive management.

Quantifying Migraine Disability

Unfortunately, there is no evidence-based cure for migraines. If left unmanaged, patients are at risk of developing increased frequency, intensity, and duration of headaches along with the corresponding debilitating effects, for example, decreased quality of life, decreased work/household productivity, and comorbidities.

S. Shah (✉)
Department of Anesthesiology & Perioperative Care, University of California Irvine, Irvine, CA, USA
e-mail: ssshah1@hs.uci.edu

M.-D. Calderon
Department of Anesthesiology and Perioperative Care, University of California Irvine Health, Orange, CA, USA

© Springer Nature Switzerland AG 2021

S. Shah (ed.), *Migraine*, https://doi.org/10.1007/978-3-030-75239-2_6

Additionally, the condition has the potential to manifest from episodic migraines (EM) into chronic migraine (CM), leaving patients severely disabled. Medication Overuse Headaches (MOH) have been recently clarified as a condition that overlaps with chronic migraine and associated comorbidities, for example, depression and anxiety, and are now to be considered a complication of chronic migraine – not an independently classifiable entity [4]. This pain is subjective by nature and it is important for clinicians to use validated assessment tools detailed in this chapter to best characterize the state of the condition.

Evidence-Based Management

Since the severity of migraines varies between each individual, one can consider the condition to fall within a spectrum ranging from episodic to chronic, with several lines of available treatment – each one with different efficacy and safety profiles. One of the most prominent choices for treating chronic migraine include onabotulinumtoxinA (OBTA) also known as Botox®. In 2010, the Phase 3 Research Evaluating Migraine Prophylaxis Therapy (PREEMPT) trials became the cornerstone of prophylactic treatment in adults. Treatments are administered every 3 months (12 weeks) with follow-up appointments every 6 weeks to monitor any improvements using validated assessment tools. The most common adverse effects associated with treatment are minor and temporary, which include neck pain, muscular weakness, ptosis, and headache [5]. According to the PREEMPT studies published in 2010, a $\geq$ 50% reduction in headache frequency from baseline [6] was considered significant. This chapter will outline the latest understood mechanism of action, assessment tools, approved dosing/administration guidelines, benefits/risks, and limitations OBTA may offer to the CM patient population.

OnabotulinumtoxinA (OBTA)

Mechanisms of OBTA

Broadly speaking, there are several lines of treatment available for migraine that utilize different mechanisms. These various pathways include suppressing excitatory nervous signaling (sodium and/or calcium receptors), inhibiting GABAergic pathways, blocking cortical spreading depression, and/or reducing the levels of calcitonin gene–related peptide (CGRP) – a neuropeptide associated in migraine pathogenesis – in the body, and downregulating neuronal sensitization [7]. Regarding the latter pathway, Botulinum toxin A is produced by the anaerobic, gram-positive bacterium *Clostridium botulinum* and one of seven different serotypes [8, 9] capable of disrupting the neuronal sensitization pathway for chronic migraine. Since manufactured OTBA did not follow the traditional development from bench to bedside before it was added to the FDA label of indications to include Chronic Migraine (CM), the mechanism of action is partially understood. The leading hypothesis suggests that OBTA attenuates neurotransmitter (gamma aminobutyric acid [GABA], glutamate, dopamine, etc.) and neuropeptide (CGRP, neuropeptide Y [NPY], etc.) exocytosis from the peripheral sensory neurons effectively reducing central sensitization – a key feature in CM [7]. While research is ongoing to accurately quantify the exact mechanisms [10–12], neurophysiological and functional imaging suggest that CM is associated with progressive brain dysfunction [13] warranting accurate assessment and timely treatment.

Assessment Tools

If a patient is referred to a headache specialist, it is important for the healthcare provider/team to administer a validated assessment tool to accurately assess the baseline migraine severity, any corresponding debilitating characteristics (e.g., quality of sleep, depression, or anxiety), and the true nature of the condition. A summary of the widely referenced and available assessment tools is listed in Table 6.1. Note, alternative surveys for headache-related disability are necessary for adolescents compared to adults, for example, school days versus workdays missed, respectively.

Reconstitution Guidelines

When administering OBTA to a patient diagnosed with Chronic Migraine, the appropriate dosing must be prepared in accordance with the approved and recommended guidelines [20] by a licensed professional. In summary, the Botox® is supplied in 100-unit or 200-unit vials that must be diluted using 2 or 4 mL of preservative-free normal saline respectively to achieve dose of 5 units per 0.1 mL, using the supplies referenced in Fig. 6.1.

Injection sites and fixed doses (155–195 U) are as follows: corrugator: 5 U on each side (10 total), procerus: 5 U, frontalis: 5 U in four sites (20 U total), temporalis: 5 U at four sites on both sides (40 U total), occipitalis: 5 U at three sites on both sides (30 U total), cervical paraspinal muscle group: 5 U at two sites on each side (20 U total), and trapezius: 5 U at two sites on both sides (30 U total). An additional 40 U OBTA could be administered to one or both sides in up to three muscle groups (occipitalis, temporalis, and trapezius) using a "follow-the-pain" strategy [6, 21, 22]. Figure 6.2 illustrates a summary of the injection sites for OBTA administration.

OBTA Administration in Adults Versus Adolescents

Recent published evidence demonstrates OBTA to be effective in children diagnosed with CM [23]. There are two distinctions: (1) using an appropriate assessment tool (e.g., PedMIDAS) scaled to children's functionality, for example missed days at school and (2) limiting the total dose is limited to 155 U. While administration of OBTA in adolescents is currently considered off-label, investigators who

Table 6.1 A list of commonly used assessment tools

Assessment tool	What is it?	Metrics and advantages	Limitation(s)
Adults			
MIDAS [14]	Migraine Disability Assessment Survey	Widely available standardized, five item questionnaire: Little or no disability: grade I (0–5 days) Mild disability: grade II (6–10 days) Moderate disability: grade III (11–20 days) Severe disability: grade IV (>21 days)	Recall bias if headaches are not tracked using daily headache diary. Not tailored to adolescents – see PedMIDAS
MSQ [15]	Migraine-Specific Quality of Life Questionnaire	14-item questionnaire: *Restrictive*: 5-point improvement *Preventive*: 5 to 8-point improvement *Emotional function*: 8- to 10-point improvement	Measured improvements may not be generalizable to other migraine treatments. Considered a tertiary variable in the PREEMPT study
HIT-6 [16]	Headache Impact Test-6	Six item self-administered questionnaire: ≥5-point change in score is considered clinically meaningful Little to no headache impact: ≤49 Some impact: 50–55 Substantial impact: 56–59 Severe headache impact: ≥60	Considered a tertiary variable in the PREEMPT study
PSQI [14]	Pittsburgh Sleep Quality Index	24-item questionnaire (total score 0–21); 18 items are scored across seven domains (0–3) Good sleep quality: <5 Poor sleep quality: >5	Considered a secondary/tertiary variable to chronic migraine
DASS-21 [14]	Depression Anxiety Stress Scale	21-item questionnaire based on three domains (normal/mild/ moderate/severe/extremely): Depression: (0–4/5–6/7–10/11–13/14+) Anxiety: (0–3/4–5/6–7/8–9/10+) Stress: (0–7/8–9/10–12/13–16/17+)	Considered a secondary/tertiary variable to chronic migraine
PHQ-9 [17]	Patient Health Questionnaire-9	Nine depression criteria questionnaire for major depressive disorder; ≥15 indicating major depression. Total score: 0–27 Minimal depressive: 0–4 Mild: 5–9 Moderate: 10–14 Severe: 20–27	Considered a secondary/tertiary variable to chronic migraine

Table 6.1 (continued)

Assessment tool	What is it?	Metrics and advantages	Limitation(s)
GAD-7 [17]	General Anxiety Disorder-7	Seven anxiety criteria for severe anxiety; ≥10 indicates generalized anxiety disorder. Total score: 0–21 Minimal anxiety: 0–4 Mild: 5–9 Moderate: 10–14 Severe: 15–21	Considered a secondary/tertiary variable to chronic migraine
Adolescents			
PedMIDAS [18]	Pediatric Migraine Assessment Disability Scale	Six item questionnaire that generates a cumulative score to rank severity of headache-related disability: None: (0–10) Mild: (11–30) Moderate: (31–50) Severe: (>50)	Does not account for other aspects of psychosocial functioning (depression, anxiety, learning difficulties, etc.)
DIHS-C [19]	Diagnostic Interview of Headache Syndromes–Child Version	Open-ended questions providing headache history, and scaled questions (1–4) assessing symptoms, severity, duration, frequency, and impairment. Survey asks both parent and child together avoiding possible underreporting	Limited to specifically migraines and not the full spectrum of headache subtypes
PAT-CP [18]	Psychosocial Assessment Tool-Chronic Pain	PAT-CP yields a total overall score ranging from 0 to 7 placing children/families into 3 risk categories (universal targeted, clinical/treatment). Six subscales ranging from 0 to 1 providing additional clinically relevant information	Subscale has low internal consistency, but still considered clinically relevant for chronic pain

have obtained appropriate regulatory approval – Investigational New Drug (IND) and local Institutional Review Board (IRB) – demonstrated in prospective double-blind randomized control trial that OBTA is effective in decreasing the frequency and intensity of migraines pending peer review. Additional multicenter studies with a larger sample size are necessary to confirm its effectiveness and generalizability to other populations.

Safety Profile

The most common side effects in subjects treated with OBTA are mild in nature and include, but are not limited to, neck pain, headache, worsening migraine, muscular

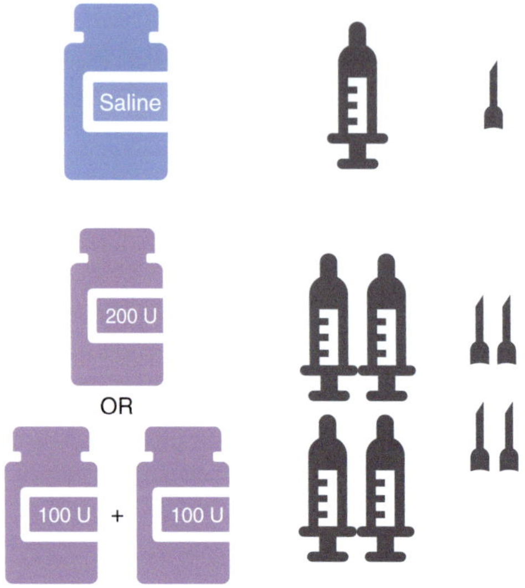

Qty.	Supplies
Reconstitution	
1	Sterile, preservative-free (0.9%) saline vial
1	5 mL syringe to draw up saline
1	21-gauge, 2-inch needle
1 OR 2	200 Unit vial of Botox® **OR** 100 Unit vial of Botox®
Adiministration	
4	30-gauge, 0.5-inch needle
4	1 mL syringe luer slip tip

Fig. 6.1 A summary of the supplies necessary to reconstitute and administer onabotulinumtoxinA (OBTA) for chronic migraine (CM)

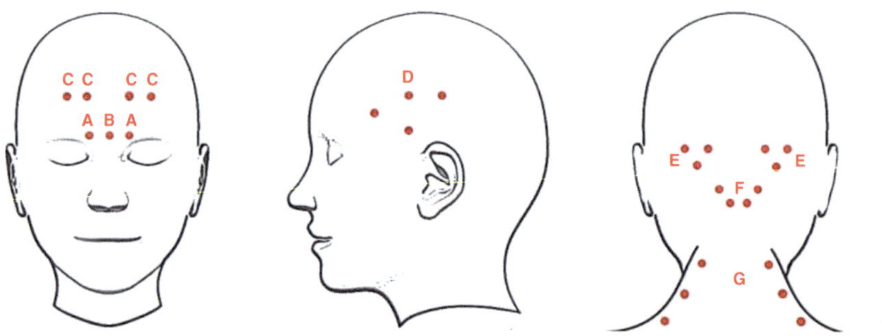

Fig. 6.2 A summary of injection sites for onabotulinumtoxinA (OBTA) administration in an adult patient diagnosed with chronic migraine (CM)

weakness, and eyelid ptosis [24]. Table 6.2 provides a summary of where OBTA fits within the host of available therapeutics available for patients diagnosed with CM [7].

Responders and Nonresponders

As previously mentioned, patients treated with OBTA for chronic migraine that do not report a ≥ 50% reduction in headache metrics are considered nonresponders.

Table 6.2 A summarized list of commonly utilized medications in patients diagnosed with chronic migraine

Migraine treatments	Dosing, frequency	Potential mechanisms
Anticonvulsants Valproate Topiramate	400–600 mg, BID 500–200 mg, QD	Blocks voltage-dependent sodium channel Blocks low-threshold calcium channels (T-type) Suppress glutamatergic neurotransmission (protein kinase C) Inhibits transcription factor pathway (NF-κB pathway) Downregulate CGRP expression Blocks voltage-dependent sodium channels and calcium channels (high-voltage-activated L-type) Inhibits glutamate-mediated excitatory neurotransmission Facilitates GABA-A mediated inhibition Inhibits carbonic anhydrase activity Reduces CGRP secretion (trigeminal neurons)
Antidepressants Amitriptyline Fluoxetine	25–75 mg, nocte (10 mg starting dose) 20 mg, QD	Inhibits serotonin/noradrenalin reuptake Facilitates endogenous pain control Blocks serotonin reuptake Blocks reversible 5-HT2C receptor
Beta (β) blockers Propranolol Metoprolol	40–120 mg, BID 25–100 mg, BID	Nitric oxide synthase inhibition Serotonergic system interaction Thalamic relay neuron inhibition Blocks central sensitization
Calcium channel blocker Flunarizine	5–15 mg, QD	Blocks voltage-gated sodium channels Reduces neuronal excitability/normalization cortical hyperexcitability D2 antagonist
Neurotoxin Onabotulinumtoxin A	155 unit at fixed sites, every 12 weeks (+ additional 40 units, "follow-the-pain")	Blocks peripheral/central sensitization Relaxes head/neck muscles

(continued)

Table 6.2 (continued)

Migraine treatments	Dosing, frequency	Potential mechanisms
Renin angiotensin system (RAS) modulating compounds Lisinopril Candesartan	20 mg, QD 16 mg, QD	Modulates vasoreactivity, alters sympathetic tone, promotes proinflammatory factor degradation Modulates endogenous opioid pathway Reduces vasoconstriction (angiotensin-mediated) Increases sympathetic discharge Releases catecholamines (adrenal) Modulates cerebral RAS (neuronal, astrocytic, & endothelial cells)
Supplements Riboflavin Coenzyme Q10 Butterbur Feverfew Magnesium	400 mg, QD 100 mg, TID or 75 mg, BID 50–75 mg, QD 6.25 mg, TID 600 mg, QD	Potential impact on mitochondria Potential impact on mitochondria Anti-inflammatory properties (inhibits cyclooxygenase-2) and vasodilation (L-type voltage-gated calcium channel inhibition) Inhibits trigeminal nucleus caudalis activation (Fox-induced) Partial TRPA1 channel antagonist Antinociceptive and anti-inflammatory properties Potential impact on enzymatic mitochondria/function

From: Sprenger et al. [7], with permission
Dosing abbreviations: *Q12H* = every 12 hours, *QD* = once a day, *BID* = twice a day, *nocte* = nightly

While the underlying mechanisms are still being investigated [25], there is evidence worth considering that will be elaborated on in the next section showing instances where such patient may experience clinical improvement after additional treatments [26, 27]. In this context, a clinician cognizant of the most recent literature may recommend supportive measures to optimize effectiveness and provide alternative modalities [28].

OBTA in Recent Literature: 2010–2020

In 2010, the PREEMPT 1 and 2 (Phase 3 Research Evaluating Migraine Prophylaxis Therapy) [6, 21] became the hallmark of clinical trials that tested the efficacy of injecting onabotulinumtoxinA (OBTA) into predetermined muscle groups throughout the head and neck of adults patients diagnosed with Chronic Migraine (CM). The results led to an amendment to include chronic migraines among the host of other FDA-approved indications. Since then, clinicians have published numerous studies highlighting the efficacy, safety, tolerability, and gaps associated the novel application of this treatment [29].

At first, there was criticism aimed at the limitations of the PREEMPT 1 & 2 trials. Potential confounders [30] such as including patients with headache medication overuse (MOH) [31] and the influence of placebo response were areas of concern that may have influenced the original findings. However, it was later clarified that the decision to include patients with MOH was done so in accordance with International Headache Society Clinical Trials Subcommittee (IHSCTS) committee and published guidelines [32]. An early case series of 35 adult patients supported OBTA effectiveness by showing that it reduces the frequency of debilitating attacks, triptan consumption, and Emergency Department visits [33]. Further study suggested that episodic migraines can manifest into chronic migraines overtime, and that MOH should be considered a complication of chronic migraine [34]. Early evidence also suggested OBTA has a better safety profile than topiramate with similar efficacy, and it became more apparent that some patients are "unresponsive" to treatment while muscle tenderness and allodynia were predictors of responsiveness to OBTA. Further investigations into the mechanism of OBTA are required to identify underlying pathophysiology at the cellular level [12].

In 2012, a retrospective study [35] showed that OBTA improved the quality of life and improved pain in subjects with chronic migraine over a 10-year period. Some clinicians speculated that the effectiveness of OBTA might increase over time and that a combination of two preventative pharmacological agents with different mechanisms of action may help reduce the impact of adverse events [11].

In 2013, clinicians investigated assessments tools for adults with migraines and [15] concluded that the Migraine-Specific Quality of Life Questionnaire (MSQ) is a valid. Early case reports started to emerge regarding management of adverse events, for example, "Mephisto Sign" when administering OBTA therapy may be avoided with an additional 2–4 U bilateral administration to the lateral most point of the frontalis muscles during primary injection.

In 2014, multicenter prospective trials showed that OBTA is effective in the long term (five cycles over 56 weeks), with muscle weakness and dysphagia being the most common adverse events without long-term toxicity [36]. Additional subanalysis of the PREEMPT trials showed continued and cumulative benefit over time [37]. With the growing number of retrospective studies showing improvements in reducing frequency and disability scoring (migraine disability assessment – MIDAS) [38], clinicians continued to seek predictive features of responsiveness, for example, ocular-type headaches. Simultaneously, questions remained about the implications on secondary outcomes, for example, cost–benefit considerations [39, 40] and treatment strategies such as offering OBTA to patients if first line of oral prophylactic medications are ineffective.

Despite the evidence supporting effectiveness of OBTA, chronic migraine was still associated with a higher burden of disease, more psychiatric comorbidity, greater use of healthcare resources, and higher total costs than episodic migraine [41] in 2015. With the pathomechanism of CM remaining to be fully understood [10], a study on cadavers discovered differences in nerve patterns – supratrochlear nerve (STN) – suggests the corresponding relationship between the muscles in the forehead (corrugator supercilii muscle) may be related to different responses to OBTA therapy [42]. Interestingly, there was a case study showing that ultrasound-guided OBTA coupled with infrared-polarized light reported significant improvement and another suggesting its effectiveness when treating patients with Hemicrania continua [43]. Another case study reported found that administration of a low dose (25 U per patient) of OBTA in regions commonly used in acupuncture showed a significant decrease in the frequency, intensity, and duration of migraines comparable to existing literature [44].

One study investigating OBTA nonresponders found that subjects may still experience clinical improvement after one or two additional treatments, suggesting a cumulative effect of OBTA [27]. Further characterizing this gap, one study supports the idea that OBTA is effective for certain types of headaches, for example, chronic migraine and trigeminal neuralgia, but not tension-type headaches [45]. Emerging evidence suggests that OBTA provides a sustained improvement in headache index and analgesic consumption in patients diagnosed with MOH [46]. Another 2-year open-label prospective study compared dosing recommendations and found superior outcomes in patients that received higher (195 U) vs. normal dose (155 U) in all efficacy measures while maintaining safety and tolerability [47].

In 2016, more evidence continues to support the applications of OBTA, extending beyond the original indications (blepharospasm, cervical dystonia, upper/lower extremity spasticity) for chronic migraine; however, it is not effective for all types of migraines – episodic migraine or chronic tension–type headaches [48]. Measurable improvements are consistent across different surveying tools during follow-up visits (HIT-6 and MSQ), supporting the improved quality of life [16]; however, there is evidence that treatment may be delayed, requiring up to three rounds of treatment before significant improvement [49]. Without a consensus on how long treatment should continue, retrospective data demonstrated that the treatment is safe and effective after five sessions [50]. A case series utilizing lasers to evoke a pain response in volunteers suggest that OBTA may modify trigeminal nociception, altering the pattern of habituation by normalizing neurotransmission [51]. Due to variations in physical anatomy, another study on cadavers proposed that injection into the temporalis muscle should be 45 mm above the zygomatic arch to avoid injecting into the tendon for optimal clinical effects [52].

In 2017, the safety and improved outcomes associated with OBTA for CM expanded to several countries (United Kingdom, Germany, Sweden, and Spain) [26] leading more than half (69.8%) of 96 headaches centers in Italy to consider OBTA a favorable option than oral prophylactic medications due to its safety profile [53]. Additional retrospective studies support that OBTA is effective in reducing headache-related disability (reduced monthly headache days/hours) with repeated administration over an 18-month period with six quarterly cycles [54]. Another cohort study found that subjects with OBTA reported a significant decrease in frequency, severity, number of analgesics, and disability scoring (MIDAS). The investigators further characterized the impact of the condition using survey tools PSQI or DASS-21 found that those with preexisting negative emotional states and poor sleep quality did not report a significant change from baseline; however, patients without negative emotional states showed an improvement in sleep quality [14]. Investigators also advise clinicians to consider preexisting conditions, muscle mass, and brow width/height before the procedure to achieve optimal outcomes [5]. Interestingly, another case series of low dose (25 U bilaterally, i.e., a total dose of 50 U) OBTA administration was effective in reducing headache days for treating intractable chronic migraine at the sphenopalatine ganglion [55]. Again, published evidence supports that even nonresponders (reporting less than 50% reduction from baseline) receiving OBTA for chronic migraine report clinically meaningful relief compared to those that received placebo [56].

It is clear that OBTA is effective for some conditions but not all. A literature review suggests preliminary evidence that OBTA's effectiveness ranges from primary headaches, trigeminal neuralgia, and chronic neuropathic pain to nociceptive and osteoarticular pain suggesting that future studies should investigate adjuvant therapy and/or physical therapies and optimal dosing. This resonates with other literature characterizing migraines that fall along a spectrum that ranges from episodic to chronic, where the severity may become progressively disabling [13] and where neurophysiological and functional imaging suggests that individuals with CM (compared to episodic) is associated with progressive brain dysfunction. Topiramate and OBTA are best suited for episodic and chronic migraines, respectively. Novel methods continue to develop where one prospective cohort study treated patients with fixed doses using a "follow-the-pain" approach to a subset of muscle groups – corrugator, and/or temporalis, and/or trapezius – totaling in 70–150 U per session. This evidence suggests the potential of OBTA's effectiveness with a more targeted approach [57]. One study challenges investigators to investigate novel inflammatory pathway in extracranial nociceptors or affected extracranial tissues highlighting the gap between OBTAs effectiveness in subjects with "imploding" headaches compared to "exploding headaches" [58].

By 2018, the extent of literature [59, 60] and longitudinal studies assessing the long-term effectiveness of OTBA treatments continue over a 3-year period [61]. The COMPEL study – an international, multicenter, open-label, long-term prospective study – reinforces the efficacy of OBTA over a 2-year period (nine treatments) [62].

Adjuvants

Recently, there are reports of subjects with amplified improvements when coupled with nonpharmacological adjuvants. One pilot study found that patients receiving OBTA therapy concurrently with low-level laser therapy (LLLT) reported improved quality of sleep in addition to the established improvements (decreased headache days, intensity, and concomitant medications) [63], while another found supplemental musculoskeletal manipulation (cervicothoracic manipulative treatment) reported decreased concomitant medications by independent examiners. Another study demonstrated that patients asked to withdraw from taking headache medications and then randomly assigned to receive OBTA or low-dose OBTA found no statistically significant difference between the two groups. The investigators argue that intentional withdrawal is efficacious/well tolerated and suggest that clinicians consider this approach before attempting more expensive therapeutics [64]. Each of these are clinically relevant improvements; however, these instances have yet to be corroborated further by scientific evidence and may not be widely generalizable to other practices at this time.

Emerging Therapeutics for CM

The latest real-world clinical data on OBTA come from the REPOSE (Real-life use of botulinum toxin for the symptomatic treatment of adults with chronic migraine, measuring healthcare resource utilization, and Patient-reported Outcomes observed in practice) and CM-PASS (CM in routine clinical practice has been a prospective, observational, multinational, post-authorization study) studies. Given that OBTA may appeal to patients with a low tolerance to oral prophylactics, these studies reiterate questions aimed at predicting likelihood of nonresponders, duration of treatment (in responders), rate of sustained benefits in patients successfully stopping therapy, and rate of relapse in those that do stop therapy [25]. Studies suggest that patient selection is a key factor in successful improvement [65] with patients with short disease duration and high serum levels of CGRP are predictors of good response to OBTA [60]. With the idea of calcitonin gene-related peptide (CGPR) is connected to migraine pathogenesis, the FDA approved a calcitonin gene-related peptide (CGPR) antagonist in 2018 [7] called erenumab. Projections estimate this novel medication to reduce migraine-related and indirect costs (productivity, functionality, etc.) suggesting it to be a more economical option compared to OBTA [66].

In 2019, results from the COMPEL study showed that OBTA was well tolerated over 2 years (nine treatment cycles) when assessed for safety and tolerability suggesting that cumulative tolerability does not occur [67]. Two different sub-analysis of the COMPEL study showed that OBTA was an effective therapeutic in patients concurrently diagnosed with allodynia (sensitization of sensory neurons) [68] or daily headache [69] with sustained improvements in depression (PHQ-9), anxiety (GAD-7), and clinically significant improved sleeping patterns [17].

Before the year 2020, there is still emerging real-world evidence supporting OBTA [70] with a good safety profile – REPOSE study over 24 months suggest the most common side effects being eyelid ptosis, neck pain, and musculoskeletal stiffness [71]. With the consistent discovery of associated improvements OBTA has to offer, such as improving photophobia and dry eye symptoms [72] in addition to CM, there remains to be overall consensus on when OBTA should be withdrawn in responders [73], while clinical recommendations for managing episodic and chronic migraines may be established in some countries [74]. A survey of Spanish neurologists' first choice of a good treatment (topiramate) in managing migraine constantly may be consistent with recommended guidelines; however there are mixed preferences on when to apply alternative treatment, for example, starting OBTA after two unsuccessful attempts with oral preventative medication [75]. History suggests that that new therapeutics endure a lag in utilization, warranting a culture of timely prevention [76] potentially by specialist headache centers to enable a multidisciplinary approach to care.

The Future of OBTA

Predicting Responsiveness, Improving Effectiveness, and Novel Treatments

Future studies will examine the potential applications of the remaining toxin formulations [8] – incobotulinumtoxinA has shown sustained efficacy in patients with refractory chronic migraine and episodic disabling migraine headaches – along with developing novel delivery methods, for example, topical administration to make improvements in safety and efficacy [9].

As the most recent GBD report suggests, evidence surrounding adolescents is limited however includes that adolescents in the analysis that were responsive to OBTA also reported decreased concomittant medication. Additionally, there is limited scientific evidence investigating migraine preventative medications in children/adolescents [77]. Since most of the published evidence is on adults, more research is warranted in children [78] to expedite the process of amending the FDA label to include a beneficial therapeutic with a history of a good safety profile to the pediatric population.

Evidence from clinical trials suggests that patients treated with OBTA fall into two categories – responders vs. no responders – suggesting that there may be underlying neurological conditions (pseudotumor cerebri) responsible for migrainous symptoms. Headache pain specialists must work in conjunction with their neurologists to rule out previously stated underlying conditions to ensure that treatment this patient population will truly benefit from such a modality. Another challenge is the matter of obtaining appropriate health coverage for the cost of treatment. At the time this literature is published, healthcare insurance providers may not consider the treatment medically necessary since the using the OBTA for migraines in the pediatric population is not listed under the FDA indications.

Existing limitations in OBTA therapy include, but are not limited to, placebo response, unequal gender groups (patients tend to be Caucasian female patients vs. male), compliance using pain journal (needs an app to randomly sample pain throughout the day to avoid sampling bias), higher resolution data to characterize features of pain (physical pain vs. emotional pain) to predict whether subjects will be benefit from treatment, and accurate reporting of concomitant medication to track changes, for example, changes in dosing and frequency. Additionally, subjects that are strong responders to OBTA therapy should exercise incremental approach to resuming everyday activities to avoid rebound.

With recent genotype analysis suggesting that two polymorphic gene variations (CALCA and TRPV1) are associated with OBTA responsiveness for CM and may play a role in predicting efficacy [79], the future studies aimed at characterizing chronic migraine may help physicians fill the gap in understanding the underlying mechanisms and optimize treatment efficacy.

Conclusion

To-date, there are three FDA-approved medications for treating migraine: (1) triptans, (2) OBTA, and (3) CGRP antagonists. OBTA in particular is an effective modality with a good safety profile for treating adult patients diagnosed with chronic migraine. Emerging evidence suggests that this modality maintains efficacy, long-term safety, and tolerability in the pediatric population.

References

1. Stovner LJ, Nichols E, Steiner TJ, Abd-Allah F, Abdelalim A, Al-Raddadi RM, et al. Global, regional, and national burden of migraine and tension-type headache, 1990–2016: a systematic analysis for the Global Burden of Disease study 2016. Lancet Neurol. 2018;17:954–76. https://doi.org/10.1016/S1474-4422(18)30322-3.
2. Olesen J, Headache Classification Committee of the International Headache Society (IHS). The international classification of headache disorders, 3rd edition. Cephalalgia. 2018;38:1–211. https://doi.org/10.1177/0333102417738202.
3. Yancey JR, Sheridan R, Koren KG. Chronic daily headache: diagnosis and management. Am Fam Physician. 2014;89:642–8.
4. Martelletti P. The journey from genetic predisposition to medication overuse headache to its acquisition as sequela of chronic migraine. J Headache Pain. 2018;19:2. https://doi.org/10.1186/s10194-017-0830-2.
5. Blumenfeld AM, Silberstein SD, Dodick DW, Aurora SK, Brin MF, Binder WJ. Insights into the functional anatomy behind the PREEMPT injection paradigm: guidance on achieving optimal outcomes. Headache. 2017;57:766–77. https://doi.org/10.1111/head.13074.
6. Dodick DW, Turkel CC, Degryse RE, Aurora SK, Silberstein SD, Lipton RB, et al. OnabotulinumtoxinA for treatment of chronic migraine: pooled results from the double-blind, randomized, placebo-controlled phases of the PREEMPT clinical program. Headache. 2010;50:921–36. https://doi.org/10.1111/j.1526-4610.2010.01678.x.

7. Sprenger T, Viana M, Tassorelli C. Current prophylactic medications for migraine and their potential mechanisms of action. Neurotherapeutics. 2018;15:313–23. https://doi.org/10.1007/s13311-018-0621-8.
8. Ion I, Renard D, Le Floch A, De Verdal M, Bouly S, Wacongne A, et al. Monocentric prospective study into the sustained effect of Incobotulinumtoxin A (XEOMIN(R)) botulinum toxin in chronic refractory migraine. Toxins (Basel). 2018;10:221. https://doi.org/10.3390/toxins10060221.
9. Cairns BE, Gazerani P. Botulinum neurotoxin A for chronic migraine headaches: does it work and how? Pain Manag. 2014;4:377–80. https://doi.org/10.2217/pmt.14.30.
10. Szok D, Csati A, Vecsei L, Tajti J. Treatment of chronic migraine with onabotulinumtoxinA: mode of action, efficacy and safety. Toxins (Basel). 2015;7:2659–73. https://doi.org/10.3390/toxins7072659.
11. Coppola G, Schoenen J. Management of acute and chronic migraine. Curr Opin Support Palliat Care. 2012;6:177–82. https://doi.org/10.1097/SPC.0b013e3283521dc3.
12. Durham PL, Cady R. Insights into the mechanism of onabotulinumtoxinA in chronic migraine. Headache. 2011;51:1573–7. https://doi.org/10.1111/j.1526-4610.2011.02022.x.
13. Aurora SK, Brin MF. Chronic migraine: an update on physiology, imaging, and the mechanism of action of two available pharmacologic therapies. Headache. 2017;57:109–25. https://doi.org/10.1111/head.12999.
14. Aydinlar EI, Dikmen PY, Kosak S, Kocaman AS. OnabotulinumtoxinA effectiveness on chronic migraine, negative emotional states and sleep quality: a single-center prospective cohort study. J Headache Pain. 2017;18:23. https://doi.org/10.1186/s10194-017-0723-4.
15. Rendas-Baum R, Bloudek LM, Maglinte GA, Varon SF. The psychometric properties of the migraine-specific quality of life questionnaire version 2.1 (MSQ) in chronic migraine patients. Qual Life Res. 2013;22:1123–33. https://doi.org/10.1007/s11136-012-0230-7.
16. Lipton RB, Rosen NL, Ailani J, DeGryse RE, Gillard PJ, Varon SF. OnabotulinumtoxinA improves quality of life and reduces impact of chronic migraine over one year of treatment: pooled results from the PREEMPT randomized clinical trial program. Cephalalgia. 2016;36:899–908. https://doi.org/10.1177/0333102416652092.
17. Blumenfeld AM, Tepper SJ, Robbins LD, Manack Adams A, Buse DC, Orejudos A, et al. Effects of onabotulinumtoxinA treatment for chronic migraine on common comorbidities including depression and anxiety. J Neurol Neurosurg Psychiatry. 2019;90:353–60. https://doi.org/10.1136/jnnp-2018-319290.
18. Woods K, Ostrowski-Delahanty S. Psychometric properties of the psychosocial assessment tool-chronic pain version in families of children with headache. J Child Neurol. 2017;32:766–73. https://doi.org/10.1177/0883073817707111.
19. Lateef T, Cui L, Heaton L, Nakamura EF, Ding J, Ahmed S, et al. Validation of a migraine interview for children and adolescents. Pediatrics. 2013;131:e96–125. https://doi.org/10.1542/peds.2012-1008.
20. Allergan. Botox reconstitution and this kit is for educational. Allergan; 2020. https://www.botoxmedical.com/Common/Assets/APC15WD15_Recon_Dilution_Instructions.pdf.
21. Diener HC, Dodick DW, Aurora SK, Turkel CC, Degryse RE, Lipton RB, et al. OnabotulinumtoxinA for treatment of chronic migraine: results from the double-blind, randomized, placebo-controlled phase of the PREEMPT 2 trial. Cephalalgia. 2010;30:804–14. https://doi.org/10.1177/0333102410364677.
22. Whitcup SM, Turkel CC, DeGryse RE, Brin MF. Development of onabotulinumtoxinA for chronic migraine. Ann N Y Acad Sci. 2014;1329:67–80. https://doi.org/10.1111/nyas.12488.
23. Calderon M-D, Der Wu W, Ma M, De Los Santos J, Canales C, Rinehart JB, Shah S. A longitudinal evaluation of the effectiveness of Botox® in pediatric patients experiencing migraines: a five-year retrospective study. Am Soc Anesthesiol. 2017. http://www.asaabstracts.com/strands/asaabstracts/abstract.htm?year=2017&index=16&absnum=5056. Accessed 10 Sept 2019.

24. Food and Drug Administration. Distant spread of toxin effect. Postmarketing reports indicate that the effects of BOTOX and all botulinum toxin products may spread from the area of injection to produce symptoms consistent with botulinum toxin effects. These may include asthenia, gener. US Food and Drug Administration; 2011. https://www.accessdata.fda.gov/drugsatfda_docs/label/2011/103000s5236lbl.pdf.
25. Frampton JE, Silberstein S. OnabotulinumtoxinA: a review in the prevention of chronic migraine. Drugs. 2018;78:589–600. https://doi.org/10.1007/s40265-018-0894-6.
26. Matharu M, Pascual J, Nilsson Remahl I, Straube A, Lum A, Davar G, et al. Utilization and safety of onabotulinumtoxinA for the prophylactic treatment of chronic migraine from an observational study in Europe. Cephalalgia. 2017;37:1384–97. https://doi.org/10.1177/0333102417724150.
27. Silberstein SD, Dodick DW, Aurora SK, Diener H-C, DeGryse RE, Lipton RB, et al. Per cent of patients with chronic migraine who responded per onabotulinumtoxinA treatment cycle: PREEMPT. J Neurol Neurosurg Psychiatry. 2015;86:996–1001. https://doi.org/10.1136/jnnp-2013-307149.
28. Wakerley BR, Davies S. Migraine management: beyond pills. Br J Gen Pract. 2018;68:464–5. https://doi.org/10.3399/bjgp18X698969.
29. Rapoport AM. New acute treatments for headache. Neurol Sci. 2010;31(Suppl 1):S129–32. https://doi.org/10.1007/s10072-010-0304-7.
30. Russell MB. Clinical trials on onabotulinumtoxinA for the treatment of chronic migraine. J Headache Pain. 2011;12:135–6. https://doi.org/10.1007/s10194-011-0333-5.
31. Martelletti P. Dispute settlement understanding on the use of Botox in chronic migraine. J Headache Pain. 2011;12:1–2. https://doi.org/10.1007/s10194-010-0288-y.
32. Aurora S, Diener H-C, Dodick D. Reply: clinical trials on onabotulinumtoxinA for the treatment of chronic migraine. J Headache Pain. 2011;12:137–8. https://doi.org/10.1007/s10194-011-0334-4.
33. Oterino A, Ramon C, Pascual J. Experience with onabotulinumtoxinA (BOTOX) in chronic refractory migraine: focus on severe attacks. J Headache Pain. 2011;12:235–8. https://doi.org/10.1007/s10194-011-0294-8.
34. Negro A, Martelletti P. Chronic migraine plus medication overuse headache: two entities or not? J Headache Pain. 2011;12:593–601. https://doi.org/10.1007/s10194-011-0388-3.
35. Robbins L. Refractory chronic migraine: long-term follow-up using a refractory rating scale. J Headache Pain. 2012;13:225–9. https://doi.org/10.1007/s10194-012-0423-z.
36. Diener H-C, Dodick DW, Turkel CC, Demos G, Degryse RE, Earl NL, et al. Pooled analysis of the safety and tolerability of onabotulinumtoxinA in the treatment of chronic migraine. Eur J Neurol. 2014;21:851–9. https://doi.org/10.1111/ene.12393.
37. Aurora SK, Dodick DW, Diener H-C, DeGryse RE, Turkel CC, Lipton RB, et al. OnabotulinumtoxinA for chronic migraine: efficacy, safety, and tolerability in patients who received all five treatment cycles in the PREEMPT clinical program. Acta Neurol Scand. 2014;129:61–70. https://doi.org/10.1111/ane.12171.
38. Lin K-H, Chen S-P, Fuh J-L, Wang Y-F, Wang S-J. Efficacy, safety, and predictors of response to botulinum toxin type A in refractory chronic migraine: a retrospective study. J Chin Med Assoc. 2014;77:10–5. https://doi.org/10.1016/j.jcma.2013.09.006.
39. Rothrock JF, Bloudek LM, Houle TT, Andress-Rothrock D, Varon SF. Real-world economic impact of onabotulinumtoxinA in patients with chronic migraine. Headache. 2014;54:1565–73. https://doi.org/10.1111/head.12456.
40. Khalil M, Zafar HW, Quarshie V, Ahmed F. Prospective analysis of the use of onabotulinumtoxinA (BOTOX) in the treatment of chronic migraine; real-life data in 254 patients from Hull, U.K. J Headache Pain. 2014;15:54. https://doi.org/10.1186/1129-2377-15-54.
41. Diener H-C, Solbach K, Holle D, Gaul C. Integrated care for chronic migraine patients: epidemiology, burden, diagnosis and treatment options. Clin Med. 2015;15:344–50. https://doi.org/10.7861/clinmedicine.15-4-344.
42. Lee H-J, Choi K-S, Won S-Y, Apinuntrum P, Hu K-S, Kim S-T, et al. Topographic relationship between the supratrochlear nerve and corrugator supercilii muscle--can this anatomical

knowledge improve the response to botulinum toxin injections in chronic migraine? Toxins (Basel). 2015;7:2629–38. https://doi.org/10.3390/toxins7072629.
43. Miller S, Correia F, Lagrata S, Matharu MS. OnabotulinumtoxinA for hemicrania continua: open label experience in 9 patients. J Headache Pain. 2015;16:19. https://doi.org/10.1186/s10194-015-0502-z.
44. Hou M, Xie J-F, Kong X-P, Zhang Y, Shao Y-F, Wang C, et al. Acupoint injection of onabotulinumtoxin A for migraines. Toxins (Basel). 2015;7:4442–54. https://doi.org/10.3390/toxins7114442.
45. Luvisetto S, Gazerani P, Cianchetti C, Pavone F. Botulinum toxin type a as a therapeutic agent against headache and related disorders. Toxins (Basel). 2015;7:3818–44. https://doi.org/10.3390/toxins7093818.
46. Guerzoni S, Pellesi L, Baraldi C, Pini LA. Increased efficacy of regularly repeated cycles with onabotulinumtoxinA in MOH patients beyond the first year of treatment. J Headache Pain. 2015;17:48. https://doi.org/10.1186/s10194-016-0634-9.
47. Negro A, Curto M, Lionetto L, Martelletti P. A two years open-label prospective study of onabotulinumtoxinA 195 U in medication overuse headache: a real-world experience. J Headache Pain. 2015;17:1. https://doi.org/10.1186/s10194-016-0591-3.
48. Simpson DM, Hallett M, Ashman EJ, Comella CL, Green MW, Gronseth GS, et al. Practice guideline update summary: botulinum neurotoxin for the treatment of blepharospasm, cervical dystonia, adult spasticity, and headache: report of the Guideline Development Subcommittee of the American Academy of Neurology. Neurology. 2016;86:1818–26. https://doi.org/10.1212/WNL.0000000000002560.
49. Vikelis M, Argyriou AA, Dermitzakis EV, Spingos KC, Mitsikostas DD. Onabotulinumtoxin-A treatment in Greek patients with chronic migraine. J Headache Pain. 2016;17:84. https://doi.org/10.1186/s10194-016-0676-z.
50. Aicua-Rapun I, Martinez-Velasco E, Rojo A, Hernando A, Ruiz M, Carreres A, et al. Real-life data in 115 chronic migraine patients treated with onabotulinumtoxin A during more than one year. J Headache Pain. 2016;17:112. https://doi.org/10.1186/s10194-016-0702-1.
51. de Tommaso M, Delussi M, Ricci K, Montemurno A, Carbone I, Vecchio E. Effects of onabotulintoxinA on habituation of laser evoked responses in chronic migraine. Toxins (Basel). 2016;8:163. https://doi.org/10.3390/toxins8060163.
52. Choi Y-J, Lee W-J, Lee H-J, Lee K-W, Kim H-J, Hu K-S. Effective botulinum toxin injection guide for treatment of temporal headache. Toxins (Basel). 2016;8:265. https://doi.org/10.3390/toxins8090265.
53. Tassorelli C, Aguggia M, De Tommaso M, Geppetti P, Grazzi L, Pini LA, et al. Onabotulinumtoxin A for the management of chronic migraine in current clinical practice: results of a survey of sixty-three Italian headache centers. J Headache Pain. 2017;18:66. https://doi.org/10.1186/s10194-017-0773-7.
54. Santoro A, Fontana A, Miscio AM, Zarrelli MM, Copetti M, Leone MA. Quarterly repeat cycles of onabotulinumtoxinA in chronic migraine patients: the benefits of the prolonged treatment on the continuous responders and quality-of-life conversion rate in a real-life setting. Neurol Sci. 2017;38:1779–89. https://doi.org/10.1007/s10072-017-3054-y.
55. Bratbak DF, Nordgard S, Stovner LJ, Linde M, Dodick DW, Aschehoug I, et al. Pilot study of sphenopalatine injection of onabotulinumtoxinA for the treatment of intractable chronic migraine. Cephalalgia. 2017;37:356–64. https://doi.org/10.1177/0333102416648328.
56. Matharu M, Halker R, Pozo-Rosich P, DeGryse R, Manack Adams A, Aurora SK. The impact of onabotulinumtoxinA on severe headache days: PREEMPT 56-week pooled analysis. J Headache Pain. 2017;18:78. https://doi.org/10.1186/s10194-017-0784-4.
57. Ranoux D, Martine G, Espagne-Dubreuilh G, Amilhaud-Bordier M, Caire F, Magy L. OnabotulinumtoxinA injections in chronic migraine, targeted to sites of pericranial myofascial pain: an observational, open label, real-life cohort study. J Headache Pain. 2017;18:75. https://doi.org/10.1186/s10194-017-0781-7.
58. Burstein R, Blake P, Schain A, Perry C. Extracranial origin of headache. Curr Opin Neurol. 2017;30:263–71. https://doi.org/10.1097/WCO.0000000000000437.

59. Herd CP, Tomlinson CL, Rick C, Scotton WJ, Edwards J, Ives N, et al. Botulinum toxins for the prevention of migraine in adults. Cochrane Database Syst Rev. 2018;6:CD011616. https://doi.org/10.1002/14651858.CD011616.pub2.
60. Bendtsen L, Sacco S, Ashina M, Mitsikostas D, Ahmed F, Pozo-Rosich P, et al. Guideline on the use of onabotulinumtoxinA in chronic migraine: a consensus statement from the European Headache Federation. J Headache Pain. 2018;19:91. https://doi.org/10.1186/s10194-018-0921-8.
61. Vikelis M, Argyriou AA, Dermitzakis EV, Spingos KC, Makris N, Kararizou E. Sustained onabotulinumtoxinA therapeutic benefits in patients with chronic migraine over 3 years of treatment. J Headache Pain. 2018;19:87. https://doi.org/10.1186/s10194-018-0918-3.
62. Blumenfeld AM, Stark RJ, Freeman MC, Orejudos A, Manack AA. Long-term study of the efficacy and safety of onabotulinumtoxinA for the prevention of chronic migraine: COMPEL study. J Headache Pain. 2018;19:13. https://doi.org/10.1186/s10194-018-0840-8.
63. Loeb LM, Amorim RP, Mazzacoratti MGN, Scorza FA, Peres MFP. Botulinum toxin A (BT-A) versus low-level laser therapy (LLLT) in chronic migraine treatment: a comparison. Arq Neuropsiquiatr. 2018;76:663–7. https://doi.org/10.1590/0004-282X20180109.
64. Pijpers JA, Kies DA, Louter MA, van Zwet EW, Ferrari MD, Terwindt GM. Acute withdrawal and botulinum toxin A in chronic migraine with medication overuse: a double-blind randomized controlled trial. Brain. 2019;142:1203–14. https://doi.org/10.1093/brain/awz052.
65. Castrillo Sanz A, Morollon Sanchez-Mateos N, Simonet Hernandez C, Fernandez Rodriguez B, Cerdan Santacruz D, Mendoza Rodriguez A, et al. Experience with botulinum toxin in chronic migraine. Neurologia. 2018;33:499–504. https://doi.org/10.1016/j.nrl.2016.09.004.
66. Lipton RB, Brennan A, Palmer S, Hatswell AJ, Porter JK, Sapra S, et al. Estimating the clinical effectiveness and value-based price range of erenumab for the prevention of migraine in patients with prior treatment failures: a US societal perspective. J Med Econ. 2018;21:666–75. https://doi.org/10.1080/13696998.2018.1457533.
67. Winner PK, Blumenfeld AM, Eross EJ, Orejudos AC, Mirjah DL, Adams AM, et al. Long-term safety and tolerability of onabotulinumtoxinA treatment in patients with chronic migraine: results of the COMPEL study. Drug Saf. 2019;42:1013–24. https://doi.org/10.1007/s40264-019-00824-3.
68. Young WB, Ivan Lopez J, Rothrock JF, Orejudos A, Manack Adams A, Lipton RB, et al. Effects of onabotulinumtoxinA treatment in patients with and without allodynia: results of the COMPEL study. J Headache Pain. 2019;20:10. https://doi.org/10.1186/s10194-018-0952-1.
69. Young WB, Ivan Lopez J, Rothrock JF, Orejudos A, Manack Adams A, Lipton RB, et al. Effects of onabotulinumtoxinA treatment in chronic migraine patients with and without daily headache at baseline: results from the COMPEL study. J Headache Pain. 2019;20:12. https://doi.org/10.1186/s10194-018-0953-0.
70. Stark C, Stark R, Limberg N, Rodrigues J, Cordato D, Schwartz R, et al. Real-world effectiveness of onabotulinumtoxinA treatment for the prevention of headaches in adults with chronic migraine in Australia: a retrospective study. J Headache Pain. 2019;20:81. https://doi.org/10.1186/s10194-019-1030-z.
71. Ahmed F, Gaul C, Garcia-Monco JC, Sommer K, Martelletti P. An open-label prospective study of the real-life use of onabotulinumtoxinA for the treatment of chronic migraine: the REPOSE study. J Headache Pain. 2019;20:26. https://doi.org/10.1186/s10194-019-0976-1.
72. Diel RJ, Hwang J, Kroeger ZA, Levitt RC, Sarantopoulos CD, Sered H, et al. Photophobia and sensations of dryness in patients with migraine occur independent of baseline tear volume and improve following botulinum toxin A injections. Br J Ophthalmol. 2019;103:1024–9. https://doi.org/10.1136/bjophthalmol-2018-312649.
73. Gago-Veiga AB, Santos-Lasaosa S, Cuadrado ML, Guerrero AL, Irimia P, Lainez JM, et al. Evidence and experience with onabotulinumtoxinA in chronic migraine: recommendations for daily clinical practice. Neurologia. 2019;34:408–17. https://doi.org/10.1016/j.nrl.2017.09.008.
74. Kouremenos E, Arvaniti C, Constantinidis TS, Giannouli E, Fakas N, Kalamatas T, et al. Consensus of the Hellenic Headache Society on the diagnosis and treatment of migraine. J Headache Pain. 2019;20:113. https://doi.org/10.1186/s10194-019-1060-6.

75. Garcia-Azorin D, Santos-Lasaosa S, Gago-Veiga AB, Viguera Romero J, Guerrero-Peral AL. Real world preventative drug management of migraine among Spanish neurologists. J Headache Pain. 2019;20:19. https://doi.org/10.1186/s10194-019-0971-6.
76. Agostoni EC, Barbanti P, Calabresi P, Colombo B, Cortelli P, Frediani F, et al. Current and emerging evidence-based treatment options in chronic migraine: a narrative review. J Headache Pain. 2019;20:92. https://doi.org/10.1186/s10194-019-1038-4.
77. Huang T-C, Lai T-H, Treatment Guideline Subcommittee of Taiwan Headache Society Taiwan Headache Society. Medical treatment guidelines for preventive treatment of migraine. Acta Neurol Taiwanica. 2017;26:33–53.
78. Shah S, Calderon M-D, Der Wu W, Grant J, Rinehart J. Onabotulinumtoxin A (BOTOX®) for ProphylaCTIC treatment of pediatric migraine: a retrospective longitudinal analysis. J Child Neurol. 2018;33:580–6. https://doi.org/10.1177/0883073818776142.
79. Moreno-Mayordomo R, Ruiz M, Pascual J, Gallego de la Sacristana M, Vidriales I, Sobrado M, et al. CALCA and TRPV1 genes polymorphisms are related to a good outcome in female chronic migraine patients treated with onabotulinumtoxinA. J Headache Pain. 2019;20:39. https://doi.org/10.1186/s10194-019-0989-9.

7 Pediatric Migraine Presentation and Treatment Algorithm

Sharoon Qaiser, Antoinette Green, and Marielle Kabbouche

Migraine Criteria

The International Classification of Headache Disorder (ICHD-3) helps to classify different headache disorders including migraine. The diagnostic criteria for children and adolescents are generally similar as adults with few exceptions [1].

Temporal Criteria

As per ICHD-3, migraine lasts between 4 and 72 h. In children and adolescents, this criterion has been revised to include shorter duration of headache lasting 2–72 h. This allowance of shorter duration of headache has many practical implementations. Time, much like pain, may be very subjective from a younger child's perspective. When asked the duration of headache, children may not be able to accurately describe. Many children only report headaches to their caregivers when the intensity reaches a moderate or severe level, and not necessarily at onset of headache.

Location Criteria

Unilateral location of migraine has been described since antiquity, and Galenus used the Latin term *hemicrania* in first century AD. Pain may not be strictly unilateral in children and adolescent presenting with migraine. ICHD-3 recognizes frontotemporal location of pain in the diagnostic criterion of migraine in adolescents

S. Qaiser · A. Green · M. Kabbouche (✉)
Department of Neurology, Cincinnati Children Hospital Medical Center (CCHMC), Cincinnati, OH, USA
e-mail: Marielle.kabbouche@cchmc.org

© Springer Nature Switzerland AG 2021

S. Shah (ed.), *Migraine*, https://doi.org/10.1007/978-3-030-75239-2_7

and children. Many younger children report more frontal pain. Location of pain also helps to identify other headache disorders including occipital neuralgias and trigeminal autonomic cephalgias, etc.

Associated Symptoms

Given polygenic nature of migraine and widely distributed genes, children may present with different phenotype of symptoms as compare to adults. These symptoms may help to aid in diagnosis. Children may have more prominent gastrointestinal symptoms when compared to adults. There is an exhaustive list of associated symptoms, including photophobia, phonophobia, nausea and vomiting, but more common symptoms seen in children include abdominal pain, lightheadedness, vertigo, etc. The most common comorbidity in children and adolescent with migraine is anxiety disorders. These comorbidities are usually overlooked. A careful assessment during each encounter should be made to identify those who suffer with anxiety and other mood disorders and provide them with resources. In general, migraine in children is similar disease as adults but may have different temporal, location, and associated symptoms. A careful history should clarify subjective terms and should remove any internal and external bias which may be inherent to any childhood disease presentation.

Migraine Equivalent or Episodic Syndromes in Children

> Migraine is a syndrome and headache is just one symptom – Andrew Hershey, MD., PhD, FAHS, FAAN

In recent years, the polygenic nature of migraine has been explored, and up to 39 genes have been associated with migraine [2]. These genes are widely expressed in the entire body and affect all major systems. As a result, children who are diagnosed with migraine in later years may present with different phenotypes in younger years. ICHD-3 guidelines in 2018, described these different phenotypes as migraine equivalent or episodic syndromes associated with migraine. According to one survey, up to 40% of children diagnosed with episodic syndromes will develop migraine as adults. Different types of migraine equivalent or episodic syndromes are discussed below.

Types of Migraine

Infant Colic

Before more complex communication skills are developed in infants, crying may be the most important communication skill and may have survival benefits, but inconsolable crying may be the most challenging thing for caregivers and may be sign of secondary cause. According to ICHD-3, infant colic is defined as “Recurrent episodes of irritability, fussing or crying from birth to 4 months of age with episodes lasting >3 hours/day, episodes >3/days in a week for over 3 weeks, in otherwise healthy infant."

Parents with migraine, have a fivefold risk of having a baby with infant colic which points toward strong genetics basis of migraine. Pathophysiology of infant colic is not clear, but it is hypothesized that GI inflammation, change in gut bacteria, or feeding techniques may cause GI distress in those who are genetically predisposed [3]. No study has proven etiological basis of infant colic. The most important thing to consider is that diagnosis of infant colic needs exclusion of other causes of inconsolable crying. Since risk of shaken baby syndrome is associated with age-related crying, hence identifying cases of infant colic may help to identify high-risk group [4].

Benign Paroxysmal Torticollis

The ability for an infant to hold their neck in first 3–4 months of life is considered an important milestone. It helps an infant to observe their surroundings, interact well with others, and may aid in their posture. According to ICHD-3, benign paroxysmal torticollis is defined as follows:

- Recurrent episodes of head tilt to either side within first year of life (most commonly after ability to hold neck) with spontaneous remission in otherwise healthy infant.
- Each episode may last for minutes to days.
- These attacks may be associated with any of the following symptoms:
  1. Pallor
  2. Irritability
  3. Malaise
  4. Vomiting
  5. Ataxia

Historically, nystagmus may be associated with this condition, but it is not listed in the diagnostic criteria. Among all periodic syndromes, this is least prevalent along with alternating hemiplegia of childhood, with an overall prevalence of <1/100,000. Few cases showed CACNA1A gene mutation but its link with hemiplegic migraine is not established. This is a diagnosis of exclusion and other differentials including focal dystonia, posterior fossa tumors, GERD, focal seizures, etc. should be considered. This clinical diagnosis is a rarity and due to the pathological differential, it is suggested to do appropriate investigations.

Benign Paroxysmal Vertigo

Common symptoms like vertigo may be difficult to communicate by children. Children may describe vertiginous symptoms as "feeling strange," "feeling frightful," "spinning sensation," or "lightheaded." In the past, paroxysmal spells of dizziness in children were thought to be related to vestibular diseases, but in 1988, ICHD included this into list of migraine equivalent in children.

According to ICHD-3, benign paroxysmal vertigo of childhood is defined as follows:

1. At least five, recurrent, brief attacks of vertigo, paroxysmal in nature and resolve spontaneously in a healthy child with normal neurological exam.
2. Each attack may last from minutes to hours without altered conscious.
3. Normal documented audiometric and vestibular testing between attacks.
4. One of the following symptoms/signs are reported:
   - Nystagmus
   - Ataxia
   - Vomiting
   - Pallor
   - Fearfulness

It is unclear about the pathogenesis of benign paroxysmal vertigo, but it may be an age-related phenotype of migraine. Majority of patients with benign paroxysmal vertigo develop migraine with aura as adults. This presents as only a periodic syndrome which requires diagnostic testing as per ICHD-3. This is diagnosis of exclusion as posterior fossa lesions, vestibular etiologies, and seizures should be included in the differential.

Alternating Hemiplegia of Childhood

Almost all periodic syndromes are self-limiting/remitting with benign course except alternating hemiplegia of childhood. Alternating hemiplegia of childhood is defined as per ICHD-3 as, "Recurrent attacks of alternating hemiplegia with paroxysmal phenomenon with onset before 18 months of age. This is an encephalopathic, neurodegenerative and progressive disease with strong genetic association with ATP1A3 gene mutation." Other genes associated with alternating hemiplegia of childhood include CACNA1A, SLC1A3, and ATP1A2 [5]. The exact relation of alternating hemiplegia in children with migraine is unknown, but it is clinically related to migraine and has similar genetic mutation as hemiplegic migraine. These known genes affect the Na+/K+ pump and their mutation may lead to channelopathy, which may result in different phenotypes.

More common presentation of symptoms is in late infancy, but few cases have been reported with onset of symptoms in neonate period. The most common muscle groups involved are upper and lower limb girdles, but there is bulbar involvement in some cases that increases the morbidity further due to feeding challenges. Paroxysmal symptoms are associated with hemiplegia and may aid to make the diagnosis. Most common paroxysmal symptoms include nystagmus, dystonia, choreoathetosis, ataxia, and autonomic dysfunction. Some of the important differentials include cerebrovascular disorder, neurodegenerative diseases, metabolic diseases, seizures, and other causes for regression.

Cyclic Vomiting Syndrome

Recurrent vomiting in otherwise healthy children who later in life develop migraine – the syndrome was described in the literature in the 1800s. In 2004, the ICHD-2 criteria gave the syndrome a specific definition and included cyclic vomiting syndrome as a migraine variant for the first time [6].

According to ICHD-3, cyclic vomiting syndrome is defined as, "At least five attacks of predictable, recurrent attacks of intense nausea and vomiting, lasting more than an hour (up to days) with complete resolution of symptoms in between attacks in an otherwise healthy child." It is important to note that if these symptoms are associated with migraine defining headache, then it is simply called migraine without aura. One hallmark of cyclic vomiting syndrome is that nausea is persistent and as opposed to migraine without aura, it doesn't resolve after vomiting. Cyclic vomiting syndrome is a diagnosis of exclusion and may require extensive gastrointestinal assessment and may result in diagnostic procedures. Among all periodic syndromes, cyclic vomiting syndrome is associated with significant morbidity including health care cost and work loss, one study showing annual cost of treatment alone averaged USD 17,000/patient [7]. Exact pathogenesis in unknown, but it is postulated that given its cyclic nature, higher centers including hypothalamus–pituitary–adrenal axis may be involved in the pathogenesis, other probable causes include mitochondrial DNA origin and autonomic dysfunction [8]. This debilitating disease is more common in children and often results in diagnostic dilemma.

Abdominal Migraine

There may be more to the tummy pains than an excuse to miss school – Sharoon Qaiser, MD

Nonacute, vague, chronic abdominal pain is a very common complaint in children and may be overlooked. Out of 39 genes associated with migraine, many are expressed in gastrointestinal system, hence, it is common to have gastrointestinal symptoms as part of migraine complex [2]. In 1922, Dr. Brams used the term "abdominal migraine" to describe the cases seen in his practice with recurrent abdominal pain and family history of migraine [9]. In 2004, ICHD included it in the list of migraine variants and described the diagnostic criteria for abdominal migraine. According to ICHD-3, it is defined as, "Recurrent paroxysmal attacks of moderate to severe, midline abdominal pain lasting 2–72 hours with associated vasomotor symptoms including anorexia, nausea, vomiting, pallor with complete resolution of symptoms in between attacks in otherwise healthy child."

Many children presenting with recurrent abdominal pain also have headache, and it may be overlooked. In case of recurrent abdominal pain and headache, diagnosis of migraine without aura should be given instead of abdominal migraine. There is no age criterion for abdominal migraine, but children usually present with symptoms around 7 years of age which coincides with early school years. The exact pathogenesis is unclear, but different hypotheses including immunogenic, altered gut motility, and hyperalgesia are given, but no hypothesis has explained higher prevalence in children. Its relation to migraine and presence of vasomotor symptoms are unclear. Abdominal migraine is a diagnosis of exclusion and require normal gastrointestinal assessment. This may lead to many unnecessary investigations or procedures.

In conclusion, migraine is a polygenic disease with wide variety of phenotypes. These phenotypes may present with different symptoms at different ages. Future studies will help to explore the pathogenesis of various migraine variants in children and may help to find target specific treatments.

Treatment Algorithm

According to one survey, 17% children are being sent home more than once from school due to medical ailments, and 47% of them have headache. Interestingly, majority of those with headache do not know what to do when they have headache [10]. A good treatment algorithm is a triad between children with headaches, their caregivers (including teachers), and health-care providers. A young child, or even an adolescent, must learn to identify headache at onset. Caregivers should learn to identify "extra headache symptoms," and health-care providers need to provide the education, treatment plan, and practical steps to remove barriers for treatment. The goal of robust headache treatment plan is to treat headaches in an outpatient setting and avoid an ER visit or inpatient stay. In the following section, we will discuss outpatient treatment algorithms for primary headaches in children especially migraine.

The treatment approach of migraine has three facets:

1. What to do when you have headache: Acute Plan
2. What to do to prevent headache and decrease the occurrences: Preventive plan
3. What to do to avoid a headache: Lifestyle changes and behavior measures

There is a flowsheet (Figs. 7.1 and 7.2) combining these three facets attached at the end of the chapter, and we will discuss them individually. We gave a special attention in the flowsheet to "medication overuse headache," and how to approach it while following the algorithm. As we must identify, treat, and eliminate this potentiating common cause of chronic headaches. According to ICHD-3, medication overuse headache is defined as worsening in preexisting primary headache with at least 15 headache days/month in conjunction with taking any single acute medication for pain for more than 15 days/month and combination of acute medication for more than 10 days/month for at least 3 months.

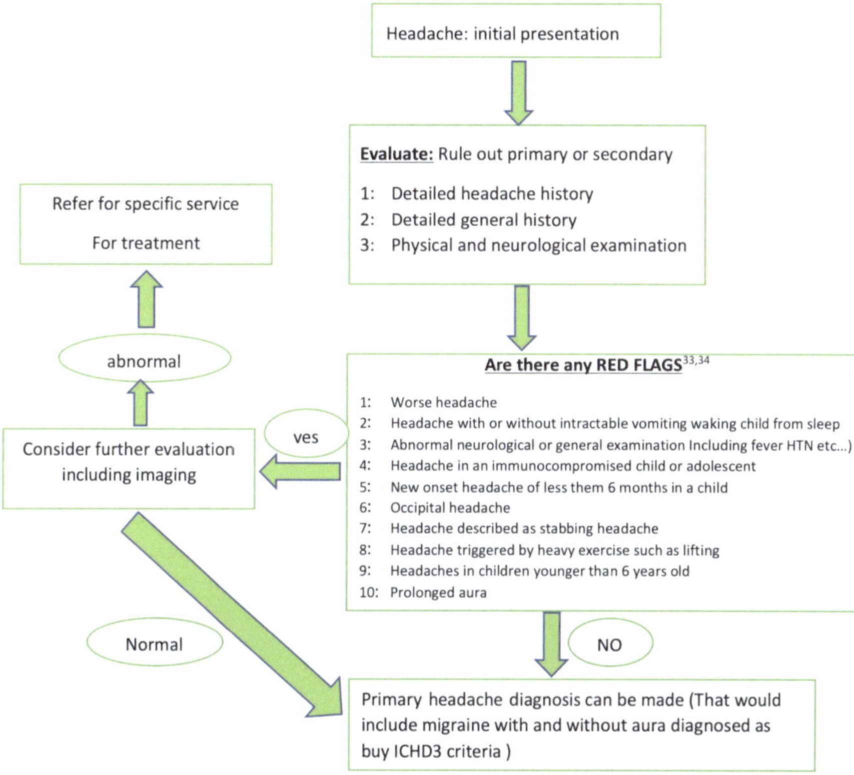

Fig. 7.1 Headache evaluation algorithm (CCHMC protocol). For any initial encounter with a child and adolescent presenting with a headache, the provider should start with a very detailed history and examination to rule out a possible secondary headache before offering any therapeutic recommendations

What to Do When You Have Headache: Acute Treatment Plan

Neurogenic edema and vasodilation are important components of pathogenesis of migraine and most acute medications target these two aspects. Interestingly, after some time, when nociceptive pathways are activated with more central sensitization, these acute medications may not effectively resolve the headache. This helps us to identify an important barrier in acute medication usage, that is, not been able to take medicine at onset of headache either due to poor access or waiting for headache to be resolved by its own. Another important barrier is the underdosing of medications. Many over-the-counter medications (i.e., nonsteroidal anti-inflammatory drugs [NSAIDs]) may be dosed based upon a dose range, but not actual per kilogram dosing standards, which results in poor efficacy and increased risk of medication overuse headache.

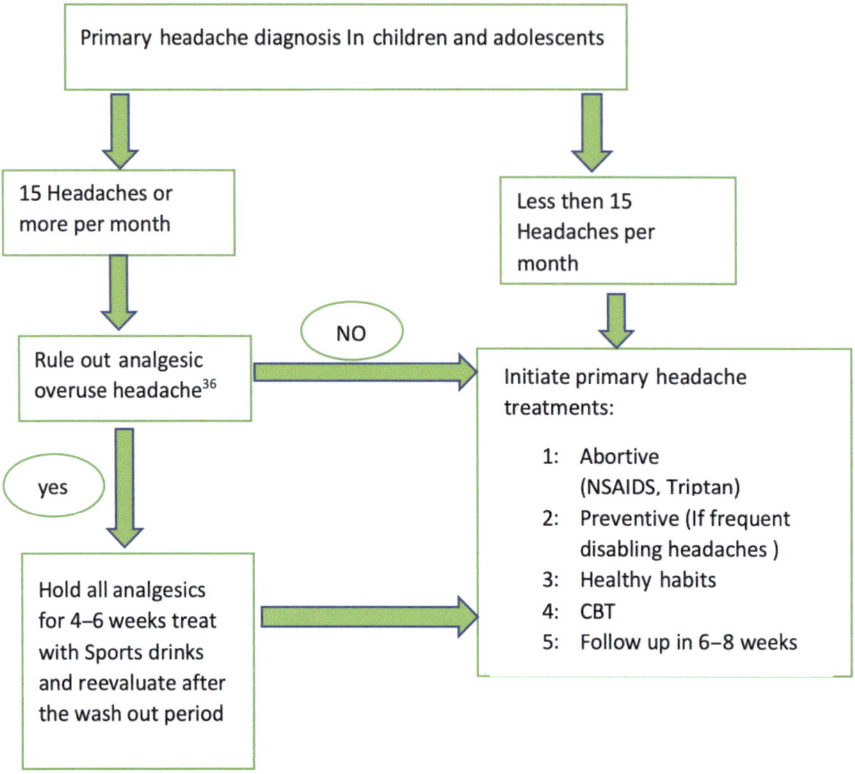

Fig. 7.2 Therapeutic algorithm for primary headache in children and adolescents (CCHMC protocol)

The goal of an acute treatment is to control the headache in 1–2 h, including the associated symptoms. Thus, the child should be able to return to their typical activity level following administration of acute medications for headache.

Nonsteroidal Anti-inflammatory Drugs (NSAIDs)

> NSAIDs work in kids — ibuprofen and naproxen sodium – *Andrew Hershey: Medscape News 2019 at Launch of migraine Guidelines*

Hippocrates documented analgesic properties of willow bark and the first NSAID (i.e., aspirin) was formulated in 1887 with its active ingredient (salicylic acid). NSAIDs are a group of medications acting through the cyclooxygenase pathway and provide analgesic and anti-inflammatory effects. There are many NSAIDs, but ibuprofen and naproxen are most commonly prescribed NSAIDs in children and adolescent for various conditions. One of the double-blind, placebo-controlled crossover studies showed that ibuprofen provided better pain control and tolerability in children with migraine when compared to acetaminophen. Hence, acetaminophen is only offered in those cases in which pain is intolerable to NSAID or have contraindication to NSAID [11].

NSAID Type There is no evidence that any specific NSAID works better. Ibuprofen, naproxen, and aspirin are commonly used NSAIDs. Ibuprofen is available in liquid and chewable forms, which may be desirable in younger children. Adolescent of ages 16 and above may be offered aspirin as well, preferably not as a combination with over-the-counter medication with caffeine and acetaminophen. Failure of one NSAID shouldn't hold back from trying other types. A child should be given different options, and he or she may decide based upon previous experience and access.

NSAID Dosing Anti-inflammatory dosing may be higher than typical antipyretic dosing. The usual recommended dosing range is 10–15 mg/kg maximum 1000 mg. It is important to take it at onset headache, and each headache should be treated. It is important to note treating not just the "bad" ones but limiting the treatments to no more than three headaches a week.

NSAID Allowance A clear NSAID allowance provides better efficacy and decreases the risk of medication overuse headache. If headache doesn't resolve in 3–4 h after taking the initial NSAID at onset of the pain, the dose can be repeated once. A child may treat up to three headaches per week using this regimen.

NSAID+ Rapid Hydration Neurogenic edema and inflammation result in electrolyte disbalance, and rapid hydration with electrolyte may help to provide some relief. It is suggested that every time when a child is required to take acute medication (NSAID), he or she must take 12–36 ounces (based upon body weight) of noncaffeinated fluid with electrolytes (e.g., sports drink) or water with salty snack. A health-care provider may help to overcome barriers of access to sports drink at school.

Triptans

Serotonin receptors are widely distributed in trigeminovascular system and provide effective target for serotonergic drugs. Triptans are a class of drugs with action at serotonin receptors 5-HT$_{1b}$ and $_{1D}$ causing vasoconstriction, hence halting the initial cascade of events in pathogenesis of migraine. Triptans were formulated in 1990s, and have been FDA approved for acute treatment of migraine. The American Academy of Neurology and American Headache Society published recent guidelines to treat acute migraine in children and include various triptans as possible treatment options [12]. The triptans can be used when the appropriately dosed NSAID is not providing relief consistently. They are usually recommended as a rescue medication.

The best described treatment for migraine is a stratified one. NSAID as a first-line drug: it is essential to educate patients that this class of medication needs to be taken at onset of a headaches for best result with sports drinks and repeat in 3–4 h no more than three times a week then reevaluate few weeks later, if some of the headaches are not responding as well as expected then a triptan can be added to those specific ones.

Triptan Timing One of the most important thing to consider is that triptans tend to work better if taken at onset of headache due to mechanism of their action. Hence, patients and guardians should be educated about the timing of taking triptan, and delay in treatment resulting in poor efficacy should not be considered as treatment failure.

Triptan Type and Concomitant Use There are many types of triptans and if one triptan does not work, it should not preclude from using different one. FDA has approved four triptans for children with migraine. Rizatriptan is approved for ages 6 and above, while almotriptan, zolmitriptan, and sumatriptan is approved for ages 12 and above. Linder et al. conducted placebo-controlled, double-blind study and provided robust evidence for almotriptan efficacy in adolescents [13]. The combination of sumatriptan and naproxen (Treximet) is approved for acute migraine treatment in adolescents and found to be superior than sumatriptan or naproxen alone [14]. Other factors involved in choosing the type of triptans include route (nasal versus oral), allergic reaction to sulfa drugs, access, and choice of prescribing physician.

Triptan Dosing Like NSAIDs, triptans are usually underdosed, and hence they do not provide adequate therapeutic response. Dosing is generally weight based and maximum dose within the weight range should be offered (Table 7.1).

Triptan Allowance Triptans can be repeated in 2 h. A careful well described plan should be given, because there may be confusion of timing of relating triptan as many children concomitantly consume NSAIDs as well. One can treat up to six headaches per month using a triptan. We usually recommend treating headache once a week using triptan in order to avoid confusion and risk of medicine overuse headache.

In summary, we should hit acute headache early and hard with NSAID + electrolyte sports drink and triptans can be used in selective cases.

Table 7.1 Dosing references for the use of some triptan for an acute migraine headache in children and adolescents

Triptan	Weight <40 kg	Weight >40 kg
Sumatriptan	50 mg 20 mg (Nasal)	100 mg 20 mg (Nasal)
Almotriptan	6.25 mg	12.5 mg
Zolmitriptan	2.5 for both oral and nasal	5 mg for both oral and nasal
Rizatriptan	5 mg	10 mg

What to Do to Prevent Headache: Preventive Treatment

> An ounce of prevention is worth a pound of cure – 'De Legibus:1240

Indication

What is acceptable number of headache days in a month. American headache society considers one to two headache days per week consistently as indication for daily preventive medication. Other indications include significant disability, ER visits, poor response to acute medication, etc. [15]. Powers et al. showed that having chronic migraine in adolescents affects quality of life in a similar way as pediatric cancer, heart disease, and rheumatoid arthritis [16]. According to one survey, 33% adolescents with migraine have indication to use daily preventive medication, but only 10% are being offered daily preventive medication [17]. We recommend daily preventive for all children and adolescents having four or more headache days per month; other things to consider include missed school days, high disability scores (PedMIDAS: Grade II), and poor response to acute treatment [18]. Once children have better control of daily headaches (<4/month), they can be weaned off from daily preventives.

Evidence

There is consistent evidence for daily preventive medication efficacy in adults for migraine, but results are variable in children. Various previous studies showed some efficacy of commonly used daily preventive medications, but modern more robust studies including Childhood and Adolescent Migraine Prevention (CHAMP) trial have failed to show any superiority of common preventive medicines (amitriptyline, topiramate, etc.) over placebo [19]. We have seen consistent high placebo response in all pediatric migraine studies. This highlights the importance of the use of preventive medication along with lifestyle changes. The American Academy of Neurology and American Headache society published their recent guidelines for migraine prevention in children and list various medication (Table 7.2) for prevention of migraine in children with variable evidence [11].

Types

Migraine is polygenic neurovascular disease with multifactorial pathogenies, hence different classes of drugs, including antiepileptics, antidepressants, antihistamines, antihypertensives, etc., are being used as preventive agents. Novel calcitonin gene-related peptide (CGRP) antibodies offer a new target specific class of drug approved for adults and being studied in children. At present, American Headache society pediatric headache expert group recommends using CGRP antibodies in post-pubertal adolescents in very selective cases [20]. These new molecules are not yet FDA approved for the use in the pediatric population, but hopefully soon. This is why we are not including these novel medicines in the algorithm mentioned below. Since no preventive is superior, decision regarding choice of preventive should be made based upon comorbidities, personal choice (patient choice), physician experience, relative contraindications, blood work, and teratogenicity.

Table 7.2 List of some preventive medications used in pediatric and adolescents with primary headaches and specifically migraine

Antiepileptics	1–4 mg/kg/day: Minimum effective dose is 100 mg/day
Topiramate [23, 24]	Typical dose is 50 mg BID or 75 mg BID
Valproic acid [25]	15–30 mg/kg divided bid
Zonisamide	100–600 mg/day
Levetiracetam	500–1500 mg BID (Weight dependant)
Antidepressants	
Amitriptyline [26, 27]	1 mg/kg qHS
Nortriptyline	1 mg/kg (10 mg–75 mg a day)
Antihypertensive Propranolol	2–4 mg/kg/day divided into BID or TID
Antihistamine Cyproheptadine	0.25–1.5 mg/kg/day divided into BID: Usually used for younger children ≤6 years of age
Neurotoxins Botulinum toxin A [21, 22, 28, 29]	155–195 units q 3 months (FDA approved for chronic migraine in adults but not in children and adolescents; only used by headache specialist for cases which failed multiple preventive therapies

The gray highlighted medications are the ones usually used as first-line preventive treatment. The rest are tried if the initial ones do not show improvement after 6 weeks on an appropriate dosing. The only preventive medication that has a placebo run study is the topiramate and is FDA approved for migraine in children and adolescents.

Titration and Dosing

Children report less side effects when medicines are titrated slowly. Although there is no study to prove the correct titration process, but we recommend 8–12 weeks titration period at 2-week interval between each change to reach the target dose. Family and patients will need to be educated about the titration and the goal of a preventive medication as well as the need to reach a full dose to assess effectiveness.

Botulinum Toxin for the Prevention of Migraine in Children

OnabotulinumtoxinA (trade name “Botox”®), an inhibitor of pain chemo-neurotransmitters, was approved by the FDA in 2010 for adult patients with the indication of chronic migraine defined as >15 headache days per month with episodes lasting >4 h per day. In adults, onabotulinumtoxinA has been shows to prevent 9 headache days a month versus 7 headache days in placebo when injected every 3 months. Significant contributions have been made to evaluate the efficacy of the toxin in the pediatric population over the last decade. A 5-year retrospective study evaluating the toxin longitudinally demonstrated safety, efficacy, and tolerability for children with migraine [21]. Most recently, in the first prospective double-blinded, placebo-controlled crossover design trial, pediatric subjects aged 8–17 that received OBTA treatment for migraine reported a significant decrease in the frequency and intensity of pediatric migraines, with a reduction in the disability scoring as well, indicating increased functionality from baseline when compared to placebo [22]. We also highlight another study which did not meet efficacy endpoints for prevention of migraine in the adolescent population [28]. These studies underscore the importance of studying the potential use of the toxin for the prevention of migraine in children in the future (Table 7.2).

What to Do to Avoid Headaches: Lifestyle Changes and Behavior Measures

The natural history of migraine is variable but according to one prospective study lasting 20 years, it was found out that 75% children with migraine continue to have headaches as adults [10]. This presents migraine as lifetime ailment (more common in females), highlighting significance of healthy lifestyle and behavior measures. The behavior measures should include an evaluation of underlying social triggers and anxiety and possible referral for biofeedback or cognitive behavioral therapy as needed. It is necessary to educate children and their family that this is a major step toward headache improvement.

We suggest the SMART approach, an approach described by Cincinnati Children's Hospital Pediatric Headache team to simplify the recommended healthy habits when presented to patients and families. The SMART table summarizes those habits (Table 7.3).

Table 7.3 SMART

S – Sleep
Children 10–12 and adolescents 8–10-h sleep
Practice sleep hygiene with regular bed and wake up times
Similar schedule over the weekend as well
Avoidance of screens before bed
M – Meal
Eating regular healthy meals without skipping any meals.
Dark green vegetables are rich source of folate and riboflavin vitamins that have been used for headache prevention [30]
Animal products are rich source of CoQ10 [31]
Dairy products are source of Vitamin D3
Avoid caffeinated drinks
Stay hydrated (8–10 glasses a day)
A – Activity
Exercise 40 min 3–4 times a week
Regular cardiopulmonary exercise helps to release beta endorphins which act as natural painkillers and increase feeling of wellbeing
R – Relaxation
Avoiding conflicts, minimize stressful situations
There are relaxations app, freely downable, which may be a helpful tool
T – Avoid proven triggers

From Cincinnati Children's Hospital Pediatric Headache team

Behavior Measures

Mind and body health have been emphasized in the treatment of chronic pain, including migraine in children. There have been few studies that have shown that is very effective in preventing headaches in the pediatric population. Powers et al. conducted a randomized control trial and found out that children receiving cognitive behavior therapy (CBT) along with daily preventive medication (amitriptyline) tend to have better outcome and improved disability score when compared to those who received preventive medication alone [32]. Other useful behavior medicine techniques include biofeedback, progressive relaxation technique, abdominal breathing technique, etc. In conclusion, no single preventive measure works absolutely, and it requires triad of preventive medication, lifestyle changes, and behavior measures.

References

1. https://ichd-3.org/
2. Schurks M. Genetics of migraine in the age of Genome Wide Association Studies. J Headache Pain. 2012;13(1):1–9.
3. Rhoads JM, Fatheree NY, Norori J, et al. Altered fecal microflora and increased fecal calprotectin in infants with colic. J Pediatr. 2009;155(6):823–8.
4. BarrabRoger RG, TrentcJulieCrossc B. Age-related incidence curve of hospitalized Shaken Baby Syndrome cases: convergent evidence for crying as a trigger to shaking. Child Abuse Negl. 2006;30(1):7–16.
5. Sweney MT, Silver K, Gerard-Blanluet M, et al. Alternating hemiplegia of childhood: early characteristics and evolution of a neurodevelopmental syndrome. Pediatrics. 2009;123(3):e534–41.
6. Heberden W. Commentaries on the history and causes of diseases, vol. 16. 3rd ed. London: Payne & Foss; 1816. p. 15–22; Cited by Hammond J. The late sequelae of recurrent vomiting of childhood. Dev Med Child Neuro.
7. Olson AD. Li BUK. The diagnostic evaluation of children with cyclic vomiting: a cost-effectiveness assessment. J Pediatr. 2002;141:724–8.
8. Zobel AW, Nickel T, Kunzel HE, et al. Effects of the high affinity corticotrophin-releasing hormone receptor 1 antagonist R121919 in major depression: the first 20 patients treated. J Psychiatr Res. 2000;34:171–81.
9. Blitzstein NL, Brams WA. Migraine with abdominal equivalent. J Am Med Assoc. 1926;86(10):675–7.
10. Buse DC, et al. The chronic migraine epidemiology and outcomes included the family burden module. Mayo Clinic Proc. 2016;91(5):596–611.
11. Hamalainen ML, et al. Ibuprofen or acetaminophen for the acute treatment of migraine in children A double-blind, randomized, placebo-controlled, crossover study. Neurology. 1997;48(1):103–7. https://doi.org/10.1212/WNL.48.1.103.
12. https://www.aan.com/Guidelines/Home/GuidelineDetail/966
13. Linder SL, Mathew NT, Cady RK, Finlayson G, Ishkanian G, Lewis DW. Efficacy and tolerability of almotriptan in adolescents: a randomized, double-blind, placebo-controlled trial. Headache. 2008;48(9):1326–36.
14. Anderson P. FDA okays sumatriptan/naproxen (Treximet) for migraine in teens. Medscape Medical News. Available at http://www.medscape.com/viewarticle/844752. Accessed 15 May 2015.
15. https://americanheadachesociety.org/wp-content/uploads/2018/05/Alan_Rapoport_-_Migraine_Prevention_Medications.pdf

16. Powers SW, et al. Quality of life in pediatric migraine: characterization of age related effects using Peds QL4.0. Cephaligia. 2004;24:120–7.
17. Lewis P, et al. Prophylactic treatment of pediatric migraine. Headache. 2004;44(3):230–7.
18. Hershey A, Powers S, Vockell A, LeCates S, Kabbouche M, Maynard M. Development of a patient-based grading system for PedMIDAS. Cephalalgia. 2004;24:844–9.
19. Powers SW, et al. Trial of amitriptyline, topiramate, and placebo for pediatric migraine. N Engl J Med. 2017;376:115–24.
20. Szperka CL, et al. Recommendations on the use of anti-CGRP monoclonal antibodies in children and adolescents. Headache. 2018;58(10):1658–69.
21. Shah S, Calderon MD, Wu WD, Grant J, Rinehart J. Onabotulinumtoxin A (BOTOX®) for prophylactic treatment of pediatric migraine: a retrospective longitudinal analysis. J Child Neurol. 2018;33(9):580–6.
22. Shah S, Calderon MD, Crain N, Pham J, Rinehart J. Effectiveness of onabotulinumtoxinA (BOTOX) in pediatric patients experiencing migraines: a randomized, double-blinded, placebo-controlled crossover study in the pediatric pain population. Reg Anesth Pain Med. 2020;46(1):41–8.
23. Lakshmi CV, Singhi P, Malhi P, Ray M. Topiramate in the prophylaxis of pediatric migraine: a double-blind placebo-controlled trial. J Child Neurol. 2007;22(7):829–35.
24. Lewis D, Winner P, Saper J, Ness S, Polverejan E, Wang S, et al. Randomized, double-blind, placebo-controlled study to evaluate the efficacy and safety of topiramate for migraine prevention in pediatric subjects 12 to 17 years of age. Pediatrics. 2009;123(3):924–34.
25. Apostol G, Lewis D, Laforet G, Robieson W, Fugate J, Abi-Saab W, et al. Divalproex sodium extended-release for the prophylaxis of migraine headache in adolescents: results of a stand-alone, long-term open-label safety study. Headache. 2009;49:45–53.
26. Kacperski J, Kabbouche MA, O'Brien HL, Weberding JL. The optimal management of headaches in children and adolescents. Ther Adv Neurol Disord. 2016;9(1):53–68. https://doi.org/10.1177/1756285615616586. PMCID: PMC4710107. PMID: 26788131.
27. Hershey A, Powers S, Bentii A, deGrauw T. Effectiveness of amitriptyline in the prophylactic management of childhood headaches. Headache. 2000;40:539–49.
28. Winner PK, Kabbouche M, Yonker M, Wangsadipura V, Lum A, Brin MF. A randomized trial to evaluate onabotulinumtoxin A for prevention of headaches in adolescents with chronic migraine. Headache. 2020;60(3):564–75.
29. Dodick DW, Turkel CC, RE DG, Aurora SK, Silberstein SD, Lipton RB, Diener HC, Brin MF, PREEMPT Chronic Migraine Study Group. Onabotulinumtoxin A for treatment of chronic migraine: pooled results from the double-blind, randomized, placebo-controlled phases of the PREEMPT clinical program. Headache. 2010;50(6):921–36.
30. Condo M, Posar A, Arbizzani A, Parmeggiani A. Riboflavin prophylaxis in pediatric and adolescent migraine. J Headache Pain. 2009;10:361–5.
31. Orr S, Venkateswaran S. Nutraceuticals in the prophylaxis of pediatric migraine: evidence-based review and recommendations. Cephalalgia. 2014;34:568–83.
32. Powers SW, et al. Cognitive behavioral therapy plus amitriptyline for chronic migraine in children and adolescents. JAMA. 2013;310(24):2622–30.
33. Tsze DS, Ochs JB, Gonzalez AE, Dayan PS. Red flag findings in children with headaches: Prevalence and association with emergency department neuroimaging. Cephalalgia. 2019;39(2):185–96.
34. Medina LS, Pinter JD, Zurakowski D, Davis RG, Kuban K, Barnes PD. Children with headache: clinical predictors of surgical space-occupying lesions and the role of neuroimaging. Radiology. 1997;202(3):819–24. https://doi.org/10.1148/radiology.202.3.9051039.
35. https://ichd-3.org/8-headache-attributed-to-a-substance-or-its-withdrawal/8-2-medication-overuse-headache-moh/

Peripheral Nerve Block for the Management of Headache and Face Pain

8

Diana Heringer, Shalini Shah, and Samer N. Narouze

Peripheral nerve blocks are valuable diagnostic and therapeutic tools in head and face pain syndromes. Moreover, they can be beneficial in intractable headache disorders. Targets of these nerve blocks include the supraorbital nerve, supratrochlear nerve, infraorbital nerve, mental nerve, greater auricular nerve, maxillary nerve, mandibular nerve, greater and lesser occipital nerves, as well as the trigeminal nerve. Equipment for these nerve blocks typically includes a total of 3–4 ml of local anesthetic drawn up in a 5 ml sterile syringe with a 25-gauge, 1.5-inch needle. A depot steroid may be added specially in cases of entrapment or inflammatory conditions. Maxillary and mandibular nerve blocks are the only exception, where a 22-gauge, 3.5-inch needle is used. Fluoroscopy C-arm can be used to confirm the position of the needle. If ultrasound guidance is desired, a high-resolution ultrasound transducer with the following specifications, 25–38 mm linear probe oscillating at 10–13 MHz, will be needed. Double-blind, randomized controlled studies are lacking. Well-designed studies are needed to ascertain the value of nerve blocks in refractory headache disorders. Due to the high vascularity of the face and the scalp, all nerve blocks render patients susceptible to local anesthetic toxicity. Subsequently, the local anesthetic dose should be cautiously calculated, especially if the plan is to perform the nerve block bilaterally. Vigilant monitoring must be established during injection. The solution is injected slowly in increments. For the same reason, there

Adapted from Costandi S, Costandi J, Souzdalnitski D, Narouze SN. Peripheral nerve block for the management of headache and face pain. In: Narouze SN, editor. Interventional management of head and face pain. New York: Springer; 2014, with permission.

D. Heringer
Department of Pain Management, University of California Irvine, Irvine, CA, USA

S. Shah (✉)
Department of Anesthesiology & Perioperative Care, University of California Irvine, Irvine, CA, USA
e-mail: ssshah1@hs.uci.edu

S. N. Narouze
Center for Pain Medicine, Western Reserve Hospital, Cuyahoga Falls, OH, USA

© Springer Nature Switzerland AG 2021

S. Shah (ed.), *Migraine*, https://doi.org/10.1007/978-3-030-75239-2_8

is increased risk of post-procedure ecchymosis and hematoma. Should this happen, manual pressure is applied to the area of the block. Applying ice packs for 15–20 min can also reduce the post-procedural pain and bleeding. Extra caution should be taken when performing the trigeminal nerve block under fluoroscopy, due to the risk of dural puncture. If cerebrospinal fluid (CSF) is aspirated and a small CSF leak is confirmed, the practitioner must weigh the risks/benefits of proceeding with the possibility of a causing a high spinal versus aborting the procedure.

Supraorbital and Supratrochlear Nerve Blocks

Indications

Supraorbital nerve block (SON) can be used in the diagnosis and treatment of facial pain in areas supplied by the supraorbital nerve (Fig. 8.1 and Table 8.1):

- Supraorbital neuralgia
- Pain due to herpes zoster in V1 distribution
- Facial bone fractures
- Facial malignancies

Similarly, the supratrochlear nerve block is a useful tool in the diagnosis and management of facial pain in areas supplied by the supratrochlear nerve whether due to entrapment neuropathy, facial bone fractures, or herpes zoster [1–3].

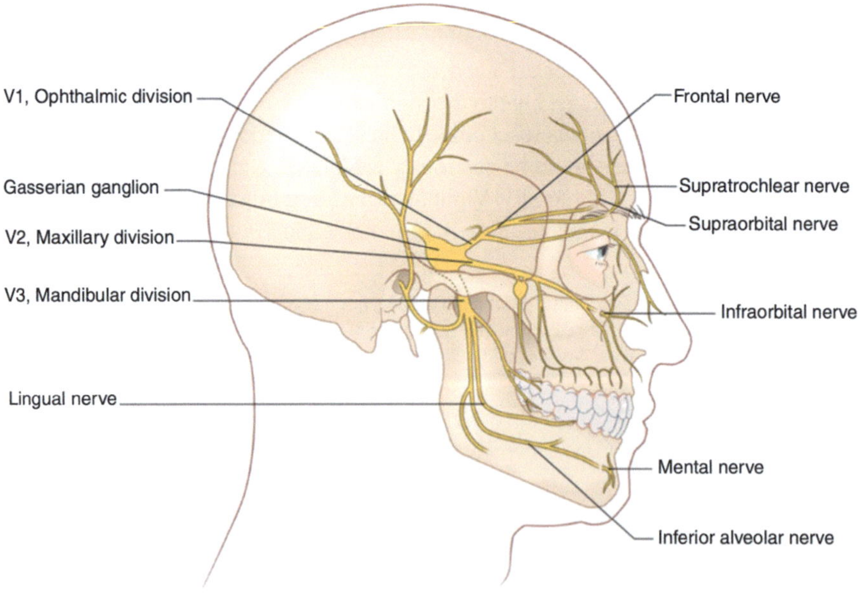

Fig. 8.1 Trigeminal nerve anatomy

Table 8.1 Peripheral nerve blocks for the management of headaches

Block type	Indications	Techniques
Supraorbital nerve, supratrochlear nerve, infraorbital nerve	Diagnosis and treatment of facial pain Supraorbital, infraorbital, or supratrochlear entrapment neuropathies Herpes zoster Facial bone fractures Malignancy	Landmark technique Ultrasound guided
Mental nerve	Diagnosis and treatment of facial pain	Landmark technique (extraoral or intraoral)
	Mental nerve entrapment neuropathies Herpes zoster Facial bone fractures Malignancy	Ultrasound guided
	Posttraumatic neuralgia Atypical facial pain Temporomandibular joint pain Herpes zoster involving external auditory meatus Pain secondary to malignancy	Ultrasound guided
Greater auricular nerve block	Diagnosis and treatment of facial pain	Landmark technique
	Posttraumatic neuralgia Postoperative neuralgias (e.g., face-lift surgery, craniotomy) Malignancies	Ultrasound guided
Greater and lesser occipital nerve block	Treatment of Occipital neuralgia Trauma to GON/LON Compression of GON/LON due to degenerative changes in the cervical spine	Landmark technique Ultrasound technique
Trigeminal nerve block	Treatment of Trigeminal neuralgia Intractable cluster headache Persistent idiopathic facial pain (atypical facial pain)	Fluoroscopic technique

Clinical Anatomy

The supraorbital nerve originates from the frontal nerve, which is the largest branch of ophthalmic division (V1) of trigeminal nerve (Fig. 8.2). The frontal nerve exits the cranium through the superior orbital fissure to run in the roof of the orbit. The frontal nerve divides into a larger lateral branch, the supraorbital nerve, and a smaller medial branch – the supratrochlear nerve. The supraorbital nerves give off nerve fibers to the vertex; thus, providing sensory innervation to the lateral portion of the forehead, the upper eyelid, and the anterior scalp. Supratrochlear nerve provides sensory innervation to the medial portion of the forehead, nasal bridge, and medial third of the upper eyelid (Fig. 8.3) [3].

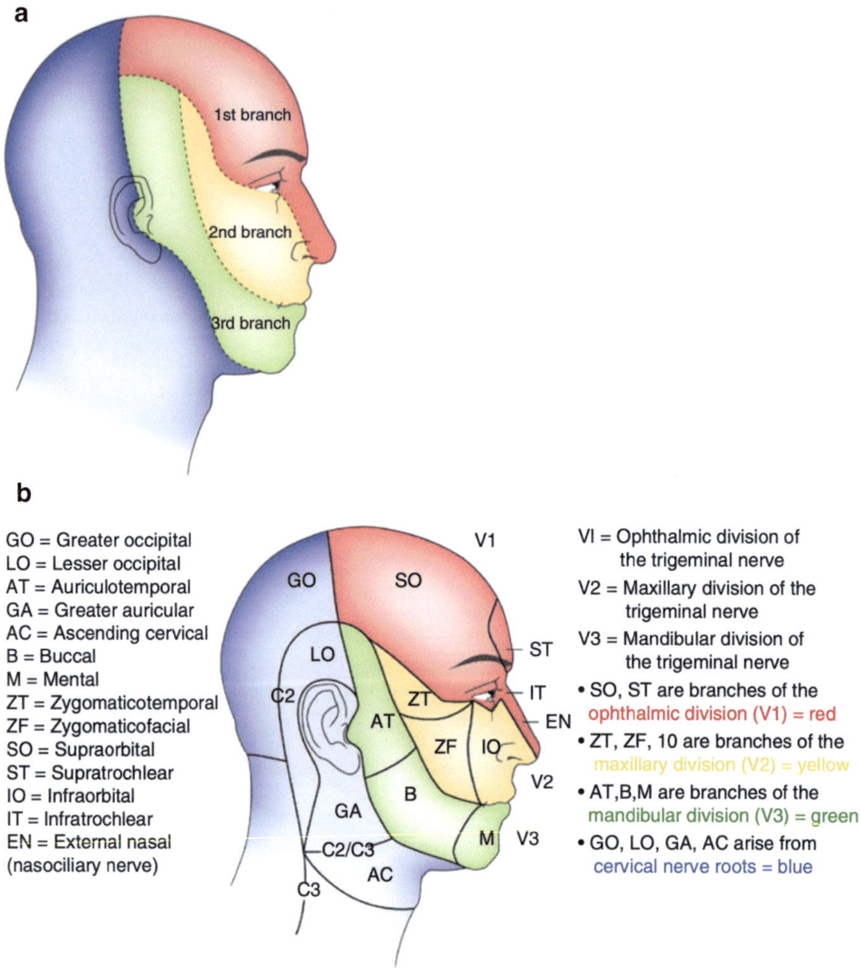

Fig. 8.2 (**a**) Trigeminal nerve distribution. (**b**) Sensory distribution of the face and scalp

Description of the Procedure

Supraorbital Nerve Block

The patient is placed in supine or seated position and is advised to report any paresthesia during the procedure along the distribution of the nerve. The supraorbital notch is identified by palpation. The skin overlying the notch is prepped with antiseptic solution. A 25-gauge, 1.5-inch needle is introduced at the level of the notch and advanced medially 15° to avoid entering the foramen and avoid inducing paresthesia (Fig. 8.4). The needle is advanced until it approaches the periosteum. If the needle slips into the foramen, it should be withdrawn and redirected medially. After negative aspiration is confirmed, 2–3 ml of the solution is injected in a fanlike

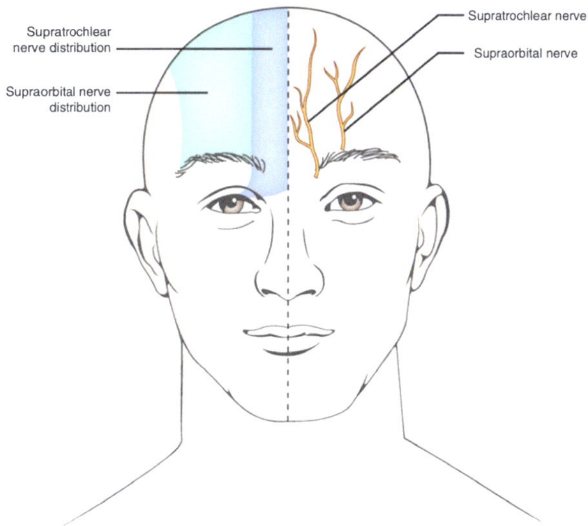

Fig. 8.3 Supraorbital and supratrochlear anatomy and sensory distribution

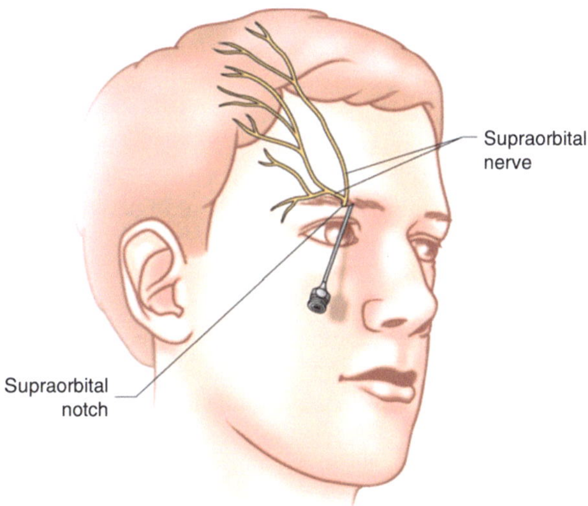

Fig. 8.4 Supraorbital nerve block technique

distribution. Meanwhile, a gauze sponge is gently applied on the upper eyelid and supraorbital tissues before, during, and after injecting the solution to prevent downward dissection of the solution in the loose areolar tissues of the upper eyelid [4, 5].

Ultrasound Technique

The patient is placed in supine or seated position. After prepping the skin with antiseptic solution, a high-resolution linear probe is placed along the supraorbital ridge in a transverse orientation. The supraorbital notch is visualized as a defect along the supraorbital ridge (Fig. 8.5a, b). The needle is then placed superior to the probe and

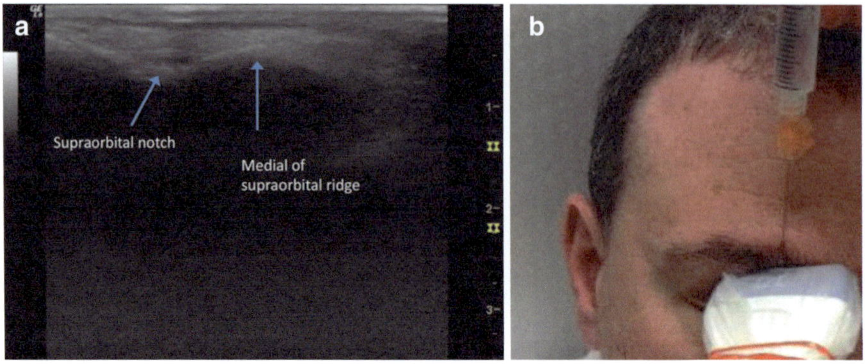

Fig. 8.5 (**a**) Ultrasound image and (**b**) probe orientation for supraorbital nerve block

advanced in an out-of-plane technique toward the supraorbital foramen. Then, 2–3 ml of the solution is injected without entering into the foramen [6, 7].

Supratrochlear Nerve Block

The patient is placed in supine or seated position and is advised to report any paresthesia during the procedure along the distribution of the nerve. The supraorbital ridge is identified by palpation. The skin at the point where the bridge of the nose adjoins the supraorbital ridge is prepped with antiseptic solution. The entry point lies laterally to the junction of the bridge of the nose and the supraorbital ridge. A 25-gauge, 1.5-inch needle is advanced medially into the subcutaneous tissues. After negative aspiration is confirmed, 3 ml of solution should be injected in a fanlike distribution (Fig. 8.6).

Ultrasound Technique

The patient is seated for this block. After prepping the skin with antiseptic solution, a high-resolution linear probe is situated at the junction of the bridge of the nose and the supraorbital ridge in a longitudinal or transverse oblique orientation. The supratrochlear notch is visualized in the same manner as for the supraorbital notch. The needle is then placed lateral to the probe and advanced in an out-of-plane technique toward the supratrochlear foramen. And 2–3 ml of the solution is then injected without entering into the foramen.

Infraorbital Nerve Block

Indications

Infraorbital nerve block serves as a useful diagnostic and therapeutic tool in the management of painful conditions of areas supplied by the infraorbital nerve [1, 2]:

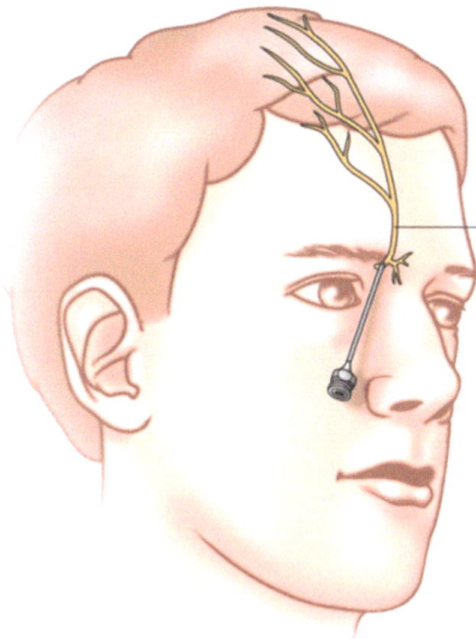

Fig. 8.6 Supratrochlear nerve block

- Infraorbital neuralgia
- Pain due to herpes zoster in V2 distribution
- Facial bone fractures
- Facial malignancies

Clinical Anatomy

The infraorbital nerve originates from the maxillary nerve and enters the orbit through the inferior orbital fissure. It then courses along the floor of the orbit in the infraorbital groove. As the nerve exits the orbit through the infraorbital foramen, it gives off sensory branches to the lower eyelid, lateral nares, and upper lip. The superior alveolar nerve, a branch of the infraorbital nerve, innervates the upper incisor, canine, and the associated gingiva (Figs. 8.1 and 8.7).

Description of the Procedure

The patient is placed in supine or seated position and is advised to report any paresthesia during the procedure along the distribution of the nerve. The infraorbital foramen is identified by palpation. The skin overlying the notch is prepped with antiseptic solution. A 25-gauge, 1.5-inch needle is introduced at the level of the notch and is advanced medially 15° to avoid entering the foramen (Fig. 8.7). The needle is advanced until it approaches the periosteum. If the needle slips accidently into the foramen, it should be withdrawn and redirected medially. After negative aspiration is confirmed, 2–3 ml of the solution is injected in a fanlike distribution. Meanwhile, a gauze sponge should be used to apply gentle pressure on the lower eyelid and infraorbital tissues before, during, and after injecting the solution to prevent downward dissection of the solution into the loose areolar tissues of the eyelid [4, 5].

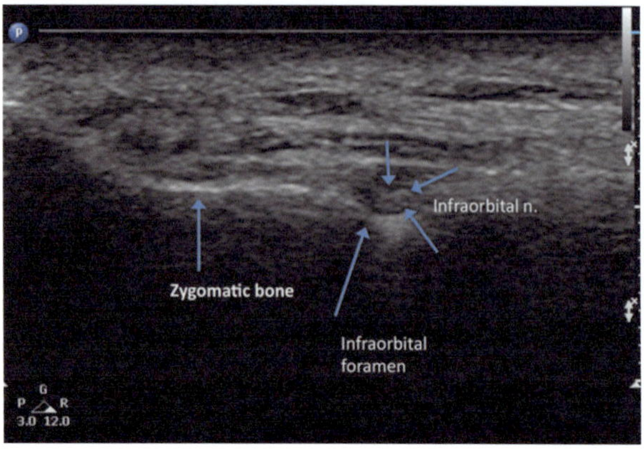

Fig. 8.7 Infraorbital nerve block technique

Ultrasound Technique

The patient is placed in supine or seated position. After prepping the skin with antiseptic solution, a high-resolution linear probe is situated along the zygomatic bone in a transverse or oblique orientation. The infraorbital notch is visualized within the maxilla (Fig. 8.8). The needle is then placed inferior to the probe and advanced in an out-of-plane technique toward the infraorbital foramen. And then 2–3 ml of the solution is injected to surround the nerve without entering into the foramen.

Mental Nerve Block

Indications

Mental nerve block serves as a useful diagnostic and therapeutic tool in the management of painful conditions of areas supplied by the mental nerve [1, 2]:

- Mental nerve neuralgia
- Pain due to herpes zoster in V3 distribution
- Facial bone fractures
- Facial malignancies

Clinical Anatomy

The mental nerve originates from the mandibular nerve. The nerve emerges from the mandible through the mental foramen at the level of the second premolar; it then turns sharply and gives off sensory branches to the medial side of the chin (Figs. 8.1 and 8.9).

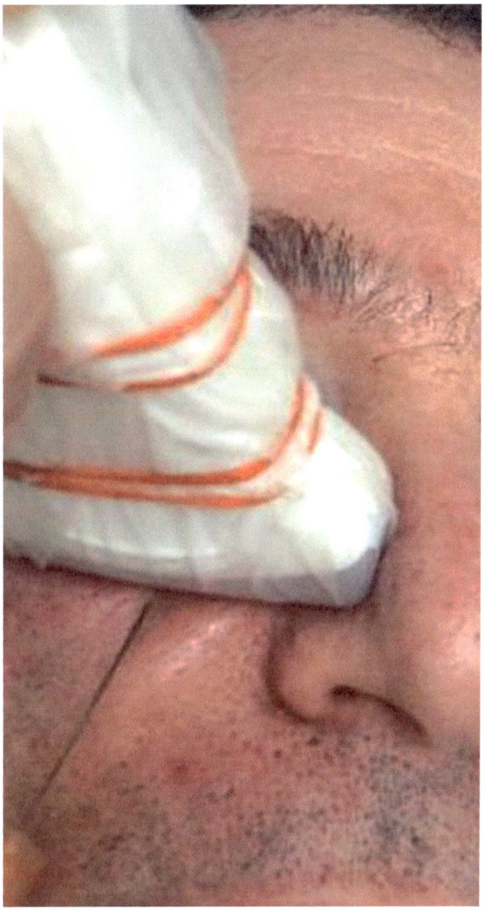

Fig. 8.8 Ultrasound image and probe orientation for intraorbital nerve block

Description of the Procedure

Extraoral Approach

The patient is placed in supine or seated position and is advised to report any paresthesia along the distribution of the nerve. The mental notch is identified by palpation. The skin overlying the notch is prepped with antiseptic solution. A 25-gauge, 1.5-inch needle is introduced at the level of the foramen and advanced medially 15° to avoid entering the foramen (Fig. 8.9). The needle is advanced until it approaches the periosteum. If the needle slips accidently into the foramen, it should be withdrawn and redirected medially. After negative aspiration is confirmed, 2–3 ml of the solution is injected in a fanlike distribution [4, 5].

Intraoral Approach

The patient is placed in supine or seated position. The mental notch is identified by palpation. The lower lip is retracted down, and cotton balls soaked in 10% cocaine

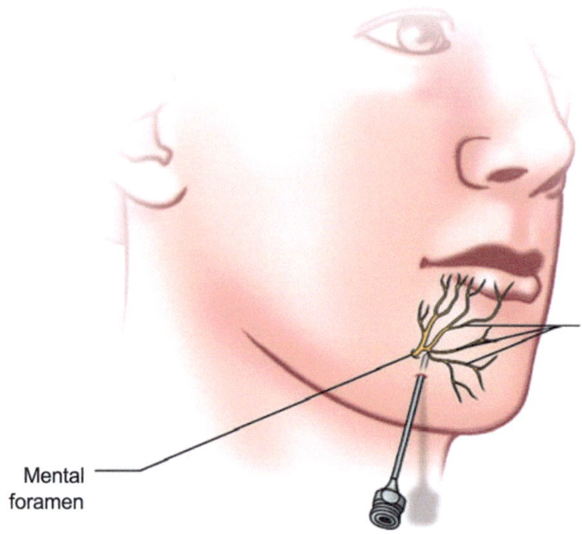

Fig. 8.9 Extraoral technique for mental nerve block

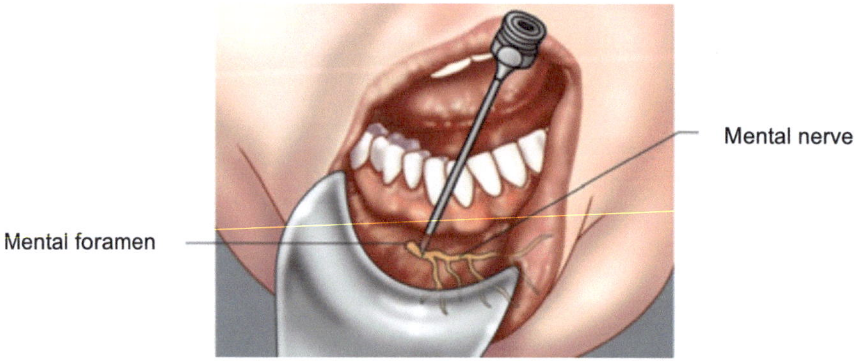

Fig. 8.10 Intraoral technique for mental nerve block

solution or viscous 2% lidocaine are placed in the alveolar sulcus close to the mental notch for adequate topical anesthesia of the mucosa. A 25-gauge, 1.5-inch needle is advanced toward the mental foramen, which may elicit paresthesia. However, there should be no paresthesia on injection. After negative aspiration is confirmed, 2–3 ml of the solution is injected in a fanlike manner (Fig. 8.10).

Ultrasound Approach

The patient is placed in supine or seated position. After prepping the skin with antiseptic solution, a high-resolution linear probe is situated along the lower border of the mandible in a transverse orientation. The mental foramen is visualized within the mandible (Fig. 8.11a, b). The needle is then placed superior to the probe and

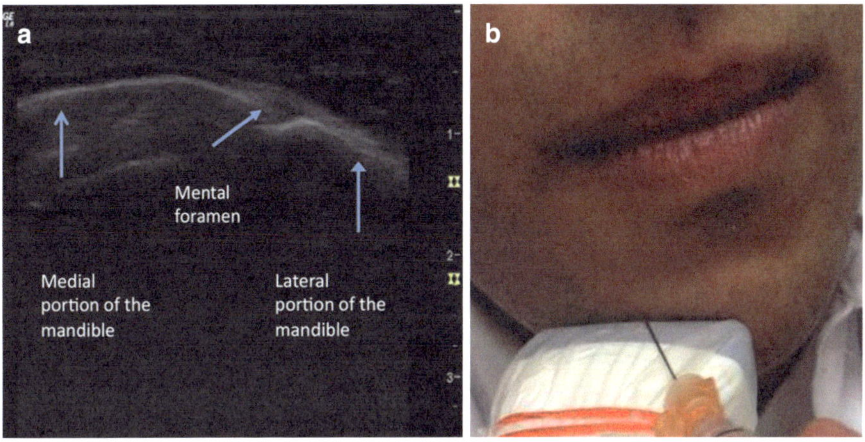

Fig. 8.11 (**a** and **b**) Ultrasound image and probe orientation for mental nerve block

advanced in an out-of-plane technique toward the mental foramen. Two to three milliliters of the solution is then injected without entering into the foramen [6, 7].

Occipital Nerve Block

Indications

The occipital nerve block is used to treat occipital headaches, otherwise known as occipital neuralgia. Beginning in 1821, the term "occipital neuralgia" was introduced to describe a headache that originates from the occipital and suboccipital region [8]. More specifically, the term indicates an irritation of the greater occipital nerve (GON) and/or lesser occipital nerve (LON). Exam is usually notable for tenderness to palpation over the irritated nerve. Common causes of occipital neuralgia include the following [8]:

- Trauma to the greater and/or lesser occipital nerves
- Compression of GON/LON or of the C2 and/or C3 nerve roots due to degenerative changes in the cervical spine
- Myofascial pain
- Tumors involving the C2 and/or C3 nerve roots

Clinical Anatomy

The GON is a branch of the dorsal ramus of the second cervical nerve, with a lesser contribution from the dorsal ramus of the third cervical nerve. The GON courses between the inferior capitis oblique and semispinalis capitis muscles and then ascends along the occiput, where it pierces the semispinalis capitis and superior portion of the trapezius muscles [8]. From here, the GON travels closely with the occipital artery and supplies innervation of the scalp from the occiput to the vertex of the skull [9].

Composed of branches from the ventral ramus of both the second and third cervical nerves, the LON ascends the back of the head by running parallel to the posterior border of the sternocleidomastoid muscle [8]. The LON then perforates the fascia at the occiput and provides cutaneous innervation to the posterolateral portion of the scalp and above the ear (Fig. 8.12).

Landmark Technique

Place the patient in a seated position with the head flexed forward. Find the occipital protuberance and then palpate the superior nuchal ridge directly above. From there, move your fingertips laterally until you identify the occipital artery, followed by the mastoid process. Envision a straight line that travels inferolateral from the nuchal ridge to the mastoid process – the GON will be one-third the distance between the nuchal ridge and mastoid process (usually medial to the occipital artery), and the LON is often two-thirds from the nuchal ridge to the mastoid process (Fig. 8.13).

Once you have mapped out your target entry points for each nerve, cleanse the scalp with either an alcohol or chlorhexidine swab. Fill a 5 cc syringe with 3.5 cc of 0.25% bupivacaine and 20 mg Kenalog and attach a 1.5-inch 25G needle. Insert the needle in an inferolateral angle starting just medial to the GON. Slowly inject 2 cc of the mixture of local anesthetic and steroid as you move the needle toward the mastoid process – a subcutaneous depot will form along the trajectory of your

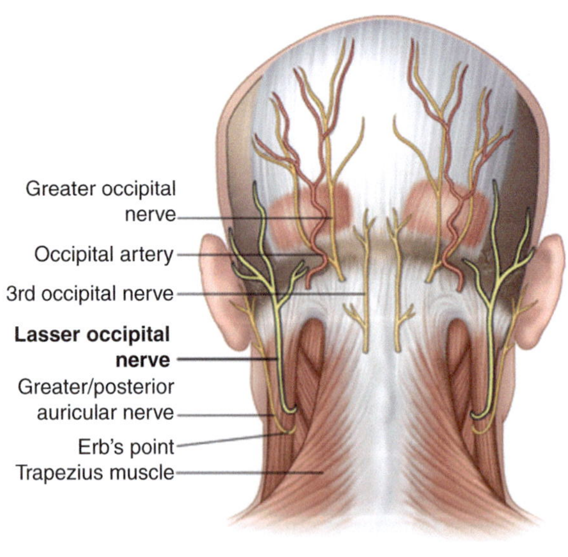

Fig. 8.12 Anatomy of the greater and lesser occipital nerves. (From Mays and Tepper [11], with permission)

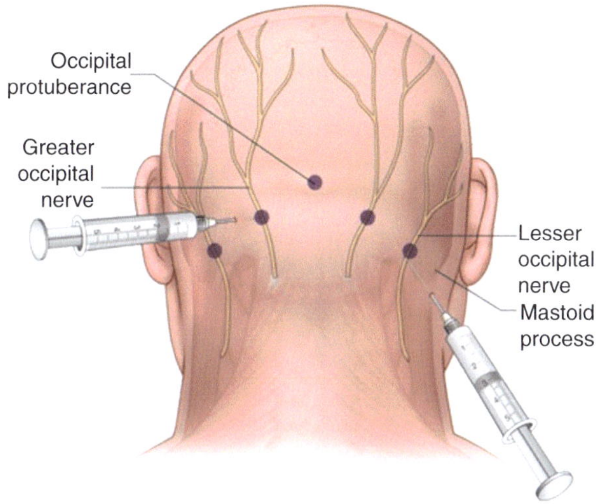

Fig. 8.13 Inferolateral trajectory for the occipital nerve block. The GON is one-third the distance from the occipital protuberance to the mastoid, and the LON is two-third this distance. Please note that the direction of the needles in this image are not advised. The block should be done in a medial to lateral orientation to avoid inadvertent injection into the foramen magnum. (From Rawner et al. [12], with permission)

needle. Once you have created a depot of medication that spans the length of the needle, remove the needle and reinsert it at the approximate location of the LON. While still aiming in the same inferolateral trajectory, deposit the remaining 2 cc in a subcutaneous depot as you traverse toward the mastoid process. Remove the needle and clean the scalp.

It is helpful to remind the patient that they may notice a "lump" on the back of their head, and that this is just the depot of medication, which will be absorbed over time. If performing a bilateral block, it is often advised that the patient has a driver or that the patient is monitored for 20–30 min post-procedure to ensure they are capable of safely driving home. Lastly, it is important to always aim the needle in a medial to lateral direction, so as to avoid inadvertent injection into the foramen magnum, which could lead to devastating side effects.

Ultrasound-Guided Technique

Place the patient in the prone position on the procedure table with head slightly flexed. Place standard monitors on the patient and observe throughout the procedure. Cleanse the skin overlying the occiput from ear to ear, as well as the neck, with a chlorhexidine solution, so as to provide yourself with a wide sterile field and drape in a sterile fashion.

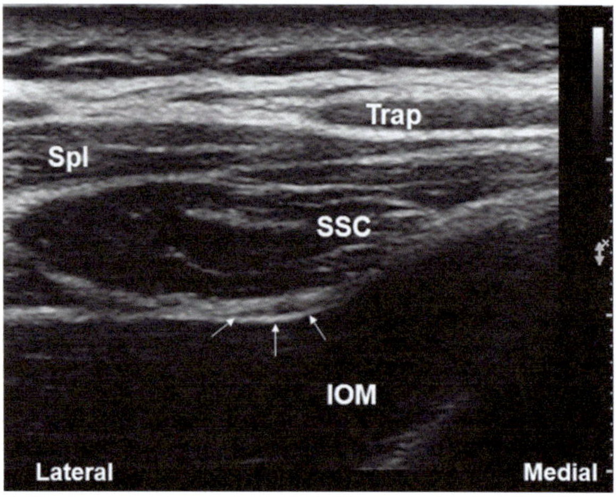

Fig. 8.14 Ultrasound image of occipital nerve block. (Courtesy of Samer Narouze, MD, PhD)

Place a sterile ultrasound cover over a liner, high frequency ultrasound probe and then begin your anatomical scan by placing the probe at the occipital protuberance. Scan caudad until atlas (C1) and axis (C2) come into view – C2 is most recognizable by its bifid spinous process [9]. From here, scan laterally until the obliquus capitis inferior muscle (OCIM) and semispinalis capitis muscle (SsCM) are visualized. The OCIM is a distinct muscle posterior to the lamina of the axis and deep to the SsCM13. The transducer should be placed obliqued along the long axis of the OCIM, with the lateral end pointing cranially toward the mastoid process [9] (Fig. 8.14). Once you have an appropriate view of the SsCM and OCIM, you will see a hypoechoic structure between these two muscles, which is the Greater Occipital Nerve (GON) [9].

Using a 27-gauge, 1.5-inch needle, the skin overlying your entry site is anesthetized with 1% lidocaine. Then with the in-plane approach (preferably), a 25-gauge, 1.5-inch needle is inserted from medial to lateral until the needle tip is positioned in the plane between the OCIM and SsCM, near the GON2. Alternatively, an out-of-plane approach can be used once the GON is centered in the midline of the ultrasound probe. Once the needle position is confirmed, deposit 2–3 cc of a mixture containing 20 mg of triamcinolone and 0.25% bupivacaine (or 0.5% lidocaine).

Trigeminal Nerve Block

Indications

Performing the trigeminal nerve block is indicated in those who have been diagnosed with trigeminal neuralgia (also known as tic douloureux) and who have failed pharmacological management. Trigeminal neuralgia is a neuropathic pain syndrome that can affect any of the three branches of the fifth cranial nerve, but most commonly affects the maxillary branch (V2) [10]. It is also the most common form of neuralgia in adults and most frequently occurs in women over the age of 40 years [8]. This block can also be used for those with intractable cluster headaches or persistent idiopathic facial pain (formerly called atypical facial pain) [8].

Clinical Anatomy

The trigeminal ganglion, also called the Gasserian ganglion, lies within a cavity of the dura mater known as Meckel's cave. The trigeminal nerve (fifth cranial nerve) consists of three divisions: the ophthalmic (V1), the maxillary (V2), and the mandibular (V3). Each branch has its own foramen through which it exits the skull: the V1 exits via the supraorbital fissure as it then passes through the orbit, the V2 branch exits via the foramen rotundum, and the V3 branch exits via the foramen ovale.

Each branch of the trigeminal nerve provides cutaneous sensation to a specific portion of the face (Fig. 8.15):

- Ophthalmic – innervates the forehead to the apex of the skull, the anterior aspect of the nose, and orbits.
- Maxillary – innervates maxilla, infraorbital region, nasal cavity, palate, upper lip, and the anterior portion of the temple.
- Mandibular – innervates the buccal mucosa, mandible (including teeth, gums, chin, lower lip, and the anterior two-thirds of the tongue), as well as the posterior portion of the temple and anterior part of the ear.

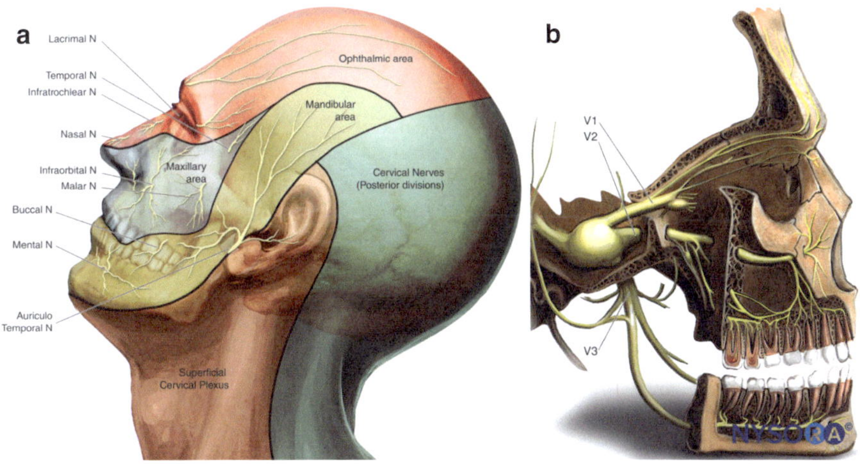

Fig. 8.15 (**a**) Dermatomes of the face corresponding to each trigeminal nerve branch. (**b**) The trajectory of each branch as it splits from the Gasserian ganglion. (Source: NYSORA.COM)

Technique

Fluoroscopy Guided

This is the preferred approach for obtaining the V2 and V3 branches of the trigeminal nerve. The approach is via the coronoid notch and the primary target is the lateral pterygoid plate. Standard monitors should be placed and observed throughout the duration of the procedure (blood pressure, pulse oximetry, heart rate). Due to the uncomfortable nature of the fluoroscopic approach, it is often recommended to provide intravenous (IV) or oral sedation to the patient. We recommend placing an IV in the preoperative area, as a safety measure prior to the procedure, as there is the risk of inadvertent spinal anesthetic administration during the block given the proximity to the dura mater.

The patient is placed supine on the procedure table and the C-arm is positioned in a lateral view such that the angles of the mandibular rami superimpose. This can be done by rotating the C-arm obliquely away from the nose approximately 20–30° and then angling the C-arm 30–35° in a caudocephalad direction [8]. The patient is asked to sublux the jaw multiple times to palpate, radiographically locate, and mark the coronoid notch. Once the patient is positioned and monitors are in place, the skin of the face should be prepped in a sterile fashion (typically with chlorhexidine solution unless otherwise indicated).

The skin overlying the notch should then be anesthetized with 1% lidocaine to create a skin wheal. Using a 22G or 25G 3.5-inch spinal needle, fluoroscopic guidance is used to direct the needle tip through the infratemporal fossa under the zygoma. As a tip, a small-angulation cephalad and slightly posterior will allow the needle to be in proximity to the lateral nasal mucosa taking extreme care not to pierce through it. The end point of the advancement of the needle is the lateral pterygoid plate. If the maxillary nerve is the final target, a slight superior and posterior angulation will elicit paresthesia into this nerve distribution (nose ridge, upper lip, gum, and face). If the mandibular nerve is targeted, a slight caudad and anterior angulation usually elicits paresthesia in its somatic distribution (lower mandible, lower lip, lower jaw, and tongue) (Fig. 8.16). Once the needle position is confirmed with fluoroscopy, aspirate for any CSF or heme. If heme is noted, the needle should be repositioned until aspiration is negative. If CSF is noted, the needle can be withdrawn until it is no longer present but bearing in mind that injection of local anesthetic has the potential of causing a high spinal block given the interruption in the dura. If the practitioner wishes to proceed in this instance, the local anesthetic should be given in approximately 0.5 cc increments with vital signs observed after each injection and all while assessing whether or not the patient's breathing patterns and mental status have changed. Aqueous formulations of steroid, that is, dexamethasone is preferred alongside preservative free 1% lidocaine. The needle should be removed and the skin cleansed and bandaged after the procedure.

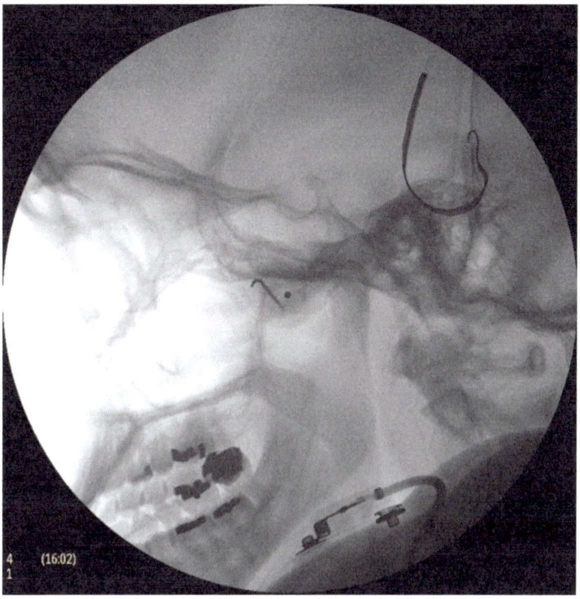

Fig. 8.16 Trigeminal fluoroscopy. (Courtesy of Samer Narouze, MD, PhD)

Pearls

- Supraorbital nerve and supratrochlear nerve blocks are usually performed simultaneously mainly to alleviate pain induced by herpes zoster of the ophthalmic division (V1) and its branches.
- Patient should be informed of the possibility of developing of small punctate facial scar especially with repeated supraorbital, supratrochlear, or infraorbital nerves blocks.
- Extra caution must be taken in an immunocompromised patient to prevent development of infections. Although it is rare, early detection is imperative to prevent deleterious fatal consequences.
- Avoid placing the needle into the mental foramen (or supraorbital/infraorbital foramina) since injecting the solution into the bony canal can cause nerve damage as a result of compression neuropathy.
- The mental nerve block is vulnerable to blunt trauma due to the acute angle as it emerges out of the mental foramen.
- Occipital nerve blocks are effective office-based procedures that can help break the pain cycle related to occipital neuralgia of either the greater or lesser occipital nerves (or both). The procedure can be done unilaterally or bilaterally, but the trajectory should always be from medial to lateral.

- Meticulous attention should be paid in patients with bony defects (e.g., craniotomy, mastoidectomy) while performing greater auricular and occipital nerve blocks to avoid deep needle insertion through the bony defects which may result in serious CNS symptoms and coma.
- We prefer to use the ultrasound-guided technique in patients with bony defects as these defects will be well visualized with ultrasound.

References

1. Headache Classification Committee. The international classification of headache disorders, 2nd edition. Cephalalgia. 2004;24:1–160.
2. Blumenfeld A, Ashkenazi A, Napchan U, Bender SD, Klein BC, Berliner R, Ailani J, Schim J, Friedman DI, Charleston L, Young WB, Robertson CE, Dodick DW, Silberstein SD, Robbins MS. Expert consensus recommendations for the performance of peripheral nerve blocks for headaches-a narrative review. Headache. 2013;53(3):437–46.
3. Evans RW, Pareja JA. Expert opinion: supraorbital neuralgia. Headache. 2009;49:278–81.
4. BCH T, Dullane D, Funicane BT. Neural blockade for the surgery to the head and neck. Chronic pain. In: Cousins MJ, Carr DB, Horlocker TT, Bridenbaugh PO, editors. Cousins and Bridenbaugh's neural blockade in clinical anesthesia and pain medicine. 4th ed. Philadelphia: LWW; 2009. p. 486–91.
5. Levin M. Nerve blocks in the treatment of headache. Neurotherapeutics. 2010;7:197–203.
6. Spinner D, Kirschner JS. Accuracy of ultrasound-guided superficial trigeminal nerve blocks using methylene blue in cadavers. Pain Med. 2012;13(11):1469–73.
7. Tsui BC. Ultrasound imaging to localize foramina for superficial trigeminal nerve block. Can J Anaesth. 2009;56(9):704–6.
8. Benzon HT, et al. Essentials of pain medicine. 4th ed. Philadelphia: Elsevier; 2018.
9. Ultrasound for Regional Anesthesia. Toronto western hospital. Greater occipital nerve block. http://www.usra.ca/pain-medicine/specific-blocks/head-neck/gon.php
10. Nader A, MD, et al. Ultrasound-guided trigeminal nerve block via the pterygopalatine fossa: an effective treatment for trigeminal neuralgia and atypical facial pain. Pain Physician. 2013;16:E537–45.
11. Mays MA, Tepper SJ. Occipital nerve blocks. In: Narouze SN, editor. Interventional management of head and face pain. New York: Springer; 2014.
12. Rawner E, Irwin DM, Trescot AM. In: Narouze SN, editor. Interventional management of head and face pain. New York: Springer; 2014.

Neuromodulation for Migraine Disorders

9

Rohan Jotwani, Ojas Mainkar, Amitabh Gulati, and Neel Mehta

The past decade has seen the emergence of neuromodulation throughout the field of chronic pain, in part due to the emphasis on minimizing the use of chronic opioids. The first reports of dorsal column stimulators started in 1967 [1]. Initial devices used tonic, low-frequency stimulation that depended on eliciting paresthesia in the region of the pain. Burst and high-frequency stimulation patterns have gained traction over the past several years based on results from key trials such as the SENZA-RCT and SUNBURST. Additionally, we have now started stimulating peripheral nerves to better target pain syndromes. Throughout the centuries, our understanding of the ability of electricity to modulate pain sensations and the sophistication of the devices utilized has unveiled new opportunities.

The first reported use of noninvasive electricity to modulate headache pain dates back to the use of electric fish to decrease pain by ancient Egyptians and Greeks as described in historical documents such as the Papyrus of Ebers [2]. Since that time, we have developed a range of new invasive and noninvasive neuromodulatory therapies specifically for migraine headaches. Occipital nerve stimulation has high-quality evidence supporting its use as a preventive therapy. Vagus nerve stimulation has had conflicting results in studies, however remains a low-risk, noninvasive

R. Jotwani · O. Mainkar · N. Mehta (✉)
Department of Anesthesiology, Pain Management,
New York-Presbyterian/Weill Cornell Medical College, New York, NY, USA
e-mail: nem9015@med.cornell.edu

A. Gulati
Department of Anesthesiology and Critical Care,
Memorial Sloan Kettering Cancer Center, New York, NY, USA

© Springer Nature Switzerland AG 2021

S. Shah (ed.), *Migraine*, https://doi.org/10.1007/978-3-030-75239-2_9

treatment option for patients. Supraorbital and supratrochlear nerve stimulation has high-quality evidence supporting its use for both prevention of migraines and as a rescue medication. Additionally, there is some literature investigating high-cervical dorsal column stimulation, transcranial direct current stimulation, and repetitive transcranial magnetic stimulation as well [3]. In this chapter, we will discuss each of these techniques in further detail.

Occipital Nerve Stimulation

The occipital nerve has long been targeted to treat medically refractory cases of occipital neuralgia and thus has been extensively studied for this purpose [3]. However, its beneficial effects in treating patients with migraines was not discovered until 1999 by accident. That year, Weiner and Reed published a case series that included 12 patients with presumed occipital neuralgia who responded to subcutaneous occipital nerve stimulation (ONS). Further functional neuroimaging studies on some of these patients suggested that the patients' pathology was more consistent with chronic migraines [4]. Since that time, there have been a handful of studies that have explored the use of ONS in treating medically refractory chronic migraines.

Anatomy

The occipital nerves are comprised of a set of nerves that together provide sensory innervation to the posterior scalp as far anterior as the vertex of the scalp. The three major nerves are the greater, lesser, and third occipital nerve. The greater occipital nerve originates from the C2 dorsal ramus with a minor contribution from the C3 dorsal ramus. The nerve then courses upwards and medially where it courses between the first and second cervical vertebrae. It then travels between the inferior capitis oblique and semispinalis capitis muscles before dissecting through the semispinalis capitis muscle in 90% of cases and the trapezius muscle in 45% of cases [5]. At this point the nerve is located 3 cm below and 1.5 cm lateral to the inion [6] and continues to run parallel to the occipital artery [5]. This artery is a key landmark for identifying the location of this nerve.

The lesser occipital nerve originates from the C2 and C3 ventral rami. It then runs along the posterior border of the sternocleidomastoid muscle and continues up the posterolateral aspects of the skull after piercing though the deep fascia. This nerve is located about 2.5 cm lateral to the occipital artery and 7 cm lateral to the external occipital protuberance [5]. The third occipital nerve is the medial branch of the C3 dorsal ramus. It courses upwards just 3 mm lateral to the inion and provides sensory innervation to the medial aspect of the posterior scalp [5].

Pathophysiology

The mechanism of action of ONS is felt to include modulation of both peripheral and central nociceptive inputs. Peripherally a field stimulation effect is created directly inhibiting afferent nociceptive signals [7]. Centrally, stimulation may increase blood flow to key structures involved in activation of migraines including the trigeminocervical complex, thalamus, and pain matrix [2, 7, 8]. Cranial positron emission tomography scans showed changes in the pain matrix which reduced ipsilateral hypothalamic activity [3]. This latter central mechanism of action has gained increased traction as analgesia has been demonstrated with subthreshold stimulation patterns.

Technique

ONS implantation can be performed under either intravenous sedation [4] or general anesthesia [6]. A vertical midline incision is made just below the inion at the level of C1. The stimulator leads are then burrowed with the help of an introducer laterally directed toward the external auditory meatus. The leads can be implanted either superficially [4] or deep [6] to the fascia and muscle layers. Neither depth has been shown to be superior to the other. The leads are then tunneled subcutaneously to the internal pulse generator, which is usually located in either the subclavicular [6], abdominal, or buttock area [4]. Appropriate lead positioning during and after implantation can be confirmed with fluoroscopy. Trial and error will need to be used to identify the stimulator electrodes along the implanted leads that maximize paresthesia in the region of the headache. As lead migration is a common complication with these devices, the internal pulse generator setting may need to be adjusted regularly.

Tonic Stimulation Studies

A majority of published studies on occipital nerve stimulation for migraines have used tonic stimulation [4, 8–11]. Literature is currently limited to five randomized control trials and eight case series. ONS appears to have a greater effect in reducing frequency of headaches than reducing severity of symptoms. Thus, ONS is best suited as a preventative therapy rather than a rescue therapy. A systematic review demonstrated a modest reduction of 2.59 days per month of prolonged, moderate to severe headaches [8]. Although this is a relatively small effect size, it may be clinically relevant as patients receiving ONS have been unresponsive to most other conventional treatments.

Currently, ONS has mostly been studied only in patients with chronic migraines refractory to at least two pharmacologic agents, who responded to either occipital nerve stimulator trials and/or nerve blocks with at least a 50% reduction in pain. The specificity and sensitivity of the stimulator or nerve block trials to predict response to a permanent stimulator appear to be low [4]. ONS outcomes are likely to improve with better patient selection criteria. This could include changing thresholds for successful trial or exclusion of patients with overuse headaches who appear to be less responsive to ONS. Three of the key trials guiding ONS use for migraines are summarized below.

PRISM Trial

The Precision Implantable Stimulator for Migraine (PRISM) study, presented at a conference in 2009, was the first randomized, controlled study featuring ONS for chronic migraines. The study accepted patients with medically refractory migraines and did not require a successful stimulation or nerve block trial prior to inclusion [8]. The results showed no difference between the stimulation group and the sham group. However, further subgroup analysis showed that after excluding patients overusing acute headache medication demonstrated a significant decrease in days with headaches (5.9 days for the ONS group versus 2.6 days in the sham group) [10].

ONSTIM Feasibility Study

The Occipital Nerve Stimulation for the Treatment of Intractable Chronic Migraine (ONSTIM) trial included patients diagnosed with chronic migraines, disease refractory to at least two classes of medication, and also having had at least a 50% reduction in pain in response to local anesthetic occipital nerve blocks. Patients were randomized to one of three groups: (2) treatment, (3) sham stimulator, and (4) medical management. The results showed that the treatment group had a 27.0% reduction in days with headaches compared to 8.8% for the sham stimulator group and 4.4% for the medical management group. Comparatively, the average reduction in overall pain intensity was just 1.5, 0.5, and 0.6 for the three groups, respectively, in a standard NRS pain scale. These findings suggested that the occipital nerve stimulation may show improvement by preventing headaches as opposed to reducing severity of the outbreaks [4].

Silberstein et al.

In 2012, Silberstein and colleagues published the results from a randomized, controlled trial of 157 patients. The study included medically refractory patients who had 50% reduction in pain with trial stimulation [8]. All the patients received an ONS and patients were randomized to either active or sham treatment. Results showed a statistically significant reduction in frequency of headache days per month compared to baseline (27.2% reduction in active treatment versus 14.9% reduction in the sham treatment). The primary endpoint of responder rate with 50% reduction in average daily pain showed no statistical difference between active treatment and sham. However, there was a statistically significant difference in percent of patients receiving a 30% reduction in average daily pain compared to baseline [10, 11].

Recent Developments with Subthreshold Stimulation

Over the past 5 years there has been an increasing interest in subthreshold stimulation throughout the neuromodulation community, which has also extended to ONS. There have been two randomized trials that have examined this possibility, which appear to show analgesic benefits. However, further studies will be needed to determine if the effect size is comparable to that of tonic stimulation.

Slotty et al.

The first study was a randomized, blinded, crossover study that assessed VAS pain scores of patients receiving one of three stimulation settings: (2) suprathreshold tonic stimulation, (3) subthreshold tonic stimulation, or (4) no stimulation. Eight chronic migraine patients who had been successfully treated with ONS with greater than 30% decrease in VAS pain scores were randomly cycled through the three stimulation settings for 1 week each. Patient VAS scores were assessed at the end of each week. Results showed an average VAS scores of 1.98 ± 1.56 for suprathreshold stimulation, 5.65 ± 2.11 for subthreshold stimulation, and 8.45 ± 0.99 for no stimulation. The difference between the suprathreshold and subthreshold groups suggests that subthreshold stimulation with non-high frequencies patterns may not be able to provide optimal analgesia although this could be due to placebo effect from inability to blind patients to suprathreshold stimulation. The difference between the subthreshold and no stimulation groups demonstrates analgesic effects with subthreshold stimulation with appropriate patient blinding [7].

Burst Occipital Nerve Stimulation

In 2019, Garcia-Ortega et al. published a retrospective case series of 12 patients with chronic migraines, many of whom demonstrated significant reduction in frequency of migraines using burst occipital nerve stimulation. Patients had an ONS implanted and then appropriate stimulation of the occipital nerves confirmed with tonic stimulation. Stimulation settings were then switch to De Ridder pattern burst stimulation. On an average, patients had a decline in days per month with migraines from 26.5 to 16.3 and a reduction in pain score by 16%. Similar to studies mentioned earlier, burst stimulation also appears to also have a greater effect as a preventive therapy than as a rescue therapy. The results are also notable for bimodal distributions of both endpoints [6]. Thus, larger studies in the future with subgroup analysis may be beneficial to identify which patients benefit most from ONS.

Complications

Lead migration and surgery site infection are the two most common complications associated with ONS, both of which are commonly accepted complications with all neurostimulation devices. The incidence of these two complications is estimated to be between 10–24% and 4–14% respectively based on data from randomized control trials and both should be considered significant as they often need surgical intervention to fix. Some procedural techniques proposed to reduce lead migration were using paddle-type leads instead of cylindrical leads, using strain–relief loops during implantation, and placing internal pulse generator in abdomen region [8]. None of these techniques have been studied in detail. However, one can be hopeful that such complications will decrease as newer devices are developed with these limitations in mind and with increased proceduralist experience. There have been no reported incidents of permanent nerve damage, although that will always remain a possibility with any interventional procedure near neural structures [8].

Clinical Applications and Future Directions

ONS is one of the most studied neuromodulation techniques for patients with chronic migraines [3]. Current literature suggests that it may provide a modest reduction in frequency of patients with chronic migraines and potentially a reduction in VAS pain scores. Preimplantation stimulation and/or nerve block trials can help determine which patients will respond successfully to ONS. Further research should be done to establish criteria to help clinicians make such decisions. Currently, ONS should be reserved for patients refractory to multiple prophylactic migraine medications and are aware of the potentially frequent complications requiring revision surgery.

Vagal Nerve Stimulation

Vagal nerve stimulation (VNS) has been used to treat refractory epilepsy and depression for many years now. Clinicians observed that patients with comorbid migraines experienced improvements in headache symptoms leading to further research into the use of VNS to treat chronic migraines. The vagus nerve is a multifunctional nerve that exits through the jugular foramen and travels down the neck inside the carotid sheath, subsequently branching off into several nerves including the auricular nerve. In addition to providing visceral innervation to many organs, it also provides general sensation from the auricle, external acoustic meatus, and dura mater of the posterior cranial fossa [3].

Since the early 2000s, numerous studies have been published on the use of VNS to treat migraines. Studies using implantable VNS have been limited to case series while studies using transcutaneous VNS have been studied with higher quality randomized, controlled trials. A majority of devices stimulate the vagus nerve as it travels in the lateral aspects of the neck. More recently, in 2015, there was a randomized trial specifically targeting the auricular branch [3, 12]. VNS has been shown to have effects on central sensitization [12] and increase blood flow to the brain [3]. Results suggest VNS may reduce frequency of migraines without any significant analgesia as a rescue medication.

Transcutaneous VNS

This technology appears to be a highly feasible, well-tolerated, and convenient therapy to prevent chronic migraines based on the EVENT study published in 2016. This was a prospective, multicenter, double-blind, sham-controlled study of transcutaneous VNS for the prevention of chronic migraine attacks. The study was designed as a feasibility study with primary end points of safety and tolerability. The study was not powered for their exploratory endpoints, which included reduction in headaches per month [12]. Patients used a stimulator that was applied to neck in the vicinity of the vagus nerve for a total of 12 min daily [3, 12, 13].

Fifty-nine patients were randomized to receive either stimulation or sham therapy for 2 months. Fifteen of the thirty patients randomized to the stimulation arm then continued into the open-label portion of the study in which all patients received the stimulation therapy for an additional 6 months. The reduction in days with headaches during the randomized portion of the study was not statistically significant (1.4 days/month for the stimulation arm versus 0.2 days/month for the sham arm). At the end of the open-label portion of the study, the patients demonstrated a reduction of 7.9 days/month compared to their baseline, which was statistically significant. However, the results are confounded by attrition bias as patients with less analgesia tended to drop out of the study during the open-label portion. Further studies with a larger sample size and potentially a longer treatment phase should be performed to guide clinical use of transcutaneous VNS [13].

Auricular VNS

The auricular nerve has also been targeted with transcutaneous stimulation using an earpiece that applies direct stimulation to the concha of the outer ear, leading to excitation of the thick, myelinated sensory A-beta fibers and in turn activation of the solitary tract nucleus. In the study, a total of 46 patients were randomized to auricular stimulation for 4 h per day for 3 months at either 25 Hz (treatment arm) or 1 Hz (control arm). Twenty-five hertz is the frequency used for VNS for treatment of epilepsy. One hertz was selected as an active control to facilitate blinding participants [14].

Surprisingly, the active control group showed a greater statistically significant reduction in headache days (7 days versus 3.3 days) and responder rate (29.4% versus 13.3%). It is unclear why stimulation of the auricular nerve responded better to the lower stimulation frequency. One hypothetical difference is that the cervical branch, which is targeted with traditional transcutaneous VNS, is a mixed nerve with both myelinated and non-myelinated fibers. Different nerves may respond differently to different types of stimulation [14]. Results from this study implore further follow-up studies looking at effects of various forms of stimulation. Currently, this device has been approved for use in Europe but not the United States [12].

Invasive VNS

Due to risk of adverse events such as infections and lead migration, a majority of research has been focused on transcutaneous VNS [14]. Literature regarding invasive VNS is limited to four case series with a total of 20 patients published between 2003 and 2009 [15–17]. A majority of these chronic migraineurs had received VNS for either depression and/or epilepsy. They were followed retrospectively to look for change in migraine symptoms before and after VNS implantation [15, 16]. Only four of the patients received the VNS specifically to treat migraines. These patients were noted to be completely debilitated from their symptoms [17].

Supraorbital and Supratrochlear Transcutaneous Nerve Stimulation

Supraorbital and supratrochlear nerve transcutaneous stimulation (STNS) is a noninvasive means of utilizing external stimulation to modulate branches of the V1 trigeminal nerve, namely the supraorbital and supratrochlear nerve branches [18]. In March 2014, the FDA-approved Cefaly, a medical device designed specifically for STNS, for the prevention of migraine [19]. Prior to and following the approval of Cefaly, a number of studies have looked at STNS as both a preventive measure in episodic and chronic migraines and as treatment during acute episodes.

Mechanism of Action

Various preclinical research and human imaging studies have sought to describe the mechanism that may explain the role trigeminal stimulation may play in attenuating migraine pathophysiology. Initially, it was proposed that trigeminal somatic afferents or visceral trigeminovascular afferents may block ascending impulses in the pain pathway, but this has been contested by Lipton et al. in studying ONS [19]. Others have proposed that STNS may exert its beneficial effect in migraine via slow neuromodulatory mechanisms involving limbic and pain control areas in the cerebral cortex [18]. An FDG-PET study in episodic migraine patients before and after 3 months of daily STNS with the Cefaly device showed a normalization of orbitofrontal hypometabolism [20]. Overall, the mechanism of action for STNS is unclear, but several plausible hypotheses are currently being studied.

Technique

The STNS device attaches externally across the forehead, starts at the level of the procerus, and extends bilaterally across the frontalis. Generally accepted and studied STNS parameters are "rectangular biphasic compensated impulses with an electrical mean equal to zero, impulse width of 250 μS, frequency of 60 Hz, maximum intensity of 16 mA with a progressive slope from 1 to 16 mA over 14 min" [18]. Alternatively, higher frequencies (120 Hz) with STNS have also been studied and have been shown to induce a sedative effect in healthy volunteers [21].

Pilot Trial

The pilot trial for the Cefaly device took place in 2009 to assess for initial safety and efficacy [22]. Ten patients were enrolled and showed a decrease of the average migraine attack frequency from 3.9 to 2.8 per month and 5 out of 8 patients were satisfied with the device [22]. Total relief without rescue medication was obtained in 13% of attacks, postponed drug intake in 20% of attacks and partial relief with additional drug treatment in 45% of attacks [22]. No major adverse events were recorded [22].

The PREMICE Trial

Following the pilot study in 2013, the Prevention of Migraine Using Cefaly (PREMICE) trial was a prospective, multicenter, double-blinded, randomized, and sham-controlled trial to better evaluate STNS and migraine prevention. Sixty-seven patients were treated with either an STNS or a sham device, with stimulation administered daily for 20 min for 3 months [23]. Primary outcome measures were changed in monthly migraine days. STNS was found to be effective in reducing monthly migraine days (6.94–4.88 days, $P = 0.023$) compared to sham, and acute medication intake was reduced by 36.7%. No major adverse events were noted [23].

The PREMICE trial was followed by Di Fiore et al. in a second study looking at prevention of chronic migraines in 23 patients prospectively over 4-month use [24]. Primary endpoints were 50% reduction in migraine days and 50% reduction in acute medication use [24]. Nineteen patients completed the study with three subjects dropping out due to adverse events, and 1 subject due to an unrelated medical issue [24]. Baseline headache days were 20.7 ± 5.7 migraine days per month and baseline acute medication use was 20.2 ± 12.4 times per month [24]. Eight subjects achieved both primary endpoints reducing to 7.6 headache days per month at month 4, and use of acute medications to 6.3 times at month 4 (no P values published) [24].

The ACME Trial

The ACute treatment of Migraine with External trigeminal nerve stimulation (ACME) trial was a single prospective, randomized, sham-controlled, double-blind study looking at the use of STNS for the acute treatment of migraine [25]. One hundred and six patients were assigned to receive either true or sham stimulation at migraine onset and treated for 1 h under similar settings as described above [25]. The primary outcome was the mean change in pain intensity VAS at 1 h. Results showed that the 1 h poststimulation group had a −3.46 ± 2.32 in VAS scores, compared to −1.78 ± 1.89 in the sham group ($P < 0.0001$) [25]. Patients who had migraine without aura also saw a statistically significant benefit with the device compared to sham (−3.3 ± 2.4 in the treatment group, −1.7 ± 1.9 in the sham group; $P = 0.0006$) [25]. The migraine with aura subgroup showed some benefit compared to sham, but results did not reach statistical significance (−4.3 ± 1.8 for the treatment group, −2.6 ± 1.9 for the sham group; $P = 0.060$) [25]. A few minor adverse events were noted including paresthesia over the stimulated area and sedation [25]. Following results from the ACME study, the FDA cleared the STNS device for the acute treatment of migraine after previously approving its use primarily for migraine prevention.

Post-marketing Survey and Complications

Following FDA approval and marketing of the Cefaly device as a treatment for headache prevention, Magis et al. published a survey from 2313 patients looking at the satisfaction and complication rate of the device [21]. The true ("per protocol") nonresponder rate was calculated to be 18.6% [21]. Of note, 1077 subjects (46.6%) returned the device and were thus considered to be dissatisfied [21]. Ninety-nine patients (4.3%) reported a total of 104 AEs [21]. The most frequent AE was intolerance to the paresthesia ($n = 31$, 1.3% of users), but also included unwanted sedation, irritation to the skin, or headache following stimulation [21].

Developing Neuromodulatory Modalities

High Cervical Spinal Cord Stimulation

Spinal cord stimulation (SCS) has been effectively used in the treatment of neuropathic pain conditions ranging from diabetic neuropathy to chronic angina pectoris;

its application for the treatment of migraine pain is currently being explored in recent studies. The placement of SCS in the high cervical region involves entering the epidural space and directing the electrodes cephalad until movement is stopped by the inferior margin of the occipital bone [26]. Stimulation in this region aims to provide analgesia and paresthesia coverage to areas of C2 as well as branches of the trigeminal, including V1 and V2 [27]. Coverage has also been noted to neck and various parts of the skull including the occipital, parietal, and frontal regions [27]. Prior to being tested in migraine headaches, placement of high cervical leads had previously been described for the treatment of cluster headaches, where it was shown to have promising results (reduction of attack strength and frequency 43% and 84%, respectively, with $N = 7$) when compared with occipital nerve stimulation by Wolter et al., albeit with a high complication rate of lead fracture or migrations [28]. A retrospective survey by De Agostino et al. of 17 patients with medically intractable chronic migraine pain who were implanted with a high-cervical SCS showed mean pain intensity was reduced by 60% ($p < 0.0001$) for 15 months (range 2–48) post implantation and with 71% of the patients experiencing a decrease of 50% or more [29]. The median number of days with migraine decreased from 28 to 9 days ($p = 0.0313$) [29]. While patients endorsed that their quality of life was significantly improved, working capacity did not significantly improved [29]. Finally, complications included three infections (13.0% of all implanted) and three lead dislocations (17.6% of all included) [29].

A second prospective, open-label trial by Arcioni studies high frequency SCS with 17 patients with 14 patients completing the trail at 6 months post-implant (one trial failure, one trial infection, one implant-site infection) [30]. Seven of the fourteen in the cohort responded with a >30% reduction in headache days and there was an overall reduction in 6.9 headache days for the entire cohort with a 12.9-day reduction specifically among the responders [30]. Larger trials exploring high cervical SCS are underway, but initial studies show that this modality may provide additional coverage and benefit not seen in alternative therapies.

Transcranial Direct Current Stimulation

Transcranial direct current stimulation (tDCS) is a noninvasive and safe technique that is hypothesized to modulate the activity of the underlying cerebral cortex through the use of a current applied through electric pads [31]. Since abnormal discharge through cortical areas has been shown to be an underlying mechanism behind migraine pathophysiology, tDCS may be able to increase habituation to this aberrant excitability [32]. A proof of concept exploratory study was done by Vigano et al. in 11 healthy and 13 episodic migraineurs by recording pattern-reversal visual evoked potentials (VEP) before and after a 15 min session (a current of 2.0 mA intensity applied for 20 min) of anodal tDCS over the visual cortex [31]. Results showed migraine attack frequency, migraine days, attack duration, and acute medication intake significantly decreased during the treatment period compared to pretreatment baseline (all $p < 0.05$) and that this benefit persisted on average 4.8 weeks after the end of tDCS [31]. Moreover, these results correlated with increased habituation to visual stimuli measured by VEP in both healthy and migraine patients [31]. A follow-up, randomized control trial with 19 patients by Rocha et al. showed similar significant decreases in a number of migraine attacks, painkiller intake, and duration of each attack with just the experimental group, but also presented conflicting evidence that these clinical improvements did not correlate with changes in cortical excitability [32].

A more recent double blind and sham-controlled trial with 42 migraine patients looking at tDCS for migraine prevention showed cathodal stimulation was associated with a significant reduction in the number of headache days (1.60, $p < 0.001$) and tablets consumption per week (0.30, $p < 0.001$) with an effect sustained over 2 weeks and with no serious side effects observed [33]. Here the researchers placed the cathode placed over the occipital cortex of the dominant side of the migraine pain and the anode electrode was placed over the supraorbital area on the opposite side [33].

This study suggests that placement of the anode and cathode pads may play a role in the efficacy of the therapy, as also suggested by Andrade et al.'s RCT, with stimulation of the left primary motor (M1) versus dorsolateral prefrontal cortex (DLPFC) versus sham with 13 patients [34]. Their results showed that not only did the DLPFC group exhibit a better performance compared to the M1 and sham participants, but also that the M1 group exhibited more adverse effects, especially headache, heartburn, and sleepiness, than did those in the other two groups [34]. Overall, tDCS represents a novel medium for noninvasive modulation requiring further investigation on the part of its mechanism of action and clinical application.

Repetitive Transcranial Magnetic Stimulation

The use of electromagnetic induction as a means of brain stimulation has been studied and utilized in the treatment of psychiatric disorders like depression for decades prior to its application to migraines. Repetitive transcranial magnetic stimulation (rTMS) utilizes an external magnetic coil to produce an electric current that is transmitted through the scalp to the cortex, much like the previously discussed tDCS [35]. Here too proof of concept studies have shown that even low-frequency stimulation with 1 Hz rTMS reduces excitability of visual cortex in normal subjects [36]. However, the same study has also shown that while the visual cortex of migraineurs is generally hyperactive and may lack functional inhibitory circuitry; rTMS has not been shown to promote inhibitory pathways in excitable cortical areas [36]. Misra et al.'s prospective randomized control trial tested three sessions of alternate day 10 Hz rTMS consisting of 600 pulses in 10 trains delivered to left frontal cortex for 51 patients versus sham [35]. Fifty (98%) patients had more than 50% reduction of headache frequency at 1 week after rTMS, persisting until the fourth week in 80% of patients [35]. Additionally, headache frequency, severity, functional disability, migraine index, and rescue medications significantly reduced at all time points, but the maximum benefit was observed in the first 2 weeks [35]. While there were no serious adverse events, the most common minor events included irritation to the facial skin and muscles, discomfort, syncope and worsening headache, or pain [35]. A follow-up trial versus sham by the same authors with a group of 100 patients showed that at 1 month, the trial group versus sham had lower headache frequency (78.7 vs. 33.3%; $P = 0.0001$) and improved VAS scores (76.6 vs. 27.1%; $P = 0.0001$) [37]. Further, functional disability also improved significantly in rTMS group ($P = 0.0001$) [37]. These studies were soon followed single pulse with TMS receiving FDA approval for treatment of migraines in 2013 as a Class II medical device.

Conclusion

Over the past decade, several neuromodulation techniques have been used to effectively treat patients with migraines. Occipital nerve stimulation has been shown to prevent occurrence of migraines. Supraorbital and supratrochlear stimulation has been shown to both prevent frequency of migraines and also treat acute exacerbations. Additionally, several newer modalities (high cervical spinal cord stimulation, transcranial direct current stimulation, and repetitive transcranial magnetic stimulation) have demonstrated promising results in preliminary studies. As the supporting literature becomes more robust, these techniques should be incorporated into the routine algorithm for the management of migraines.

References

1. Fishman M, Antony A, Esposito M, Deer T, Levy R. The evolution of neuromodulation in the treatment of chronic pain: forward-looking perspectives. Pain Med. 2019;20(Supplement_1):S58–68.
2. Stillings D. Mediterranean origin of electrotherapy. Biolelectricity. 1983;2:181–6.
3. Antony A, Mazzola A, Dhaliwal G, Hunter C. Neurostimulation for the treatment of chronic head and facial pain: a literature review. Pain Phys J. 2019;22:447–77.
4. Saper J, Dodick D, Silberstein S, McCarville S, Sun M, Goadsby P. Occipital nerve stimulation for the treatment of intractable chronic migraine headache: ONSTIM feasibility study. Cephalalgia. 2010;31(3):271–85.
5. Cohen-Gadol A, Kemp W III, Tubbs R. The innervation of the scalp: a comprehensive review including anatomy, pathology, and neurosurgical correlates. Surg Neurol Int. 2011;2(1):178.
6. Garcia-Ortega R, Edwards T, Moir L, Aziz T, Green A, FitzGerald J. Burst occipital nerve stimulation for chronic migraine and chronic cluster headache. Neuromodulation. 2019;22(5):638–44.
7. Slotty P, Bara G, Kowatz L, Gendolla A, Wille C, Schu S, et al. Occipital nerve stimulation for chronic migraine: a randomized trial on subthreshold stimulation. Cephalalgia. 2014;35(1):73–8.
8. Chen Y, Bramley G, Unwin G, Hanu-Cernat D, Dretzke J, Moore D, et al. Occipital nerve stimulation for chronic migraine—a systematic review and meta-analysis. PLoS One. 2015;10(3):e0116786.
9. Schwedt T. Occipital nerve stimulation for chronic migraine—interpreting the ONSTIM feasibility trial. Cephalalgia. 2010;31(3):262–3.
10. Silberstein SD, Dodick DW, Saper J, et al. Safety and efficacy of peripheral nerve stimulation of the occipital nerves for the management of chronic migraine: results from a randomized, multicenter, double-blinded, controlled study. Cephalalgia. 2012;32:1165–79.

11. Dodick DW, Silberstein SD, Reed KL, et al. Safety and efficacy of peripheral nerve stimulation of the occipital nerves for the management of chronic migraine: long-term results from a randomized, multicenter, double-blinded, controlled study. Cephalalgia. 2014;35:344–58.
12. Halker Singh R, Ailani J, Robbins M. Neuromodulation for the acute and preventive therapy of migraine and cluster headache. Headache. 2019;59(S2):33–49.
13. Silberstein S, Calhoun A, Lipton R, Grosberg B, Cady R, Dorlas S, et al. Chronic migraine headache prevention with noninvasive vagus nerve stimulation. Neurology. 2016;87(5):529–38.
14. Straube A, Ellrich J, Eren O, Blum B, Ruscheweyh R, et al. J Headache Pain. 2015;16(1):543.
15. Proietti Cecchini A, Mea E, Tullo V, Curone M, Franzini A, Broggi G, et al. Vagus nerve stimulation in drug-resistant daily chronic migraine with depression: preliminary data. Neurol Sci. 2009;30(S1):101–4.
16. Lenaerts M, Oommen K, Couch J, Skaggs V. Can vagus nerve stimulation help migraine? Cephalalgia. 2008;28(4):392–5.
17. Mauskop A. Vagus nerve stimulation relieves chronic refractory migraine and cluster headaches. Cephalalgia. 2005;25(2):82–6.
18. Riederer F, Penning S, Schoenen J. Transcutaneous Supraorbital nerve stimulation (t-SNS) with the Cefaly® device for migraine prevention: a review of the available data. Pain Ther. 2015;4(2):135–47.
19. Lipton RB, Buse DC, Serrano D, et al. Examination of unmet treatment needs among persons with episodic migraine: results of the American Migraine Prevalence and Prevention (AMPP) Study. Headache. 2013;53:1300–11.
20. D'Ostillo K, Thibaut A, Laureys S, et al. Cerebral FDG uptake changes after supraorbital transcutaneous electrical stimulation with the Cefaly(R) device in patients with migraine. Poster at international headache conference, Valencia, Spain, 14–17 May 2015.
21. Magis D, Sava S. d' Elia TS, et al. Safety and patients' satisfaction of transcutaneous supraorbital neurostimulation (tSNS) with the Cefaly® device in headache treatment: a survey of 2313 headache sufferers in the general population. J Headache Pain. 2013;14:95.
22. Gérardy P, Fabry D, Fumal A, Schoenen J. A pilot study on supra-orbital surface electrotherapy in migraine. Cephalalgia. 2009;29:134.
23. Schoenen J, Vandersmissen B, Jeangette S, Herroelen L, Vandenheede M, Gérard P, Magis D. Migraine prevention with a supraorbital transcutaneous stimulator: a randomized controlled trial. Neurology. 2013;80(8):697–704.
24. Di Fiore P, Bussone G, Galli A, et al. Transcutaneous supraorbital neurostimulation for the prevention of chronic migraine: a prospective, open-label preliminary trial. Neurol Sci. 2017;38:201–6.
25. Chou DE, Shnayderman Yugrakh M, Winegarner D, Rowe V, Kuruvilla D, Schoenen J. Acute migraine therapy with external trigeminal neurostimulation (ACME): a randomized controlled trial. Cephalalgia. 2019;39:3–14.
26. Wolter T, Kiemen A, Kaube H. High cervical spinal cord stimulation for chronic cluster headache. Cephalalgia. 2011;31(11):1170–80.
27. Wolter T, Kaube H, Mohadjer M. High cervical epidural neurostimulation for cluster headache: case report and review of the literature. Cephalalgia. 2008;28(10):1091–4.
28. Wolter T, Kaube H. Neurostimulation for chronic cluster headache. Ther Adv Neurol Disord. 2012;5(3):175–80.
29. De Agostino R, Federspiel B, Cesnulis E, Sandor PS. High-cervical spinal cord stimulation for medically intractable chronic migraine. Neuromodulation. 2015;18(4):289–96.
30. Arcioni R, Palmisani S, Mercieri M, Vano V, Tigano S, Smith T, Fiore MR, Al-Kaisy A, Martelletti P. Cervical 10 kHz spinal cord stimulation in the management of chronic, medically refractory migraine: a prospective, open-label, exploratory study. Eur J Pain. 2016;20(1):70–8.
31. Viganò A, D'Elia TS, Sava SL, Auvé M, De Pasqua V, Colosimo A, Di Piero V, Schoenen J, Magis D. Transcranial Direct Current Stimulation (tDCS) of the visual cortex: a proof-of-concept study based on interictal electrophysiological abnormalities in migraine. J Headache Pain. 2013;14(1):23.

32. Rocha S, Melo L, Boudoux C, Foerster Á, Araújo D, Monte-Silva K. Transcranial direct current stimulation in the prophylactic treatment of migraine based on interictal visual cortex excitability abnormalities: a pilot randomized controlled trial. J Neurol Sci. 2015;349(1–2):33–9.
33. Ahdab R, Mansour AG, Khazen G, El-Khoury C, Sabbouh TM, Salem M, Yamak W, Ayache SS, Riachi N. Cathodal transcranial direct current stimulation of the occipital cortex in episodic migraine: a randomized sham-controlled crossover study. J Clin Med. 2020;9(1):60.
34. Andrade SM, de Brito Aranha RE, de Oliveira EA, de Mendonça CT, Martins WK, Alves NT, Fernández-Calvo B. Transcranial direct current stimulation over the primary motor vs prefrontal cortex in refractory chronic migraine: a pilot randomized controlled trial. J Neurol Sci. 2017;378:225–32.
35. Misra UK, Kalita J, Bhoi SK. High frequency repetitive transcranial magnetic stimulation (rTMS) is effective in migraine prophylaxis: an open labeled study. Neurol Res. 2012;34(6):547–51.
36. Brighina F, Piazza A, Daniele O, Fierro B. Modulation of visual cortical excitability in migraine with aura: effects of 1 Hz repetitive transcranial magnetic stimulation. Exp Brain Res. 2002;145(2):177–81.
37. Misra UK, Kalita J, Bhoi SK. High-rate repetitive transcranial magnetic stimulation in migraine prophylaxis: a randomized, placebo-controlled study. J Neurol. 2013;260(11):2793–801.

Surgical Treatment of Chronic Migraine Headaches

10

Melissa Kanack and Raj M. Vyas

Surgical improvement of migraine headaches was serendipitously discovered and first described by an academic plastic surgeon, Bahman Guyuron, in 2000 [1]. Many of his patients anecdotally reported relief of chronic migraine headaches after undergoing resection of corrugator supercilii muscles as part of an aesthetic procedure for forehead rejuvenation. A retrospective review by Guyuron then confirmed that 79.5% of patients with a reported history of migraines had significant improvement in headache symptoms following this surgical procedure. Numerous subsequent prospective studies and anatomic investigations have established the evidence-based foundation of modern migraine surgery, which focuses on careful patient selection followed by selective decompression of craniofacial sensory nerves identified as "triggers" for migraine headache. This chapter reviews the relevant anatomy, pathophysiology, patient/surgical site selection, operative techniques, perioperative care, and outcomes assessment of surgery to relieve chronic migraine headaches.

M. Kanack
Department of Plastic Surgery, University of California Irvine, School of Medicine, Irvine, CA, USA

R. M. Vyas (✉)
Department of Plastic Surgery, University of California Irvine, Orange, CA, USA
e-mail: rajv1@hs.uci.edu

© Springer Nature Switzerland AG 2021

S. Shah (ed.), *Migraine*, https://doi.org/10.1007/978-3-030-75239-2_10

Anatomy and Pathophysiology

Four major trigger sites comprise the primary targets for migraine surgery [2]. The frontal trigger site is made up of both the supraorbital and supratrochlear nerves (SON, STN) (Fig. 10.1). These are both branches of the first division of the fifth cranial nerve (V1). The temporal trigger site refers to the zygomaticotemporal branch of the trigeminal nerve (ZTBTN), which is a branch of the second division of the fifth cranial nerve (V2). The occipital trigger site primarily involves the greater occipital nerve and can also include the third occipital nerve. Finally, the intranasal (rhinogenic) trigger site involves irritation of the intranasal terminal branches of the first division of the trigeminal nerve (V1). Several minor trigger sites have also been identified, including the auriculotemporal nerve and the lesser occipital nerve. Irritation of these nerves – via compression from muscles, fascial bands, bony foramina, and/or blood vessels – is thought to lead to release of pro-inflammatory neuropeptides contributing to the development of a migraine headache [3, 4]. In the case of the rhinogenic trigger site, sinusitis, nasal allergies, or points of contact between the nasal septum and turbinates are thought to similarly irritate intranasal sensory nerves. These trigger site nerves – branches of the fifth cranial nerve and occipital nerve – are peripheral craniofacial nerves with direct to brainstem/upper cervical spine messaging.

Preoperative Evaluation and Selection of Optimal Candidates for Migraine Surgery

Migraine surgery is reserved for patients with a diagnosis of chronic migraine headache who either fail or seek to avoid pharmacologic interventions for treatment of their headaches. Patients should be evaluated in conjunction with their neurologists. Careful preoperative identification of trigger sites is paramount and a 1-month headache journal is critical for capturing headache frequency, severity, duration,

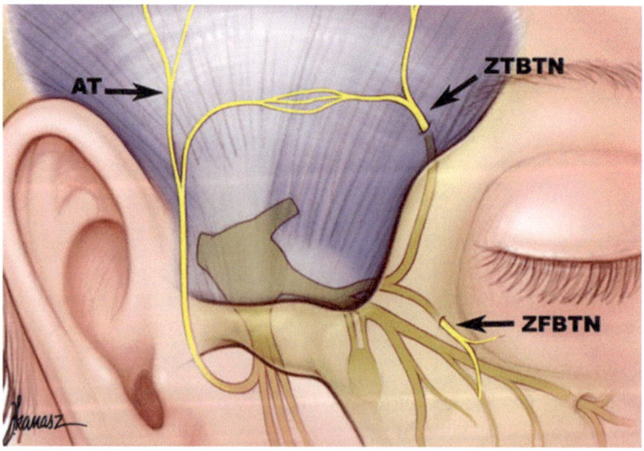

Fig. 10.1 Anatomy of the temporal trigger site, showing the zygomaticotemporal branch of the trigeminal nerve (ZTBTN), auriculotemporal nerve (AT), and the zygomaticofrontal branch of the trigeminal nerve (ZFBTN). (From Guyuron et al. [28], with permission)

associated symptoms, and – most importantly – precise location of headache onset [5]. (See appendix, for example, headache journal and headache questionnaires.) Patients are instructed to use a single finger to specify where his or her migraine headaches *start*… *Not* to where they spread or settle [2]. A Doppler can be used to confirm the presence of vasculature in the trigger area that might be contributing to nerve compression.

Specific "constellations of symptoms" have been reported in the literature for each of the main migraine trigger sites [4]. Frontal headaches involve pain above the eyebrow and usually start in the afternoon. Patients may experience eyelid ptosis on the affected side during the headache and often demonstrate strong corrugator supercilii muscle activation with frowning (vertical or oblique glabellar furrows or wrinkles). Temporal headaches often occur in the morning and are associated with nocturnal teeth clenching or grinding. Patients may have tenderness of the temporalis or masseter muscles. Occipital headaches are not associated with onset at any specific time of day and can be triggered by strenuous exercise or strained neck positioning. Tight neck muscles are usually subjectively reported. Occipital migraines must be differentiated from occipital neuralgia; the former involves spread upward into the scalp, temporal areas, and forehead while the latter radiates to the neck and back. Rhinogenic headaches usually involve pain behind the eye and classically waken the patient from sleep at night or in the morning. Patients can experience rhinorrhea on the affected side during the headache episode. Some experts believe rhinogenic migraines are akin to "cluster headaches" in etiology and symptoms. Like cluster headaches, rhinogenic migraine can be triggered by nasal allergies, changes in seasonal weather, and/or dependent positioning. Frontal, temporal, and occipital migraines may also be triggered by stress, diet, drugs, hormone cycles, activity, and environmental sensory triggers such as light, noise, and certain smells. Asking patients about their symptom patterns in addition to where their headaches start anatomically further helps the clinician characterize potential trigger sites for decompression.

Once suspected trigger sites have been identified, anesthetic nerve blocks and/or botulinum toxin A can be used for confirmation. Nerve blocks are useful if the patient is seen in office with an acute migraine headache that has not spread significantly, or when there is persistent tenderness at a trigger site. Local anesthetic is injected at the suspected trigger site, and the trigger site is confirmed when relief is obtained within 5–10 minutes after injection [2]. Botulinum toxin A injection is believed to relieve migraine headaches by paralyzing musculature that surrounds and compresses peripheral nerves at target sites [5, 6]. As many patients who present for evaluation for migraine surgery will have already had treatment with botulinum toxin injections, it is important to differentiate between diagnostic and therapeutic injections. Therapeutic injections are typically performed by neurologists and involve diffuse, high-dose injections of toxin into multiple nonspecific face, scalp, and neck sites [7]. Diagnostic botulinum toxin injections are performed by plastic surgeons seeking to verify surgical targets and these injections specifically target muscles at sites of suspected nerve and vessel compression. Preoperative response to botulinum toxin A injection has been found to be a significant predictor of successful surgical intervention, with 90.3% of patients with a positive injection response obtaining relief following surgery, compared to only 72.3% of patients who did not responded to botulinum toxin injections [5]. One study did show, however, that with careful history and diligent attention to the preoperative headache journal, appropriate surgical candidates can be equally well identified without relying on response from diagnostic botulinum toxin injections [4].

Non-contrast CT scans are useful in rhinogenic migraines to identify areas of contact between the nasal septum and turbinates as well as presence or absence of concha bullosa and sinus inflammation [8] (Fig. 10.2). Imaging is not commonly utilized for the other trigger sites.

All patients should be prospectively studied and therefore must complete validated migraine questionnaires at time of initial evaluation, after diagnostic botulinum toxin injection, and at regular intervals following migraine surgery. Calculation of a Migraine Headache Index (MHI) score – a multiple of intensity, frequency, and duration of migraine headaches – is paramount [9]. Additional options include the Migraine Disability Assessment (MIDAS) [10] and Migraine Specific Quality of Life (MSQ) questionnaires [11]. During the evaluation period, patients can stay on abortive and preventative migraine medications with the exception of caffeine-containing medications. Use of narcotic pain medications preoperatively has been associated with poorer postoperative outcomes, and patients who take narcotic medications should be encouraged to wean these prior to surgery [12]. If the patient has undergone treatment with botulinum toxin injections, surgery is scheduled for at least 3–4 months after the last injection to ensure that the paralysis has worn off and to facilitate muscle identification and activation during surgery.

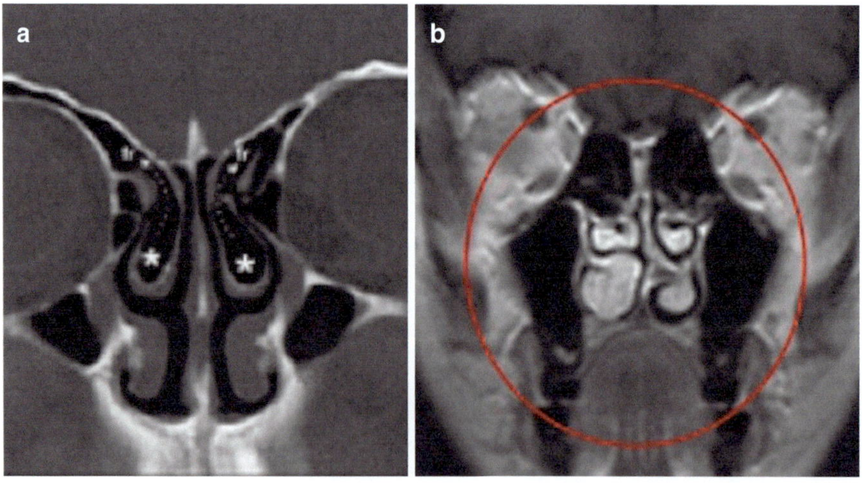

Fig. 10.2 (**a**) Non-contrast CT scan demonstrating concha bullosa (starred in image). (**b**) MRI demonstrating turbinate enlargement (right side) and septal deviation resulting in contact between the septum and turbinate (left side)

Surgical Options

Frontal Trigger Site

Surgical treatment of the frontal trigger site involves addressing four potential causes of compression of the supraorbital and supratrochlear nerves: bone, fascia, muscle, and vessels. The surgical approach typically involves a trans-palpebral approach through an upper eyelid incision (Fig. 10.3). The supraorbital and supratrochlear nerves lie within the glabellar muscles, which include the corrugator supercilii, depressor supercilii, and procerus. These nerves are dissected under loupe or microscope magnification in order to preserve sensory function while the surrounding musculature is resected [13]. If patients are undergoing simultaneous decompression of the temporal trigger site, an endoscopic approach can be considered to simultaneously address all surgical targets. If the supraorbital and

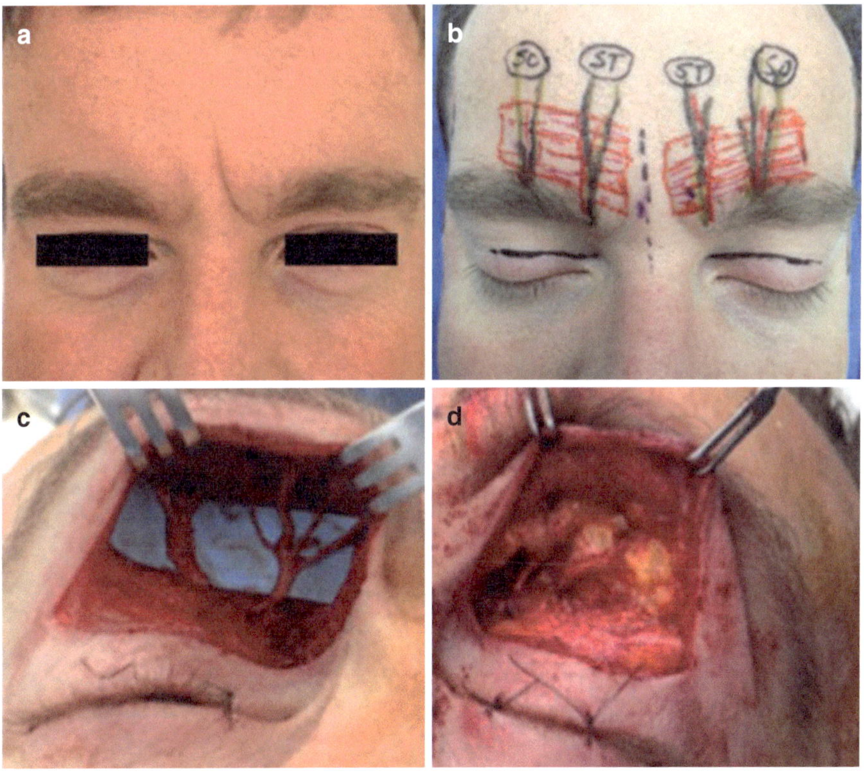

Fig. 10.3 (**a**) Preoperative image of a patient with chronic frontal migraines. Note strong corrugator supercilii activation at rest. (**b**) Planned upper eyelid incision and schema of supratrochlear (ST) and supraorbital (SO) neurovascular bundles. (**c**) Corrugator muscles resected with microdissection and preservation of supraorbital and supratrochlear neurovascular bundles. (**d**) Fat grafts placed to cushion the neurovascular bundles and restore brow contour

supratrochlear vessels are found to be closely associated with these nerves, they are carefully ligated [14]. If the nerves exit the orbit through a true foramen (unusual) instead of a notch (more common), a foraminotomy can be performed with a small 2 mm osteotome; fibrous bands across the notch should also be transected if present [15]. Fat grafts are harvested from the patient and used to restore supraorbital contour and cushion the decompressed trigger sites nerves.

Temporal Trigger Site

For treatment of temporal migraines, a small portion (3 cm) of the zygomaticotemporal branch of the trigeminal nerve is either decompressed or resected where it emerges from the temporalis muscle. Studies show similar outcomes from decompression versus resection [16]. Care must be taken to preserve the frontal branch of the facial nerve (which lies just deep to the superficial temporal fascia) by approaching the ZTBTN at the level of the deep layer of the deep temporal fascia (Fig. 10.4). This is typically done via an endoscopic approach similar to that used for an endoscopic brow lift [13] or with a small incision in the temporal scalp. An open approach utilizing the same transpalpebral incision that is used for the frontal trigger site has also been described for the temporal trigger site [17].

Occipital Trigger Site

The occipital trigger site is addressed through an open approach using either a vertical posterior scalp midline incision below the occipital protuberance or via a transverse incision at the posterior hairline. The greater occipital nerve is typically identified approximately 3 cm inferior and 1.5 cm lateral to the occipital protuberance and is accompanied by the occipital vessels [18]. The semispinalis capitis muscle and trapezius fascia are implicated in compression of the GON and portions of these muscles are resected. There is a low threshold to ligate occipital vessels that cross over or spiral around the GON (Fig. 10.5). While these are the most common

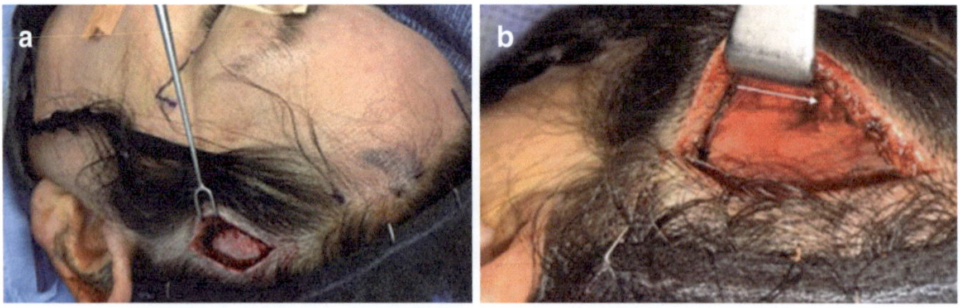

Fig. 10.4 (**a**) Temporal scalp incision for decompression of the ZTBTN. (**b**) Exposure of the ZTBTN (arrow) emerging from deep temporal fascia/muscle

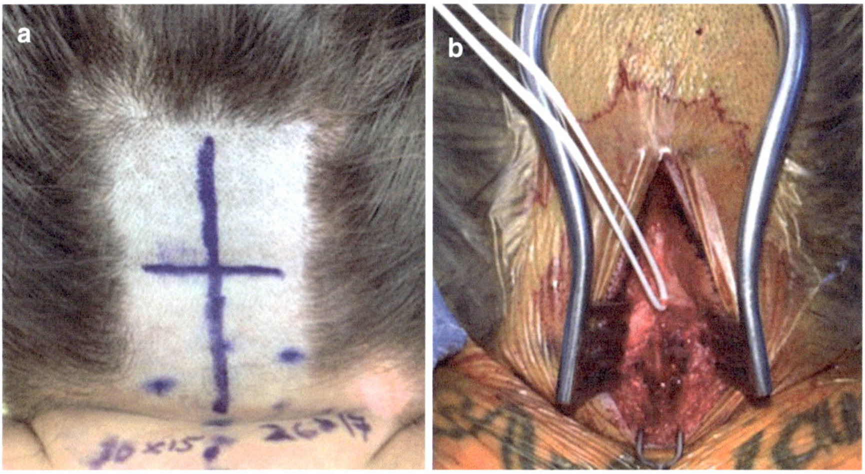

Fig. 10.5 (**a**) Patient in prone position. Vertical line marks posterior midline and horizontal line is drawn between external auditory canals. From intersection of these lines, right GON is 26 × 17 mm inferolateral and left GON is 30 × 15 mm inferolateral. Vertical incision is made below intersection to identify and decompress bilateral GONs. (**b**) Exposure of the GON (white vessel loop)

sites of nerve compression and release, other potential sites of compression including deeper musculature have been well described in cadaver studies, and should be considered for extended decompression [19, 20]. Finally, adipofascial flaps are elevated on each side of the incision and sewn together to create a soft pad upon which the decompressed GONs are laid to rest.

Rhinogenic Trigger Site

Treatment of rhinogenic migraines focuses on separating "contact points" between the nasal septum and lateral nasal architecture. The patient's preoperative CT scan will dictate the procedure performed to address sites of intranasal contact and/or turbinate pathology. These procedures can include septoplasty to address a deviated septum or septal spurs, turbinate outfracture, and submucous resection of involved turbinates to address hypertrophy or other anomalies contributing to intranasal mucosal contact and irritation [8]. Failure of surgery for rhinogenic migraines may result from contact points that were missed during the initial procedure or inadequate turbinate resection.

Postoperative Care

Migraine surgery is typically performed as an outpatient procedure. Patients should be seen in the first week postoperatively for evaluation of the incision and suture/staple removal as needed. Reported complications associated with surgery include temporary nasal dryness and/or rhinorrhea in treatment of rhinogenic headaches and scalp itching and minor hair loss for the other surgical procedures; there is also a risk of temporary or permanent numbness or paresthesia in the distribution of the decompressed nerve [13]. Temporary frontal branch paresis has also been reported after surgery for temporal migraines, most often from neuropraxia during operative retraction. The most common reasons for failure of migraine surgery include failure to identify all trigger sites or incomplete decompression of the trigger site. Chronic opioid use prior to migraine surgery also predicts decreased response [12]. There may be emergence of secondary trigger sites following decompression of the patient's primary site that then require similar evaluation and management [21]. In the senior author's practice, patients are seen at 1 and 3 weeks postoperatively and begin filling out their first postoperative headache journal and questionnaire at the second postoperative visit. Patients are then seen every 3–6 months for follow-up with continued headache journals as needed. Follow-up MHI scores are calculated at each visit starting at the 6-month postoperative visit.

Long-Term Outcomes

To confirm their initial retrospective findings, Guyuron's group performed a prospective placebo-controlled trial comparing trigger site decompression to sham surgery. Compared to 57.7% of patients in the placebo group, 83.7% of patients who underwent trigger site decompression experienced at least a 50% decrease in headache frequency, severity, and/or duration 1 year after surgery [22]. At 1 year, 57.1% of patients who underwent decompression reported complete headache relief compared to 3.8% of the placebo group. In a 5-year follow-up study to this cohort of patients, 88% reported a positive response to migraine surgery with 29% demonstrating continued complete elimination of headaches [9]. Other groups have reported on their migraine surgery results with response rates ranging from 68% to 95% [3]. Schoenbrunner, Khansa, and Janis [23] found that migraine surgery was cost-effective in comparison to botulinum toxin injection for migraine headaches requiring treatment beyond a period of 6.75 years.

Special Populations: Adolescent Migraine Surgery

There is an estimated 8% prevalence of migraines in pediatric patients [24]. Compared to treatment options for adult patients, there are fewer pharmacologic options for migraine prevention in pediatric and adolescent patients. While use of botulinum toxin A has not been approved by the FDA for use in a pediatric population, several studies have found it to be efficacious in treatment of adolescent migraines [25, 26]. Surgical management should be considered for adolescent patients with severely debilitating migraines that have failed medical management. These patients should undergo the same thorough preoperative workup and identification of trigger sites with the judicious use of botulinum toxin. Surgical decompression of trigger sites has shown statistically significant improvement without significant complications in a small population of pediatric patients ranging in age from 9 to 18 years [27].

References

1. Guyuron B, Varghai A, Michelow BJ, Thomas T, Davis J. Corrugator supercilii muscle resection and migraine headaches. Plast Reconstr Surg. 2000;106(2):429–34.
2. Guyuron B, Nahabet E, Khansa I, Reed D, Janis JE. The current means for detection of migraine headache trigger sites. Plast Reconstr Surg. 2015;136(4):860–7.
3. Kung TA, Guyuron B, Cederna PS. Migraine surgery: a plastic surgery solution for refractory migraine headache. Plast Reconstr Surg. 2011;127(1):181–9.
4. Liu MT, Armijo BS, Guyuron B. A comparison of outcome of surgical treatment of migraine headaches using a constellation of symptoms versus botulinum toxin type A to identify the trigger sites. Plast Reconstr Surg. 2012;129(2):413–9.
5. Lee M, Monson MA, Liu MT, Reed D, Guyuron B. Positive botulinum toxin type a response is a prognosticator for migraine surgery success. Plast Reconstr Surg. 2013;131(4):751–7.
6. Silberstein S, Mathew N, Saper J, Jenkins S. Botulinum toxin type A as a migraine preventive treatment. Headache: J Head Face Pain. 2000;40(6):445–50.
7. Shuhendler AJ, Lee S, Siu MM, Ondovcik MS, Lam MK, Alabdullatif MA, et al. Efficacy of botulinum toxin type a for the prophylaxis of episodic migraine headaches: a meta-analysis of randomized, double-blind, placebo-controlled trials. Pharmacotherapy: J Human Pharmacol Drug Ther. 2009;29(7):784–91.
8. Lee M, Erickson C, Guyuron B. Intranasal pathology in the migraine surgery population: incidence, patterns, and predictors of surgical success. Plast Reconstr Surg. 2017;139(1):184–9.
9. Guyuron B, Kriegler JS, Davis J, Amini SB. Five-year outcome of surgical treatment of migraine headaches. Plast Reconstr Surg. 2011;127(2):603–8.
10. Lipton RB, Stewart WF, Sawyer J, Edmeads JG. Clinical utility of an instrument assessing migraine disability: the migraine disability assessment (MIDAS) questionnaire. Headache: J Head Face Pain. 2001;41(9):854–61.
11. Jhingran P, Osterhaus JT, Miller DW, Lee JT, Kirchdoerfer L. Development and validation of the migraine-specific quality of life questionnaire. Headache: J Head Face Pain. 1998;38(4):295–302.
12. Impact of Preoperative Narcotic Use on Outcomes in Migraine...: Plastic and Reconstructive Surgery [Internet]. [cited 2020 Mar 10]. Available from: https://cdn.journals.lww.com/plasreconsurg/Fulltext/2014/07000/Impact_of_Preoperative_Narcotic_Use_on_Outcomes_in.26.aspx.
13. Guyuron B, Kriegler JS, Davis J, Amini SB. Comprehensive surgical treatment of migraine headaches. Plast Reconstr Surg. 2005;115(1):1–9.
14. Gatherwright JR, Wu-Fienberg Y, Guyuron B. The importance of surgical maneuvers during treatment of frontal migraines (site I): a prospective, randomized cohort study evaluating foraminotomy/fasciotomy, myectomy, and arterectomy. J Plast Reconstr Aesthet Surg. 2018;71(4):478–83.
15. Chepla KJ, Oh E, Guyuron B. Clinical outcomes following supraorbital foraminotomy for treatment of frontal migraine headache. Plast Reconstr Surg. 2012;129(4):656e–62e.
16. A Prospective randomized outcomes comparison of two temple m...: plastic and reconstructive surgery [Internet]. [cited 2020 Mar 10]. Available from: https://journals.lww.com/plasreconsurg/Fulltext/2015/07000/A_Prospective_Randomized_Outcomes_Comparison_of.25.aspx.
17. Gfrerer L, Maman DY, Tessler O, Austen WG Jr. Nonendoscopic deactivation of nerve triggers in migraine headache patients: surgical technique and outcomes. Plast Reconstr Surg. 2014;134(4):771–8.

18. Mosser SW, Guyuron B, Janis JE, Rohrich RJ. The anatomy of the greater occipital nerve: implications for the etiology of migraine headaches. Plast Reconstr Surg. 2004;113(2):693–7.
19. Janis JE, Hatef DA, Reece EM, McCluskey PD, Schaub TA, Guyuron B. Neurovascular compression of the greater occipital nerve: implications for migraine headaches. Plast Reconstr Surg. 2010;126(6):1996–2001.
20. Janis JE, Hatef DA, Ducic I, Reece EM, Hamawy AH, Becker S, et al. The anatomy of the greater occipital nerve: part II. Compression point topography. Plast Reconstr Surg. 2010;126(5):1563–72.
21. Punjabi A, Brown M, Guyuron B. Emergence of Secondary trigger sites after primary migraine surgery. Plast Reconstr Surg. 2016;137(4):712e.
22. Solomon S. A placebo-controlled surgical trial of the treatment of migraine headaches. Plast Reconstr Surg. 2010;125(3):1041–2.
23. Schoenbrunner AR, Khansa I, Janis JE. Cost-effectiveness of long-term, targeted onabotulinumtoxina versus peripheral trigger site deactivation surgery for the treatment of refractory migraine headaches. Plast Reconstr Surg. 2020;145(2):401e–6e.
24. Abu-Arafeh I, Razak S, Sivaraman B, Graham C. Prevalence of headache and migraine in children and adolescents: a systematic review of population-based studies. Dev Med Child Neurol. 2010;52(12):1088–97.
25. Chan VW, McCabe EJ, MacGregor DL. Botox treatment for migraine and chronic daily headache in adolescents. J Neurosci Nurs. 2009;41(5):235–43.
26. Shah S, Calderon M-D, Wu WD, Grant J, Rinehart J. Onabotulinumtoxin a (BOTOX®) for prophylactic treatment of pediatric migraine: a retrospective longitudinal analysis. J Child Neurol. 2018;33(9):580–6.
27. Guyuron B, Lineberry K, Nahabet EH. A retrospective review of the outcomes of migraine surgery in the adolescent population. Plast Reconstr Surg. 2015;135(6):1700–5.
28. Guyuron B, et al. The zygomatictemporal branch of the trigeminal nerve: an anatomical study. Plast Recon Surg. 2005;115(1):273–7.

Dietary Modification and Migraine Relief 11

Kim Hecht and Lilian Au

Food Triggers

The treatment of migraines often encompasses pharmacological and lifestyle modifications, including diet. Patients commonly report dietary factors as triggers for headaches. The International Classification of Headache Disorders III states that the ingestion of different substances can cause headache immediately or within 12 hours of ingestion and resolve after 72 hours after ingestion [1]. Commonly reported triggers are caffeine, alcohol, aged cheeses, chocolate, biogenic amines, and food preservatives with nitrites, nitrates, monosodium glutamate, or artificial sweeteners such as aspartame and gluten [2–4]. Scientific evidence for dietary triggers continues to be debated, but the recognition and elimination of food or additives that provoke headaches may be beneficial for many patients. Food diaries or IgG food antibody testing may provide additional support in determining specific dietary triggers.

Caffeine

Caffeine is extensively consumed throughout the world. It is found in coffee, tea, soda, energy drinks, and chocolate in addition to being a component of combination analgesic medications. Caffeine's effects on the body are dose dependent and use between 50 and 200 mg can increase alertness, energy, memory as well as improve mood [5]. At dosages greater than 300 mg, it can cause anxiety, insomnia, and irritability [6, 7]. The mechanism by which caffeine acts on the central nervous system is through antagonizing adenosine (A1 and A2A) receptors [8]. Through antagonizing

K. Hecht (✉) · L. Au
Susan Samueli Integrative Health Institute, University of California Irvine Health, Costa Mesa, CA, USA
e-mail: khecht@hs.uci.edu

© Springer Nature Switzerland AG 2021

S. Shah (ed.), *Migraine*, https://doi.org/10.1007/978-3-030-75239-2_11

adenosine receptors, caffeine intrinsically provides analgesia, decreases excitatory neurotransmitter release and cerebral vasodilation – which may be potential mechanisms by which it relieves headaches when consumed in combination medications and cause headaches upon withdrawal [9, 10].

Migraines triggered by caffeine occur in around 6.2% [3] to 14.5% [2] of patients. Caffeine overuse has been found in chronic headache in children who consumed about 190 mg of caffeine daily and resolved after discontinuation of caffeine [11]. Lee et al. utilized an observational study of migraine patients with daily caffeine consumption where patients self-selected whether they would completely abstain from caffeine [12]. No differences were found in headache intensity or headache days in the abstinence versus non-abstinence group, but participants in abstinence group had significantly greater efficacy of medication usage.

Headaches are more commonly associated with caffeine withdrawal. Various studies have found caffeine withdrawal headaches occur with sudden termination from daily low-to-moderate consumption of caffeine [13–15]. It is defined as a headache that appears with discontinuation of caffeine following consumption of greater than 200 mg of caffeine daily for more than 2 weeks, developing within 24 hours of discontinuation, and resolves within 7 days of cessation of caffeine [1]. The headaches are characterized as bilateral, throbbing headaches and can be accompanied by nausea [1]. Individuals who regularly consume caffeine are recommended to consume less than 400–500 mg/day and not vary their consumption habits [16]. Others who cannot maintain a consistent routine are recommended to drink decaffeinated coffee [16].

Caffeine in combination with acetaminophen and/or aspirin has been shown to be effective in prevention and treatment of migraines [17–19]. Caffeine may provide pain relief by improving plasma concentrations and decreasing the plasma clearance of the other analgesic medications [10, 18]. Chronic use of caffeine in medications may increase the frequency and intensity of headaches, which in turn leads to more medication usage [20]. Medication overuse headache is defined as a headache occurring on 15 or more days per month in a patient with a pre-existing primary headache that develops after overuse of headache medications for more than 3 months [20]. High medication usage is defined as the use of ergotamines, triptans, opioid, and combination medications 10 days or greater per month or the use of simple analgesics for 15 days or more per month for greater than 3 months [20]. Headaches often improve after overuse stops [1].

Chocolate

Chocolate has been reported to trigger migraines in 2–22% of migraineurs [16]. The potential mechanism by which chocolate is thought to induce migraines is through increased nitric oxide generation leading to vasodilation of blood vessels, or through the release of the neurotransmitter phenylethylamine causing vasodilation then vasoconstriction of blood vessels [21]. Chocolate is also known to contain substances that may also be beneficial for migraineurs such as magnesium, riboflavin, and tryptophan [21]. It remains uncertain whether chocolate is an actual trigger for migraines as only 3 double-blind placebo studies have been performed to date [22–24]. Gib et al. found 41.7% (5/12) of participants developed migraines after eating chocolate versus 0% (0/8) in the placebo group, although the results did not reach statistical significance [22]. Marcus et al. examined 81 females with chronic recurrent headaches and performed 4 trials in each subject [23]: two trials were with carob and two trials were with chocolate. No difference was found between the two groups with respect to incidence of headache. Moffett et al. examined 25 participants in one study, and 15 participants from the first study also participated in the second study [24]. Participants were given two samples, one chocolate and placebo sample at different times. In both studies performed by Moffett et al., there were no differences between chocolate versus placebo. Fifteen participants had headache in the first study, 8 after chocolate ingestion and 5 after placebo ingestion. Eleven participants had no headache after either sample. In the second study, 5 participants had headaches occurred after chocolate only, 3 after placebo only, and 1 participant developed headache after ingesting chocolate and placebo. Six participants had no headache after either sample. Currently, the evidence is lacking with regard to chocolate being a migraine trigger.

Biogenic Amines

Biogenic amines such as histamine, tyramine, and phenylethylamine (PEA) are naturally found in food and beverages and are frequently reported as migraine triggers. They can be found in raw products or produced through the fermentation process [16].

Foods with high histamine content include aged cheeses, fish such as tuna or sardines, vegetables such as spinach, processed meats, strawberries, tomatoes, fermented foods, and some alcoholic beverages [25]. It is also thought that decreased activity of the diamine oxidase (DAO) enzyme may also contribute to elevated histamine and is associated with increased migraines [26, 27]. A histamine-free diet was examined in patients with food intolerances and chronic headaches, where 19 of 45 patients studied had chronic headaches [28]. Headache attacks decreased from 3.1 (±2.3) attacks per week to 1.1 (±1) attack per week ($p < 0.001$), and 6 patients had 50–75% reduction of analgesic medication usage. Izquierdo-Casas et al. conducted a double-blind randomized study examining DAO supplementation versus placebo for 1 month in 100 patients with episodic migraines and documented DAO deficiency [29]. Patients were given 4.2 mg of porcine kidney protein extract with 7% of DAO and enzymatic activity of 10,000 HDU/ml before breakfast, lunch, and dinner or placebo capsules. Researchers found reduction in pain hours from pre-to-post supplementation in the treatment group from 6.1 to 4.7 hours and decreased used of triptans in the treatment arm versus the placebo arm. There was no statistical significance in pain hours between the treatment versus placebo group as the placebo group also had a decrease of pain hours that was nonsignificant and may be due to the short duration of the trial.

Foods high in tyramine include cheese, wine, beans, sausage, and yeast extract [30]. Higher serum level tyramine, dopamine, and noradrenaline have been found in patients with chronic migraines compared to controls [31]. In a review of biogenic amines and headaches from 2003, 12 studies found equivocal results on the ingestion of tyramine and headaches, whereas 5 studies found no exacerbation of migraines with tyramine [32].

PEA is found in various animal products, wine, and chocolate [33]. As discussed under the chocolate section, PEA is thought to mediate migraines potentially through inducing vasodilation and then vasoconstriction of blood vessels [21]. Thirty-six patients with self-reported chocolate-induced migraines were given lactose and PEA capsules to find out if migraines were triggered [34]. No difference was found between the groups, but the participants that did complain of headache, and it was noted 12 hours after ingesting PEA.

Alcohol

Approximately 23% of participants from 42 studies completed between 1984 and 2014 cited alcohol as a trigger for migraines [35]. The variety of alcoholic beverages make it challenging to generalize its effects on migraine [35]. Wine, beer, and whiskey contain more vasoactive bioactive amines than bourbon, gin, rum, or vodka [35]. Wine and beer also contain sulfites and phenolic flavonoids [35]. Littlewood et al. performed a small randomized study on 19 patients to migraines comparing frequency of migraine attacks with ingesting red wine versus vodka [36]. They found 82% of subjects had migraine with consumption of 300 ml of red wine versus 0% with 300 ml of vodka. With respect to the delayed headache or "hangover," alcohol metabolites such as acetate may be the precipitating factor [37]. Those that have alcohol dehydrogenase enzyme 2 allelic variant may be at increased risk of migraine with alcohol usage [38].

Nitrites/Nitrates

Nitrites and nitrates are preservatives found in cured or processed meats such as hot dogs, bacon, sausage, and lunch meats. The trigger was considered when a single-blind case study was performed on a patient who was noted to have multiple migraines triggered with nitrites as compared to no headaches triggered by placebo [39]. No further provocative studies have tested nitrites, but plasma nitrite levels have been found to be elevated in migraine patients during migraine attacks as compared to normal [40]. In a diary study of 326 migraine patients, 2.4% reports nitrites as a potential trigger [41].

Aspartame

Aspartame is an artificial sweetener that is very commonly seen as an ingredient in many foods including chewing gum, sugarless candy, cough drops, yogurt, diet soda, meal replacement shakes, vitamins, and medications. Its consumption has been associated with headaches, anxiety, depression, sleep disturbances, memory loss, and learning impairments [42–44]; 8.2% reported aspartame as a dietary trigger in one study of 171 patients in the Montefiore Medical Center Headache Unit [42]. The metabolism of aspartame leads to the formation of phenylalanine, aspartic acid, and methanol [45]. Methanol is turned into formaldehyde and formic acid which are known toxic substances that may increase oxidative stress [46]. Jacob and Stechschulte found five patients with self-reported history of migraines after aspartame consumption had allergic reactions to formaldehyde on patch testing [47]. Although many experiments document various adverse neurological effects of aspartame [46], the studies on aspartame and its relationship to headaches in humans have found mixed results.

Two randomized control studies discovered associations between aspartame and headaches. Koehler et al. examined aspartame versus placebo capsules in 11 migraine patients in a crossover study [48]. Patients were given aspartame 300 mg capsules versus placebo capsules 4 times a day for a 4-week period with 1 week in between group changes. They found headaches were significantly more frequent in the aspartame versus placebo group. A different crossover study was conducted by Van Den Eden et al. where 32 patients were placed on aspartame 300 mg 3 times a day versus placebo with 1-week washout in between [49]. They found increased percentage of days with headache in the aspartame group with 33% versus placebo group with 24%.

Two studies did not find headaches were induced by aspartame. Lindseth et al. examined the adverse neurobehavioral effects of a high (25 mg/kg/day) versus low (10 mg/kg/day) aspartame diet in healthy adults [43]. Participants were placed on either diet for 8 days with 2-week washout in between. Outcomes related to cognition, depression, mood, and headache were measured. The study found increased depression and irritability in the high-aspartame diet group, but no increased incidence of headaches. The other negative study was conducted by Schiffman et al. examining 40 individuals with self-reported headaches from the consumption of aspartame who were given 3 doses of aspartame versus placebo over 4 hours in a crossover design (1987) [50]. Eight individuals developed headache while receiving aspartame but not placebo, 12 individuals developed headache while receiving placebo but not aspartame, and 6 individuals developed headaches in both trials. No significant difference was found between aspartame versus placebo trials.

Monosodium Glutamate (MSG)

MSG is a food additive used as a flavor enhancer in many processed foods such as soups, snack foods, seasoning salts, and sauces. MSG has been reported to cause various symptoms such as dizziness, abdominal discomfort, and headaches. Obayashi and Nagamura conducted a systematic review of studies examining whether MSG provoked headaches [51]. They divided the studies into two groups, one group where MSG was added to food, and the other where MSG was consumed as a liquid. The integrity of the blinding of patients was also assessed as beverages containing approximately 1.3% MSG or more should be distinguishable from a placebo beverage. In the studies where MSG was added to food, three of six studies deemed properly blinded did not find a difference in headache incidence between MSG versus placebo [52–54]. The studies that involved MSG dissolved in liquid at 1.125–12% found MSG led to headache in 4 of 7 provocation studies [55–59]. A problem with the Baad-Hansen study where MSG was found to provoke headaches was the sodium content and osmotic pressure in the placebo beverage did not match the MSG beverage [58], whereas the negative study from Rosenblum and colleagues did have an osmotically equivalent placebo [55]. Given the equivocal results of multiple studies, it currently remains inconclusive whether MSG provokes headaches.

Gluten

Gluten-related disorders comprise of celiac disease, non-celiac gluten sensitivity (NCGS), and food allergies when gluten is a trigger for primarily gastrointestinal symptoms but may also cause headache or other neurological symptoms as well. Celiac disease affects 1% of general population and results from an immune response to gliadin molecules in gluten which damages the intestinal mucosa [60]. The gastrointestinal symptoms of celiac disease and NCGS are abdominal pain, diarrhea, constipation, and bloating [60–62]. Neurological symptoms such as hypotonia, developmental delay, learning disorders, ADHD, headache, and cerebellar ataxia have also been seen in pediatric patients with celiac disease [61]. Patients with celiac disease will test positive for IgA antibodies to tissue transglutaminase (TTG) and IgG antibodies to gliadin [60]. Diagnosis is generally confirmed with small bowel biopsy showing villous atrophy, but in children where biopsy is not recommend, diagnosis can be confirmed if TTG concentration is 10 higher than the upper limit of normal with positive endomysial antibodies and HLS-DQ2 or HLA DQ 8 [60]. Patients with NCGS will test positive for anti-gliadin IgG but not TTG [60].

Zis et al. performed a systemic review and meta-analysis of headache associated with celiac disease and found a pooled prevalence of headache in adults with celiac disease to be 26%, and in children and adolescents it was 18.3% [63]. Those that suffer from celiac disease and migraines have been found to have occipital and occipitoparietal calcifications and white matter changes on neuroimaging [64–67].

Adults with celiac disease and migraines placed on gluten-free diet have reduced headache frequency from 51.6% to 100% [65, 68]. Children with celiac disease also have improvement of headaches from 69.2% [69] to 100% [70, 71]. Upon reintroduction of gluten, headaches did return in 13% of pediatric patients [72] and 23% in adults [73] that knew they were consuming gluten. In patients with NCGS, one study of 78 children with NCGS found 32% had headaches when not on a gluten-free diet [74]. Gluten may be a food trigger in migraines and headaches for individuals that suffer from gluten-related disorders.

IgG Food Sensitivity Testing and Elimination Diet

Many individuals who suffer from migraine report headache symptoms with eating particular foods or additives as discussed in the previous section on food triggers, which are possibly related to delayed food hypersensitivities. Delayed food hypersensitivities, also known as food sensitivities, are commonly seen in other conditions such as urticaria, angioedema, eczema, and irritable bowel syndrome [75–77]. A food allergy generally causes a systemic immune reaction to the food proteins that may result in urticaria, anaphylaxis, asthma, diarrhea, or vomiting [78]. As opposed to food allergies which are mediated by IgE antibodies and typically cause mast cell activation, IgG food hypersensitivities may cause delayed reactions from chronic antigen exposure that trigger various immune mediators as well as lead to permeability of the small intestinal wall [78, 79]. The delayed reactions can be very similar to IgE-mediated allergy symptoms such as asthma, hives, nausea, vomiting, and diarrhea, but may also cause other symptoms including fatigue, weakness, joint pain or swelling, memory or behavioral disturbances [78]. These food sensitivities may also play a role in migraine symptoms that IgG food antibody testing may be able to elucidate [80].

There are uncertainties regarding the validity of IgG food antibody testing as there may be false negatives and/or false positive results in addition to lack of standardization in methodology [78]. Furthermore, normal subjects and allergic subjects may both be found to have elevated IgG titers to various food antibodies [81]. Lack of statistical difference in IgG food antibody testing has also been seen in other conditions thought to be related to food sensitivity such as in subjects with inflammatory bowel disease versus control subjects [82]. Nevertheless, studies have found differences in IgG antibody titers between controls and individuals suffering from migraines [83]. Multiple studies have also found reductions in migraine severity, frequency, and/or duration with completing an elimination diet based upon IgG food antibody testing and return of symptoms with stopping the diet [83–87]. The various studies that utilized IgG food antibody testing to determine an elimination diet and its effectiveness in reducing migraines are discussed in the following paragraphs.

Arroyave Hernandez et al. examined 108 foods through IgG antibody testing in 56 patients with migraine versus control and found that patients with migraine had between 6 and 30 positive foods versus no more than 4 in the control group [83].

The migraine group was then placed on a specific diet based on their IgG food sensitivity testing for 1–6 months, and 43 patients reported resolution of migraine on the elimination diet. The limitations of this study were that there was no placebo diet or comparison to an alternate diet and the duration of the elimination diet greatly varied between patients.

In a proof-of-concept, non-controlled study conducted by Rees et al., IgG food antibody levels were measured in 61 patients with headaches that lasted less 15 days/month or chronic migraines with frequency of 15 headaches or more/month [84]. The most common foods associated with elevated IgG titers were cow's milk (85.2%), yeast (60.7%), egg white (55.7%), egg yolk (32.8%), wheat (31.1%), gliadin (24.6%), corn (24.6%), and cashews (19.6%). Patients were then placed on an elimination diet. Twenty-two patients changed their diets for 1 month, while 39 patients underwent the diet for 2 months. Patients reported benefit on a 6-point scale with 0 = no benefit and 5 = high benefit. After 1 month, 27.5% of patients found considerable benefit, and after 2 months 38.2% reported considerable benefit (score = 4 or 5). Unfortunately, over 60% of patients who reintroduced foods associated with elevated IgG antibody level into diets had relapse of symptoms.

Alpay et al. conducted the first randomized, double-blind controlled crossover study examining an elimination diet based upon IgG food antibody testing for 266 food antigens in 30 individuals with migraines [85]. Participants initially completed a baseline headache diary for 6 weeks documenting headache attack frequency, headache days, attack duration in hours, pain severity based on visual analog scale, and medication intake. In the second phase, patients were either placed in a 6-week elimination diet or provocation diet for 6 weeks. There was a 2-week period of normal diet between before the third phase which involved completing the opposite diet. Patients were given diets by a dietician and were asked to only eat the foods recommended. Participants in the elimination diet phase had significant reduction in number of migraine attacks, number of headache days, use of acute medication, and total medication compared to baseline and to provocation. There was no difference seen in attack severity or duration between the three phases.

A later study conducted by Mitchell et al. did not find improvement of migraine frequency after an elimination diet based upon IgG food sensitivity testing [88]; 167 patients with migraines randomized to the elimination diet or a sham diet for 12 weeks. Results showed a 24% reduction in headache days over 4 weeks that did not reach statistical significance. There was a 17% attrition rate from the study that may have contributed to the lack of significance. The attrition rate may provide insight into true patient behavior, as patients may not be able to adhere to a restricted diet in clinical practice. It was noted by the authors that the study lacked dietary support as compared to the Alpay et al. study [85] which may have been a factor in the attrition rate. Another weakness was that only 52% of those in the true elimination diet group returned their daily food diary. In contrast, participants in the Alpay group were given a very specific diet and asked not to eat other foods not recommended which would have made it easier to avoid eating foods had elevated IgG antibody titers and would not require a food diary [85]. This may be similar to patients seen in clinical practice, as patients that may have challenges adhering to the diet because of difficulty with self-managing all of the foods and ingredients to avoid.

A few studies have looked at patients that suffer from both IBS and migraines. IBS and migraine share many similarities as both conditions predominantly affect women, are comorbid with other illnesses such as fibromyalgia, depression and anxiety, and are chronic in nature [89]. Chang et al. did a meta-analysis of 6 studies and found that in those suffering from IBS, 25–50% reported migraine or headache symptoms versus 4–19% of controls [90]. In 2012, Aydinlar et al. published a study that was very similar to the Alpay et al. [85] investigation in protocol except that patients had migraine and IBS [86]. Twenty-one patients participated in a double-blind, randomized controlled, crossover study. The study examined 270 food allergens and half of the patients were randomized to either the elimination or provocation diet prepared by 2 dieticians for 6 weeks. Participants were then placed on 3-week usual diet and then switched to the opposite diet for 6 weeks. The elimination diet provided benefits for multiple symptoms and quality of life. Results showed significant improvement in migraine attack count, duration maximum attack severity, number of migraine attacks that needed acute medication, and total medication intake. Participants also had statistical improvements in IBS symptoms of pain-bloating severity and number of bowel movements/week. Patients also reported higher happiness at home and work. The provocation diet was associated with worsening of attack count as well as increased use of acute medication. Given the improvements while on the elimination and the aggravation of symptoms while on the provocation diet, the authors of this study affirmed that the elimination diet is an "active" treatment.

Recently, Xie et al. examined the effects of an elimination diet based on IgG food antibody testing with or without probiotics or just probiotics on symptoms of both migraines and IBS, analgesic usage, and serotonin levels in 60 patients [87]. The probiotic product utilized contained *Bifidobacterium infantis*, *Lactobacillus acidophilus*, *Enterococcus faecalis*, and *Bacillus cereus*. Patients in the elimination diet with probiotics had reduced migraine days at 7 and 14 weeks, while patients on the elimination diet without probiotics had reduced migraine days at 14 weeks. There was no significant improvement in migraine days in the probiotic only group. The use of triptan medications were not altered in any of the groups, but patients in the elimination diet with probiotics utilized less analgesics at 7 weeks, while those in the elimination diet only and probiotic only groups had less analgesic usage at 14 weeks. Bowel habits improved in all groups at 14 weeks, but severity of abdominal distention only improved in the elimination diet with probiotic group at 14 weeks. Serotonin levels were significantly increased in the elimination diet with or without probiotics at 14 weeks. The results indicate that the addition of probiotics to an elimination diet improves migraine days quicker than the standard elimination diet by itself, and it also has the added benefit of reducing bloating as opposed to the other groups. The fact that serotonin levels were increased with the elimination diet with or without probiotics may point to one mechanism why migraines are improved on the IgG-based elimination diet.

Patients with migraines that report aggravation of symptoms with eating certain foods may benefit from IgG food sensitivity testing and an elimination diet as seen by the studies discussed above. Dietician support and high motivation by patients are also important in the success of the therapy.

Comprehensive Diets

Low-Fat Diet

Individuals that suffer from migraines tend have higher cholesterol levels than their non-migrainous counterparts [91–93]. A retrospective study on cholesterol level in migraine patients conducted by Tana et al. found a correlation between migraine intensity and total and LDL cholesterol [92]. Part of the Zabut aging study involved measuring cholesterol levels in adults with migraines over 50 and found those that had migraines had higher total cholesterol than non-migraineurs, and the findings were also more prominent in males [91]. Onderwater et al. observed lower levels of HDL status in males [94]. Gelaye et al. measured cholesterol levels in pregnant females with and without migraines and discovered elevated LDL and total cholesterol levels in the migraine group [93]. Other studies have shown higher levels of free fatty acids during migraine episodes [95] as cited by [96].

Given the association between high lipid levels and migraines, three studies thus far have examined the low-fat diet and its potential for reducing migraines. Bic et al. performed a non-controlled open label study of 54 patients with migraines and reduced their fat intake by more than 50% from an average of 66 gram per day to 28 grams per day over a 28-day period [96]. Migraine frequency was decreased from an average of 6 days per month to 1 day per month after the diet. The second study was a crossover study that compared a low-fat vegan diet and elimination diet to placebo supplement for 16 weeks in each group with 4-week washout in between [97]. The placebo supplement contained 10 mcg of alpha-linoleic acid and 10 mcg of vitamin E. The investigators did not see statistical differences between the groups for headache intensity, duration, or frequency which they attributed to lack of complete crossover and having four participants drop out. Some participants that began in the vegan diet group continued to avoid meat and fish during the washout period and also during the supplement period. In examining the data on those that completed the study, Bunner et al. did find a significant decrease in headache intensity and duration in the diet group and significantly decreased headache number and days in the supplement group. In a sub-analysis of only the first 16 weeks of the study, the authors found a significant decrease in headache number, intensity, days, and use of headache medications in the diet group. The third study that evaluated lipids and migraines was a crossover study involving 83 persons with episodic or chronic migraine were randomized to a low or normal lipid diets and then crossed over to the opposite diet [98]. The low-lipid diet restricted lipids to <20% of their total daily energy intake versus 25–30 in the normal-lipid diet. The results were that those consuming the low-lipid diet had significantly lower attack frequency and intensity than those consuming the normal-fat diet. Overall, the low-fat diet shows benefit in reducing migraines and may be useful for those with elevated cholesterol.

Low Glycemic Index Diet

Many are aware of the benefits of the low glycemic index diet for those with pre-diabetes and diabetes as it reduces blood sugar, free fatty acid levels, inflammation, and weight [99]. The glycemic index (GI) measures how quickly the consumption of a specific type of carbohydrate increased blood glucose levels. Foods that raise blood sugar the quickest are classified in glycemic index group and have GI > 70 [99]. Foods that are digested slower are classified in the low glycemic index group and have GI < 70 [99]. In the low GI diet, individuals are recommended to eat foods on the lower end of the glycemic index such as apples, vegetables such as raw carrots and avoid foods on the higher end such as pastries, bagels, bread, pasta, juices, and sugary carbonated soda [100]. One study has explored the effect of low glycemic index diet on migraines. Evcili et al. examined 350 patients with migraines, who were placed in either low GI index diet or prophylactic medication group (propranolol, flunarazine, amitriptyline, and topiramate) [100]; 344 patients completed the study, and 1 month after dietary restriction, frequency of attacks were reduced significantly in both groups and mean pain score was reduced in only the medication group. After 3 months, the low GI diet reached statistical significance in reducing the mean pain score and the benefit continued in the medication group. Overall, the low GI diet was as helpful in reducing headache intensity and frequency as the medication group, but effects of pain intensity relief were not seen until after 3 months.

Ketogenic Diet and Modified Atkins Diet

The ketogenic diet was first utilized in the treatment of children with non-refractory epilepsy, but its use has also been investigated in patients with migraines, Alzheimer's, Parkinson, brain cancer, polycystic ovarian syndrome, and for weight loss [101–103]. This section will review the different ketogenic diets, contraindications, laboratory evaluations, potential side effects, discontinuation of the diet, and review the prospective studies examining the ketogenic diet in the prevention and treatment of migraines.

What Is the Ketogenic Diet?

The ketogenic diet is a high-fat, low-carbohydrate diet that mimics a fasting state through severely limiting glucose and increasing the production of ketone bodies (B-hydroxybutyrate and acetoacetate) in the liver through the breakdown of fatty acids [104]. The ketone bodies are then converted to acetyl-CoA in the Krebs cycle to produce energy [104]. The diet consists 55–60% of calories from fat, 30–35% of calories from protein, and 5–10% of calories from carbohydrates [105]. Typically, carbohydrates are restricted to less than <50 mg/day [104].

Classic Ketogenic Diet

In the classic ketogenic diet, first used in children to manage non-refractory epilepsy, the total calories and mg of fat, protein, and carbohydrates are determined by age, height, and weight [106]. The classic regimen is 1 g/kg protein with 10–15 g/day carbohydrates, and the outstanding recommended calories are fat [106]. The ratio of fats-to-carbohydrates are generally 4:1, but may start off as 3:1 [106]. Fat consumption primarily comes in the form of long-chain triglycerides [105].

Medium-Chain Triglycerides

A modified form of the ketogenic diet that began in the 1960s involved the addition of medium-chain triglyceride oil [107]. It produces more ketones than long-chain fatty acids and is more easily absorbed by the liver, which allows for more calories to be derived from protein and carbohydrates on this diet [106]. In an animal model, medium- and long-chain triglycerides were found to reduce propagation of cortical spreading depression related to migraine auras [108].

Modified Atkins Diet

The modified Atkins diet also severely restricts carbohydrates to 10 gram/day in children and 15–20 grams/day in adolescents and adults [105, 109]. The majority of diet's remaining calories are from fat without specific limitations in protein [105, 109]. Of note, the recommended dietary allowance of protein in a young adult male or female is 0.75 g/kg/day [110]. Children are also given multivitamins and calcium supplementation in this diet [105].

Very Low-Calorie Ketogenic Diet (VLCKD)

The VLCKD has been used for rapid weight loss in obese individuals and has been shown to produce greater weight loss than a nonketogenic low-calorie diet [103]. Several of the studies discussed below conducted by DiLorenzo and his group of investigators used the VLCKD as a potential therapy for migraines in overweight patients [111, 112]. The diet consists of a total caloric intake of 600–800 kcal/day.

The range of carbohydrate intake is approximately 30–50 g/day, 10–20 g/day of lipids, 0.8–1.2 g/kg of protein for ideal body weight, or approximately 75 g/day of protein and micronutrients to fulfill the dietary reference intake [110–112].

Other Considerations in Ketogenic Diet

Sugar-free options should be carefully examined as additives such as maltodextrin, sorbitol, starch, or fructose contain hidden carbohydrates [106]. Carbohydrates in medications may also need to be accounted for as well [106]. Children with epilepsy undergoing the ketogenic diet are given multivitamin supplements to prevent vitamin and mineral deficiencies [105, 106]. In all the studies discussed below utilizing the ketogenic diet and modified Atkins diet for migraines, participants were given multivitamins [111–113].

Contraindications

Absolute contraindications include carnitine deficiency, fatty acid metabolic deficiencies, pyruvate carboxylase deficiency, and porphyria [105, 106]. Aggravation of various medical conditions may be experienced on this diet and may be contraindicated in those suffering from kidney stones, hyperlipidemia, liver disease, gastroesophageal reflux, constipation, cardiomyopathy, and chronic metabolic acidosis [105]. In one study on migraine utilizing the VLCKD, exclusion criteria also included psychiatric history, pregnancy, or lactation, type I diabetes, use of corticosteroids, use of non-K+ sparing diuretics, and kidney and liver failure [112].

Laboratory Evaluation

Urine ketones are checked regularly throughout the initial weeks to ensure ketosis [105]. Typical serological tests checked every 3–6 months and include urine calcium creatinine, urinalysis, fasting lipid panel, electrolytes, and complete blood count [106]. Adults in the modified Atkins diet from Di Lorenzo et al. study had the following labs checked: "alanine aminotransferase, aspartate aminotransferase, gamma glutamic transpeptidase, lactic dehydrogenase, alkaline phosphatase, bilirubin, blood urea nitrogen, and creatinine" [113].

Maintenance

Studies examining the ketogenic diet in participants with migraines did not examine the diet for longer than 1–3 months.

Potential Side Effects of the Diet

Multiple side effects may be experienced, and health-care providers should be monitoring for various issues. General consumers reported feeling fatigue, headache, dizziness, gastrointestinal discomfort, and heartbeat alterations early on in starting the ketogenic diet that improved after 4 weeks [114]. Approximately 25% of children that began the ketogenic diet experienced one or more episodes of hypoglycemia in the first week [115]. Acidosis may happen during the beginning of the diet and during illnesses [106]. Common gastrointestinal side effects from the classic diet include constipation and worsening of reflux, whereas in the MCT version, individual may experience diarrhea and abdominal cramps [103, 106]. Fatigue commonly occurs with the ketogenic diet, and sometimes carnitine is recommended if there are no further changes to the composition of the diet [103, 106]. Renal calculi happen in 5–6% of children due the elevated secretion of calcium [116–118]. There is also a concern that the ketogenic diet with ingestion of topiramate or other carbonic anhydrous inhibitors may also increase risk of nephrolithiasis [106]. Uric acid may also be elevated [103]. Elevations in total cholesterol, triglycerides, and apolipoprotein B can also be found [119–122]. Patients at risk for hyperlipidemia may benefit from adding MCT oil [107]. Osteoporosis or osteopenia can follow the ketogenic diet [123]. Deficiencies in vitamin D, calcium, copper, selenium, and zinc can occur without appropriate supplementation [106].

Rare Complications

A few cases of death have been reported from children developing acute pancreatitis while on the ketogenic diet [124, 125]. Cardiomyopathy related to selenium deficiency is a concern as 20–50% of children on ketogenic diet were tested and found to have selenium deficiency [126–128].

Discontinuation of Ketogenic Diet

Discontinuation of the diet can be done by gradually lowering the ratio of fats to carbohydrates to 2:1 or 2.5–1 [106].

Prospective Studies on Ketogenic Diet and Modified Atkins Diet

Obesity and insulin resistance have been seen in patients with migraines [129, 130]. Many of the studies discussed below that examined the ketogenic diet and migraines were performed on overweight or obese individuals and have been found to reduce headache frequency, severity, and medication use [111–113, 131].

In a non-randomized open-label study of 96 overweight female migraineurs, participants were placed in either the very low-calorie ketogenic diet (VLCKD) for

1 month or standard low-calorie diet [131]. The participants that were randomized to the VLCKD group spent 1 month eating less than 800 kcal/day with 30 g/day derived from carbohydrates, 15 g/day derived from lipids, and 1.0–1.2 g/kg/day of protein. During the second month, participants in the VLCKD were placed in a transitional diet with nutritional integrators; in the third month, participants continued the transitional diet without nutritional integrators; and finally in the fourth through sixth month, participants were placed on a standard low-calorie diet. The other group was placed on a standard low-calorie diet for 6 months. The participants in the standard low-calorie diet group had 1200–1500 kcal/day that contained 46% carbohydrates, 24% protein, and 30% lipids. Results showed that participants in the VLCKD group had less frequent headache attacks, less headache days, and medications use during the 1st month that slightly worsened during the transitional and standard diet as attack frequency returned to baseline, but headache days and medication usage was still less than from baseline, whereas participants in the standard low-calorie group had significantly decreased headache attacks, headache days, and medication use after the 3rd month of dieting. Overall, improvements in headaches continued after stopping the diet and lasted for the duration of the 6-month study. Diet-induced weight loss stemming from the standard low-calorie diet did not results in the same benefits for reducing migraines as the VLCKD.

In 2018, Di Lorenzo and his group investigated the modified Atkins diet in drug-resistant cluster headache patients [113]. Cluster headaches generally cause one-sided headaches that can occur up to 8×/day and last up to 180 minutes and continue for weeks or months. The clinical study was open label and consisted of only one arm. Eighteen patients were placed on a 3-month diet where they received a modified Atkins diet consisting of 15 g/day of carbohydrates, 0.7–1.2 g/kg/day of protein and high fat derived from the weight of carbohydrates and protein together. In the first month, patients were only allowed 10 of carbohydrates/day. Patients were to avoid rice, grains, cereals, legumes, and starchy vegetables. Lipids were given the form of medium-chain triglycerides, omega-3, and long-chain triglycerides with nutraceutical integrators. At the conclusion of the study, 11 patients experienced no more headaches, and 4 patients had 50% improvement in the number of attacks.

In another study by Di Lorenzo et al., multimodal evoked potentials that were evaluated in 18 participants with migraines were either randomized to a VLCKD or normal calorie modified Atkins diet [111]. Multimodal evoked potentials were used to study brain excitability. At baseline, migraine patients did not habituate to the visual or somatosensory stimulation as compared to healthy controls. Overweight participants in the VLCKD ate less than 800 kcal/day and were placed on four protein shakes, one daily meal of meat or fish which consisted of 30 g/day of carbohydrates 15 g/day of lipids and between 1.0–1.2 g/kg of protein. Normal weight patients in the modified Atkins diet arm had 15 g/day of carbohydrates, 0.9 g/kg/day of protein, and the rest of the diet was fat in the form of food and medium-chain triglycerides and long-chain triglyceride supplements. After completion of the diet, patients in both diet groups had significantly improved migraine frequency and duration as well as normalization of reduced visual evoked potentials and somatosensory evoked potential habituation deficit. Migraine frequency in both groups improved from an average of 4.1–1.3 attacks/month and duration of 50.7–15.8 hours/month. This indicates that the improvements seen in participants in the ketogenic diet group may be due to improved balance of cortical excitation and inhibition events.

Di Lorenzo and his group further studied whether very low-calorie nonketogenic (VLCnKD) diets contained the same number of calories could produce similar benefits as VLCKD did in obese patients that suffered from migraines (2019) [112]. In a limited study with double-blind, controlled crossover design, they randomized 35 participants to VLCKD or VLCnKD for 1 month. Those in the VLCKD group had significantly less migraine days, migraine attacks, and higher responder rate than VLCnKD group, but did not have a significant difference in medication usage. A nonketogenic low-calorie diet was not as effective at preventing migraines even though there was similar weight loss and glycemic profile in both groups.

Overall, the ketogenic diet and modified Atkins diet are very promising approaches to mitigating migraines and headaches. Further studies still need to be conducted on more participants and for longer durations of time.

Nutrients/Nutraceuticals B2, B6, B9, B12, Vitamin D, Magnesium, COQ10, Polyunsaturated Fatty Acids (PUFAS)

Although the etiology of migraines is unknown, there are various factors that may play a role in the pathogenesis of migraines from genetics, environmental exposures, and nutrient deficiencies [132]. Other new approaches for improving and preventing migraine symptoms include nutraceuticals such as the use of vitamins (B2, B6, B9, B12, and D3), minerals (magnesium), and antioxidants (CoQ10) in the prophylaxis of headaches and migraines [133, 134]. Certain nutraceutical therapies have been shown to reduce the frequency and severity of episodes, minimize attacks, and have minimal adverse effects. The mechanisms of action are associated with essential cofactor pathways, mitochondrial function and stabilization, anti-inflammatory response in the pain pathway, and improved antioxidant status. There is evidence that supplementation to correct nutrient deficiencies have prophylactic and therapeutic benefits [135].

Vitamin B2 (Riboflavin)

Mitochondrial deficits resulting in insufficient oxygen metabolism and impairment in brain energy metabolism have been found to be associated with migraine pathophysiology in children and adults [136]. Riboflavin or vitamin B2 is an essential cofactor in oxidative metabolism and precursor to the flavin compounds involved in mitochondrial function and electron transport chain of the Krebs cycle as well as membrane stabilization and maintenance of ATP cellular functions [137–139]. As low riboflavin levels and dysfunction in mitochondrial phosphorylation are suspected in some patients, riboflavin has been evaluated in clinical trials that has shown efficacy and tolerability in migraine prophylaxis [140–142].

Many studies using vitamin B2 have shown it to be effective in migraine prevention. Summarized are randomized controlled trials of low- and high-dose riboflavin treatments, which assessed for improvement in migraine symptoms, severity, and reduction in frequency of attacks. Initial studies by Shoenen et al. reported improved migraine symptoms and decreased migraine attacks from supplementation of 400 mg daily dose of B2 in 49 adult migraine patients with or without aura [142, 143]. Boehnke et al. [141] also found 400 mg daily dose of B2 to be efficacious in migraine symptoms and attacks. Based on riboflavin studies evaluating moderate dose (50 mg/day) by Brujin et al. [144] and high dose (200 mg/day) by MacLennan et al. [145], riboflavin has not been shown to have significant effects on migraine symptoms and frequency in pediatric patients. However, a recent study by Athaillah et al. found a high dose (400 mg/day) of riboflavin treated in 98 adolescents between ages 12 and 17 years for 3 months was significant in decreased frequency, disability, and duration of migraines [146].

The combination of pharmaceutical therapy and nutritional supplementation have been recommended for migraine prevention. Sandor et al. looked at combination therapy of beta-blockers and high-dose riboflavin (400 mg/day) to assess two separate mechanisms of action in migraine pathophysiology [147]. Biochemical shifts affecting cortical information processing in the central nervous system and mitochondrial energy reserves in the brain are hypothesized as potential factors in activating the trigeminovascular system that trigger migraine attacks. Both beta-blocker and riboflavin therapy showed improvement in migraine symptoms with the latter having therapeutic efficacy and no CNS adverse effects. Nambiar et al. also compared lower dose riboflavin (100 mg/day) to propranolol (80 mg/day) for 3 months and both treatment groups showed reduction in migraine frequency, duration, and severity of migraine headaches with no significant difference in study groups [148]. Rahimdel et al. evaluated riboflavin (400 mg/day) compared to sodium valproate (500 mg/day) for 3 months and findings showed decreased frequency, duration, and migraine severity but with no significant differences in both groups [149]. Both studies comparing riboflavin to pharmacological agents did find significant fewer side effects and similar efficacy in vitamin B2-supplemented groups. Gaul et al. evaluated the efficacy of combination nutritional therapy in a double-blind, placebo-controlled trial with riboflavin (400 mg/day), magnesium (600 mg/day), and CoQ10 (150 mg/day). Findings were significant for decreased number of migraine days per month and migraine intensity compared to placebo [150].

Low and high doses of riboflavin have been shown to be safe, efficacious, and well tolerated for migraine prophylaxis in some adults. However, riboflavin studies in children and adolescents are inconclusive as a recommendation for migraine treatment. Further studies on riboflavin therapy and additional data are needed to clarify and refine its therapeutic position in migraine headache prophylaxis.

Cobalamin (B12), Folic Acid (B9), and Pyridoxine (B6)

Homocysteine is a molecule that is synthesized from methionine and involves the methylenetetrahydrofolate reductase (MTHFR) enzyme along with B-vitamin cofactors, cobalamin (B12), folic acid (B9), and pyridoxine (B6) [151–153]. The MTHFR gene has been studied in its relationship to the metabolism of homocysteine [154]. Deficiencies in the enzyme or vitamin cofactors have been associated with hyperhomocysteinemia and considered as a hypercoagulable state. Homocysteine-related endothelial dysfunction and its relationship to hypercoagulability-inducing factors have been associated with cerebrovascular and cardiovascular events such as increased risk of stroke, peripheral occlusive artery disease, and heart disease [155]. Multiple studies have indicated a possible link between MTHFR gene polymorphisms, reduced enzyme activity, elevated homocysteine levels, and increased migraine risk [155, 156].

Many studies did not find elevated plasma homocysteine levels in patients with migraines, although Isobe et al. found that cerebrospinal fluid homocysteine levels to be higher in subjects with migraines with auras as compared to controls [152]. The total concentration of homocysteine in the cerebrospinal fluid was higher in migraine subjects with aura by 376% compared to 41% increase in migraine subjects without aura. However, when B6, B9, and B12 serum concentrations were measured, the findings did not reflect on the change in homocysteine concentrations.

Various studies that supplemented with vitamin B6, B9, and/or B12 to determine if their homocysteine-lowering effects may have benefit in the effectiveness of reducing migraine disability, frequency, and severity are discussed in the following paragraphs.

In a randomized control trial, Lea et al. examined a 6-month trial of daily vitamin supplementation with 2 mg of folic acid, 25 mg of vitamin B6, and 400 μg of vitamin B12 in 52 patients that had migraines with auras and associated with a MTHFR gene variant [157]. There was an overall decrease in the frequency and pain severity as well as lowering of homocysteine levels by 39% compared to baseline was observed in the experimental group versus the control group. Marked findings from the study reported significant reduction in the prevalence of migraine disability from 60% compared to 30% at baseline and improved health-related quality of life for patients from vitamin supplementation therapy.

Menon et al. performed a randomized controlled, double-blinded placebo-controlled trial in 162 female patients with migraines with auras and found 20% reduction in homocysteine and decrease in frequency in migraine disability and pain severity with folic acid 2 mg, vitamin B6 25 mg, and B12 400 μg daily for 6 months [158]. Serum levels of vitamins were also increased in the supplement-treated group compared to placebo. Dietary consumption of B6, B12, and folate also was not significant after the 6-month follow-up. Homocysteine and/or MTHFR gene variants may be a factor in vascular alterations, which when modified through supplementation decreases migraine frequency and severity. Menon et al. also performed a later randomized control trial in 300 female subjects that had migraines with aura and found no benefit from 1 mg of folate, 25 mg of B6, and 400 μg of B12 in disability, frequency, severity, or reduced homocysteine levels [159]. Patients with MTHFR mutation may not respond to lower dose folic acid supplementation because the mutation limits the enzymatic synthesis of folic acid. Those patients may benefit from methylated form of folate or its precursor folinic acid.

Several studies utilized higher doses of B6 and folic acid alone or in combination. Di Rosa et al. gave adolescents between 8 and 18 years (median age 12) with migraines without aura folic acid 5 mg daily for 6 months and found 10 out of 16 patients had complete elimination of headaches, 75% reduction in 5 out of 16 patients, and 50% reduction in 1 out of 16 patients [160]. Plasma levels of homocysteine were normalized after 6 months of treatment compared to elevated baseline levels in 100% of the patients. However, there were no differences that were statistically significant in the reduction of migraine attacks compared to serum homocysteine levels at baseline or post-treatment, and homocysteine reduction during the treatment. Askari et al. conducted a 6-month double-blind, randomized control study examining higher doses of B6 (80 mg) and folic acid (5 mg) daily or folic acid (5 mg) alone [161]. Findings among the 95 migraine patients with aura show significant decrease in migraine characteristics (headache frequency, severity, and headache diary results) from combination treatment of both pyridoxine and folic acid versus folic acid group alone compared to placebo. However, plasma B6 and B9 levels were not measured at baseline and at the end of the clinical trial. Sadeghi et al. also examined a small cohort of 66 patients with migraine with aura that were treated with 60 mg of pyridoxine alone [162]. Findings showed similar effectiveness in reducing severity, duration, and headache diary results with no significant therapeutic effect on the frequency of attacks. This study also had limitations as it did not measure plasma B6 levels and homocysteine levels to be able to determine vitamin B6 deficiency or effect on lowering homocysteine overall.

Vitamin supplementation may reduce migraine disability, frequency, and severity. Therapeutic dosing of vitamin B6, B9, and B12 may benefit cofactor and methylation pathways in homocysteine metabolism and reduction as seen by the studies discussed above. However, larger clinical trials elucidating vitamin supplementation and MTHFR gene polymorphisms in association with homocysteine levels should be further investigated as effective and preventative migraine treatments.

Vitamin D

Vitamin D is a fat-soluble vitamin found in two forms (D2 and D3) and plays an important role in numerous functions in the body from decreasing inflammation, modulating immune function, and controlling the neuromuscular system. Vitamin D's proposed mechanisms of action for its anti-inflammatory and antioxidant effects include its modulation of T-helper cell function, reduction of cytokine release, inhibition of nitric oxide synthase, suppression of prostaglandin E2, and neuroactive steroid properties [163, 164]. Although the role of vitamin D has not been clearly identified in migraine chronicity, it has been suggested that vitamin D deficiency is linked to promoting inflammatory pain mechanisms associated with migraine pathophysiology. Vitamin D status is assessed by determining 25 (OH) serum concentrations and as a biomarker to dietary and physiologic levels synthesized by the skin's exposure to UV radiation [165]. Among previous clinical trials and studies, there is higher prevalence of vitamin D insufficiency and deficiency found in common in patients with migraines [166–169]. Summarized are randomized controlled trials from serum vitamin 25(OH) measurements before treatment and results from vitamin D supplementation in ranges between 1000 and 10,000 IU daily or 50,000 IU weekly, which may reduce frequency and duration of migraine attacks in correlation to vitamin D levels.

Gazerani et al. conducted a randomized, double-blinded, placebo-controlled trial and found insufficient serum 25(OH)D levels in 48 adults between 18 and 65 years of age [170]. The study compared treatment with vitamin D3 100 μg/day (or 4000 IU/day) to placebo over 24 weeks. Findings showed significant increase in 25(OH)D levels in the first 12 weeks and decreased migraine frequency but no effect on migraine severity or pain sensitivity levels. Serum 1,25(OH)2D levels were also measured but showed no significant change after vitamin D3 treatment, and no adverse effects were observed in the study. Buettner et al. performed a randomized, double-blind, placebo-controlled trial of simvastatin 20 mg plus vitamin D3 1000 IU twice daily in 57 adults with episodic migraine to placebo over 12-week baseline and 24-week intervention period [171]. The use of statin therapy in headache prevention has been hypothesized to repair endothelial dysfunction and reduce vascular disease associated with migraine pathophysiology [171]. Serum 25(OH)D levels were measured before and after treatment. Findings demonstrated an increase in serum 25(OH)D levels and significant decrease in number of migraine days and higher responder rate overall. Mottaghi et al. investigated serum 25(OH)D and C-reactive protein (CRP) levels in 65 migraine patients between 10 and 61 years old and treated with a 50,000 IU dose per week for 10 weeks in a randomized, double-blind, and placebo-controlled clinical trial [172]. About 81.5% of the participants were vitamin D deficient or insufficient. There were significant findings in decreased mean headache frequency and mean headache diary results compared to placebo but no effect on headache severity, duration, or association between CRP levels with migraine pathology. However, Knutsen et al. found no significant effect on pain measures (occurrence, anatomical location, degree of musculoskeletal pain by visual analog scale, and headache frequency) in 157 adult patients from a randomized, double-blind, placebo-controlled, parallel-group trial with lower doses of vitamin D3 at 25 μg/day (1000 IU/day) or 10 μg/day (400 IU/day) over 16 weeks compared to placebo [173].

Several pediatric trials also found association of deficient and insufficient serum 25(OH)D levels with migraine headaches and significant responses to vitamin D therapy. Kilic et al. conducted a retrospective study and found migraine frequency, duration, and PedMIDAS scores were significantly higher in pediatric migraine patients with vitamin D deficiency and insufficiency [174]. A total of 92 pediatric patients between 6 and 18 years old with deficient and insufficient vitamin D levels were supplemented with vitamin D3 and compared to pediatric patients with normal

25(OH)D levels who did not receive supplementation. The study found vitamin D therapy in doses of 2000 IU/day for 2 months and maintenance dose of 600–1000 IU/day for 6 months was significant in shortening migraine duration, lowering frequency, VAS, and PedMIDAS scores completed to baseline values in the case-control study. Cayır et al. studied 53 children between 8 and 16 years of age and found a combination therapy with vitamin D (800 IU/day with mildly deficient 25(OH)D levels and 5000 IU/day with severely deficient 25(OH)D levels) plus amitriptyline over 6-month treatment reduced migraine frequency in pediatric patients [175].

Vitamin D supplementation in adult and pediatric migraineurs with insufficient and deficient 25(OH)D levels may reduce migraine symptoms, frequency, and duration. However, previous studies have conflicting results with vitamin D assessment and its role in the management and treatment of migraines. Further studies are necessary to establish consistency in clinical trials and confirm the use of vitamin D3 therapy for migraine prophylaxis.

Magnesium

Magnesium is an abundant mineral that plays an important role in brain physiology and supports various neurochemical processes in the body [138]. It is postulated that magnesium deficiency may influence migraine pathophysiology associated with the following: neurogenic inflammation, neuronal dysfunction, platelet aggregation, cerebral vasoconstriction, and altered mitochondrial metabolism resulting in cortical spreading depression [176–178]. Therefore, multiple randomized controlled trials have investigated the use of exogenous magnesium in intravenous or oral forms to target the biological and physiological mechanisms of migraine pathogenesis. Summarized are trials evaluating the treatment of acute migraine attacks with intravenous magnesium and oral supplementation for migraine prophylaxis.

Intravenous magnesium in various forms for intervention has been evaluated in multiple clinical trials as potential treatment for patients with acute migraine. Shahrami et al. evaluated the effects of intravenous magnesium sulfate (1gm) and combined dexamethasone (8 mg) and metoclopramide (10 mg) in emergency room patients with acute migraines [179]. Two treatment groups were divided from 70 patients and assessed for severity of migraine at 20-minute, 1-hour, and 2-hour intervals after IV infusions. Results were significant in decreased pain severity across all three time intervals in the IV magnesium sulfate group and as an effective and rapid-acting migraine treatment compared to the dexamethasone/metoclopramide group. Earlier randomized controlled trials have also found IV magnesium as an effective medication in the acute treatment for migraine pain and associated symptoms (nausea, photophobia and phonophobia). Bigal et al. investigated the effects of magnesium sulfate, 1000 mg intravenously, compared to 0.9% normal saline in 60 migraine patients with and without aura divided randomly into two treatment groups [180]. Both groups were assessed after 30 minutes, 1 hour, and 24 hours after infusion. Results were significant in decreased intensity of associated symptoms (photophobia and phonophobia) in the migraine with aura and without aura groups but not nausea. Findings in the migraine with aura group receiving IV magnesium sulfate were also significant in improved pain assessments and all associated migraine symptoms compared to placebo controls. There are limited studies with intravenous magnesium as an intervention in acute pediatric migraine treatments in emergency departments. A retrospective study by Martinez et al. investigated IV magnesium sulfate 1000 mg/dose in 23 pediatric and adolescent patients (≤18 years old) who were given 4 doses over 15 minutes [181]. Results after 4 doses showed improved pain relief from about 48% of migraine attacks, and IV therapy was well tolerated among the patients. Pediatric patients who received IV magnesium treatment in the study had previously failed other intravenous acute migraine interventions.

Köseoglu et al. investigated the effects of 600 mg/day dose of magnesium citrate in 30 adult migraine patients without aura between 20 and 55 years old for a 3-month period [182]. Results indicated a significant decrease in frequency and severity of migraine attacks as well as an increase in cortical blood flow in the inferolateral frontal, inferolateral temporal, and insular regions of the brain captured by computerized tomography scans after magnesium treatment, while these changes were not observed in the placebo group. This suggests that oral magnesium treatment may be effective in counteracting the vascular and neurogenic mechanisms in migraine pathophysiology. Peikert et al. also evaluated the effects of 600 mg/day of oral magnesium (trimagnesium dicitrate) in 81 adults patients aged 18–65 years old with migraine [183]. After 9–12 weeks of treatment, overall frequency of migraine attacks, number of days with migraine, and drug intervention for symptomatic migraine treatment were significantly reduced compared to the placebo group. Common side effects of high-dose magnesium are gastrointestinal symptoms including diarrhea and gastric irritation but are mostly well tolerated in treatment groups. Among limited pediatric studies, Wang et al. conducted a randomized double-blind, placebo-controlled trial on the efficacy of oral magnesium for the prevention and treatment of pediatric migraines [184]. In the study, 119 children and adolescents between 3 and 17 years old were randomized to receive 9 mg/kg of magnesium oxide in 3 divided doses or placebo over 12–16 weeks. Results indicate a significant reduction in the number of headache days but inconclusive in the prevention of frequent pediatric migraine headaches.

Among various studies, findings show IV magnesium reduced acute attacks, pain, and associated migraine symptoms. Data from randomized clinical trials support intravenous magnesium therapy as a potential and effective treatment for patients with migraine with aura, or as adjuvant therapy for migraine patients with and without aura. Oral magnesium findings show decrease in overall frequency and intensity of migraine. Based on available studies, IV and oral magnesium therapy for acute and preventative migraine treatment remains unclear for children but maybe effective in acute migraine treatment and migraine prophylaxis for adults. Further larger and prospective studies will need to determine the efficacy of the use of magnesium in the acute and prophylactic treatment of pediatric migraines.

Coenzyme Q10 (CoQ10)

CoQ10 or ubiquinone is a lipophilic antioxidant and essential cofactor of ATP production through the electron transport train. Its function is to protect against impaired antioxidant status, mitochondrial dysfunction and degeneration, and preserve energy metabolism, which have been suggested to improve the clinical manifestations of migraines [185, 186]. The cofactor also counteracts endothelial dysfunction by stimulating endothelial release of nitric oxide and exerts anti-inflammatory properties as well [187]. The following randomized controlled trials are summarized using CoQ10 as a preventative nutrient and therapeutic agent for migraine treatment.

Rozen et al. assessed the efficacy of CoQ10 in 32 adults with episodic migraines and treated with a dose of 150 mg daily dose for 3 months [186]. There was a significant reduction in average number of days with migraine compared to baseline and decreased frequency of attacks with no adverse side effects. Shoeibi et al. treated adult migraine patients with CoQ10 100 mg/day and preventative medications such as sodium valproate compared to placebo for 3 months [188]. Findings showed reduction in symptoms (nausea, phonosensitivity, and photosensitivity) with significant decreases in both frequency and severity of headaches. Higher doses of CoQ10 were also found to be effective and well tolerated with minimal side effects. Sandor et al. evaluated a CoQ10 dose of 100 mg three times daily for 4 months in 42 patients and found significant reduction in migraine attack frequency, days with nausea, and number of headache days [185]. Dahri et al. also treated with high dose (400 mg/day) in 84 women with episodic migraine compared to placebo and found similar significant results of supplementation on duration of attacks, frequency, and severity [189]. A later study by Dahri et al. also measured serum CoQ10 concentration and inflammatory markers associated with migraine pathophysiology at baseline with 400 mg/day dosing for 3 months in 45 women [190]. CoQ10 supplementation did significantly increase CoQ10 serum levels and reduce calcitonin gene-related peptide (CGRP) and tumor necrosis factor-α (TNF-α) but no difference in serum interleukins (IL-6 and IL-10). Findings also showed significant improvement in duration, frequency, and severity of migraine attacks compared to placebo.

Among pediatric studies, CoQ10 supplementation in children and adolescents with migraine were effective and well tolerated with minimal side effects. Slater et al. treated 120 children and adolescents with 100 mg/day dose for 3 months and results showed significant reduction in frequency migraine attacks and improved trend in duration and severity [191]. Hershey et al. measured serum CoQ10 levels in children and adolescents at baseline and found 510 out 1550 patients were below the reference range of <0.5 μg/mL [192]. Of these patients, 252 patients with deficient serum levels were treated with CoQ10 between 1 and 3 mg/kg per day. At follow-up around 3 months, the serum CoQ10 levels had significantly increased (1.20 ± 0.59 μg/mL) with improvement in headache frequency and disability based on PedMIDAS assessment.

CoQ10 has potential therapeutic effects for migraine prophylaxis and treatment for children and adults. CoQ10 deficiency may be common in pediatric migraines and determining deficient serum levels and consequent treatment may result in clinical improvement with therapeutic supplementation. Future studies analyzing the methodology and therapy will be required to assess efficacy and confirm observations in pediatric and adult studies.

Phytomedicine

Butterbur

The use of phytomedicine, or plant-based medicinal formulations, has shown benefits in the treatment and prevention of migraines [193, 194]. Specific medicinal herbs and plants contain active constituents that have antioxidant, anti-inflammatory, and anti-nociceptive effects, which can influence the physiologic processes and biochemical pathways associated with migraine pathophysiology [195].

Petasites hybridus (*P. hybridus*), or commonly known as butterbur, is a member of the Asteraceae family and a purified extract from the rhizome and stems of the perennial shrub that is native to Europe [196]. The active constituents are two sesquiterpene substances in the form of petasin and isopetasin, known to have anti-spasmodic activity, vasodilatory, and anti-inflammatory properties [197]. Petasin reduces spasms in smooth muscle and vascular endothelium. Isopetasin inhibits the lipoxygenase pathways, acts as a leukotriene inhibitor, and modulates prostaglandin metabolism, thus reducing inflammation in blood vessel walls with a marked affinity for cerebral blood vessels [198, 199]. However, there are safety concerns regarding hepatotoxic pyrrolizidine alkaloids from raw and unprocessed butterbur extracts causing sinusoidal obstruction syndrome (formerly known has hepatic veno-occlusive disease) and hypersensitivity reactions to plants within the Asteraceae family [200]. Based on these anti-spasmodic, anti-inflammatory, and vasodilatory properties and with safety concerns aside, these indications have been studied in multiple clinical trials as a potential treatment alternative for migraine prevention.

Summarized below are randomized control trials in adults and children with migraine diagnoses meeting the criteria according to the International Headache Society classifications and using the standardized, registered butterbur root extract, Petadolex®.

Three randomized, double-blind, placebo-controlled trials studied the efficacy and tolerability of butterbur extract for migraine prophylaxis. Grossman and Hanns treated 60 patients with a butterbur extract of 50 mg twice daily dose over 12 weeks and examined migraine frequency, intensity, and duration of attacks with accompanying symptoms [194]. The frequency of attacks decreased by 60% compared to baseline and with excellent tolerance by the experimental group. Diener [201] reproduced the Grossman and Hanns study [194] and found 50 mg twice a day dose was also well tolerated among the 33 patients treated. There was a significant reduction in mean attack frequency from 3.4 to 1.8 after 3 months, and the responder rate (improvement of migraine frequency ≥50%) was 45% in the experimental group compared to 15% in the placebo group. Lipton et al. conducted a three-arm, parallel- group randomized trial with 245 adults between ages 18 and 65 [202]. The study compared migraine frequency attacks per month with a dose of 75 mg twice daily of *P. hybridus* extract, 50 mg twice daily of *P. hybridus*, and placebo over a 4-month period. Marked findings reported reduction of migraine attack by 48% for the 75 mg arm, 36% reduction in the 50 mg arm, and 26% in the placebo group. Lipton also found a higher responder rate of 68% for patients in the 75 mg arm compared to 49% in the placebo arm. In the 4 months of treatment, the 75 mg twice daily dose was found to be more effective than placebo compared to 50 mg twice daily dose and was well tolerated overall with minimal gastrointestinal adverse effects.

Due to the hepatotoxic properties of *Petasites hybridus*, there are limited pediatric studies in its use as a treatment therapy overall. Two preliminary pediatric studies looked at the efficacy and safety of butterbur extract, Petadolex®, compared to the previous adult studies. In a prospective study of 108 children and adolescents between ages 6 and 17 years old, Pothman and Danesch treated patients with 50–150 mg of butterbur extract depending on age over 4 months [203]. Children aged 6–9 years received 25 mg twice daily for 2 months and an optional 25 mg three times daily if needed to achieve a response. Adolescents between ages 10 and 17 years received 50 mg twice daily for 2 months and also an optional 50 mg three times daily if needed as well. Findings report about 81.6% improvement in well-being with at least a 50% reduction in the frequency of migraine attacks during the 4 months of treatment. There was an overall reduction in migraine frequency among the children (67%) and adolescent (62%) groups. The responder rate was about 85.7% in the children's group and 74.1% in the adolescent's group. There was a 63% reduction in attack frequency and 77% responders in the total sample population. The mean duration of migraines decreased from 10 hours to 6.5 hours. Similarly, Oelkers et al. assessed the efficacy of butterbur extract treatment and music therapy in 58 primary school children between ages 8–12 years in a prospective, randomized, placebo-controlled study [204]. The pediatric patients either received butterbur root extract, music therapy, or placebo over 12 weeks with follow-up. Oelkers et al. [204] treated with the same butterbur extract dosing to the Pothman and Danesch [203] study for both children and adolescent groups. During post-treatment, there was a higher reduction in the frequency of migraines with music therapy (65.7%) compared to butterbur (36.1%) and placebo (28.8%), and the difference was significant between music therapy and placebo. In the 6-month follow-up, music therapy (63.2%) and butterbur (58.7%) were significant in decreasing migraine frequency at baseline compared with placebo. There was no difference in responder rates post-treatment and 6-month follow-up.

Overall, the results and minimal adverse events from pediatric studies are consistent with the results of the randomized controlled butterbur extract studies in adults. Butterbur root extract may also be offered as a potential and well-tolerated migraine prophylaxis for children and adolescents suffering from migraines.

Although it has shown effectiveness in most randomized controlled studies in adults, Butterbur has limited data and results in pediatric trials based on study design. In addition, the potential risk of hepatotoxicity related to its preparation has been the cause of concern for further recommendation in its use for migraine prevention. Although the use of herbal treatments may present as potential alternatives in the treatment of migraines, high-quality clinical trials are necessary to further examine the effectiveness, efficacy, and safety as treatments for migraines [205].

References

1. Headache Classification Committee of the International Headache Society (IHS). The international classification of headache disorders, 3rd edition. Cephalalgia. 2018;38(1):1–211.
2. Fukui PT, Gonçalves TRT, Strabelli CG, et al. Trigger factors in migraine patients. Arq Neuropsiquiatr. 2008;66:494–9.
3. Mollaoğlu M. Trigger factors in migraine patients. J Health Psychol. 2013;18(7):984–94.
4. Marmura MJ. Triggers, protectors, and predictors in episodic migraine. Curr Pain Headache Rep. 2018;22(12):81.
5. Nehlig A. Effects of coffee/caffeine on brain health and disease: what should I tell my patients? Pract Neurol. 2016;16(2):89–95.
6. Botella P, Parra A. Coffee increases state anxiety in males but not in females. Hum Psychopharmacol. 2003;18(2):141–3.
7. Nardi AE, Valenca AM, Nascimento I, Freire RC, Veras AB, de-Melo-Neto VL, et al. A caffeine challenge test in panic disorder patients, their healthy first-degree relatives, and healthy controls. Depress Anxiety. 2008;25(10):847–53.
8. Fredholm BB, Battig K, Holmen J, Nehlig A, Zvartau EE. Actions of caffeine in the brain with special reference to factors that contribute to its widespread use. Pharmacol Rev. 1999;51(1):83–133.
9. Sawynok J. Caffeine and pain. Pain. 2011;152(4):726–9.
10. Shapiro RE. Caffeine and headaches. Curr Pain Headache Rep. 2008;12(4):311–5.
11. Hering-Hanit R, Gadoth N. Caffeine-induced headache in children and adolescents. Cephalalgia. 2003;23(5):332–5.
12. Lee MJ, Choi HA, Choi H, Chung CS. Caffeine discontinuation improves acute migraine treatment: a prospective clinic-based study. J Headache Pain. 2016;17(1):71.
13. Lader M, Cardwell CC, Shine P, Scott N. Caffeine withdrawal symptoms and rate of metabolism. J Psychopharmacol. 1996;10(2):110–8.
14. Rubin GJ, Smith AP. Caffeine withdrawal and headaches. Nutr Neurosci. 1999;2(2):123–6.
15. Silverman K, Evans SM, Strain EC, Griffiths RR. Withdrawal syndrome after the double-blind cessation of caffeine consumption. N Engl J Med. 1992;327(16):1109–14.
16. Martin VT, Vij B. Diet and headache: part 1. Headache. 2016;56(9):1543–52.
17. Derry CJ, Derry S, Moore RA. Caffeine as an analgesic adjuvant for acute pain in adults. Cochrane Database Syst Rev. 2014;(12):CD009281.
18. Diener HC, Pfaffenrath V, Pageler L, Peil H, Aicher B. The fixed combination of acetylsalicylic acid, paracetamol and caffeine is more effective than single substances and dual combination for the treatment of headache: a multicentre, randomized, double-blind, single-dose, placebo-controlled parallel group study. Cephalalgia. 2005;25(10):776–87.
19. Goldstein J, Silberstein SD, Saper JR, Elkin AH, Smith TR, Gallagher RM, et al. Acetaminophen, aspirin, and caffeine versus sumatriptan succinate in the early treatment of migraine: results from the ASSET trial. Headache. 2005;45(8):973–82.
20. Diener H, Holle D, Solbach K, Gaul C. Medication-overuse headache: risk factors, pathophysiology and management. Nat Rev Neurol. 2016;12(10):575–83.
21. Nowaczewska M, Wiciński M, Kaźmierczak W, Kaźmierczak H. To eat or not to eat: a review of the relationship between chocolate and migraines. Nutrients. 2020;12(3):608.

22. Gibb CM, Davies PT, Glover V, Steiner TJ, Rose FC, Sandler MS. Chocolate is a migraine-provoking agent. Cephalalgia. 1991;11(2):93–5.
23. Marcus DA, Scharff L, Turk D, Gourley LM. A double-blind provocative study of chocolate as a trigger of headache. Cephalalgia. 1997;17(8):855–62.
24. Moffett AM, Swash M, Scott DF. Effect of chocolate in migraine: a double-blind study. J Neurol Neurosurg Psychiatry. 1974;37(4):445–8.
25. Silla Santos MH. Biogenic amines: their importance in foods. Int J Food Microbiol. 1996;29(2–3):213–31.
26. Garcia-Martin E, Martinez C, Serrador M, Alonso-Navarro H, Ayuso P, Navacerrada F, et al. Diamine oxidase rs10156191 and rs2052129 variants are associated with the risk for migraine. Headache. 2015;55(2):276–86.
27. Meza-Velázquez R, López-Márquez F, Espinosa-Padilla S, Rivera-Guillen M, Ávila-Hernández J, Rosales-González M. Association of diamine oxidase and histamine N-methyltransferase polymorphisms with presence of migraine in a group of Mexican mothers of children with allergies. Neurologia. 2017;32(8):500–7.
28. Wantke F, Götz M, Jarisch R. Histamine-free diet: treatment of choice for histamine-induced food intolerance and supporting treatment for chronic headaches. Clin Exp Allergy. 1993;23(12):982–5.
29. Izquierdo Casas J, Comas Basté O, Latorre Moratalla ML, Lorente Gascón M, Duelo A, Soler-Singla L, et al. Diamine oxidase (DAO) supplement reduces headache in episodic migraine patients with DAO deficiency: a randomized double-blind trial. Clin Nutr (Edinb). 2019;38(1):152–8.
30. McCabe BJ. Dietary tyramine and other pressor amines in MAOI regimens: a review. J Am Diet Assoc. 1986;86(8):1059–64.
31. D'Andrea G, D'Amico D, Bussone G, Bolner A, Aguggia M, Saracco MG, et al. The role of tyrosine metabolism in the pathogenesis of chronic migraine. Cephalalgia. 2013;33(11):932–7.
32. Jansen SC, van Dusseldorp M, Bottema KC, Dubois AE. Intolerance to dietary biogenic amines: a review. Ann Allergy Asthma Immunol. 2003;91(3):233–40.
33. Borkum JM. Migraine triggers and oxidative stress: a narrative review and synthesis. Headache. 2016;56(1):12–35.
34. Sandler M, Youdim MB, Hanington E. A phenylethylamine oxidising defect in migraine. Nature. 1974;250(464):335–7.
35. Davis-Martin RE, Polk AN, Smitherman TA. Alcohol use as a comorbidity and precipitant of primary headache: review and meta-analysis. Curr Pain Headache Rep. 2017;21(10):42.
36. Littlewood JT, Gibb C, Glover V, Sandler M, Davies PT, Rose FC. Red wine as a cause of migraine. Lancet. 1988;1(8585):558–9.
37. Maxwell CR, Spangenberg RJ, Hoek JB, Silberstein SD, Oshinsky ML. Acetate causes alcohol hangover headache in rats. PLoS One. 2010;5(12):e15963.
38. Garcia-Martin E, Martinez C, Serrador M, Alonso-Navarro H, Navacerrada F, Agundez JA, et al. Alcohol dehydrogenase 2 genotype and risk for migraine. Headache. 2010;50(1):85–91.
39. Henderson WR, Raskin NH. "Hot-dog" headache: individual susceptibility to nitrite. Lancet (British Edition). 1972;2(7788):1162–3.
40. Neyal M, Geyik S, Çekmen M, Balat A, Neyal A. Elevated plasma total nitrite levels may be related to migraine attacks. Gaziantep Med J. 2014;20(4):299–30.
41. Peris F, Donoghue S, Torres F, Mian A, Wöber C. Towards improved migraine management: determining potential trigger factors in individual patients. Cephalalgia. 2017;37(5):452–63.
42. Lipton RB, Newman LC, Cohen JS, Solomon S. Aspartame as a dietary trigger of headache. Headache. 1989;29(2):90–2.
43. Lindseth GN, Coolahan SE, Petros TV, Lindseth PD. Neurobehavioral effects of aspartame consumption. Res Nurs Health. 2014;37(3):185–93.
44. Rycerz K, Jaworska-Adamu JE. Effects of aspartame metabolites on astrocytes and neurons. Folia Neuropathol. 2013;51(1):10–7.

45. Humphries P, Pretorius E, Naude H. Direct and indirect cellular effects of aspartame on the brain. Eur J Clin Nutr. 2008;62(4):451–62.
46. Choudhary AK, Lee YY. Neurophysiological symptoms and aspartame: what is the connection? Nutr Neurosci. 2018;21(5):306–16.
47. Jacob SE, Stechschulte S. Formaldehyde, aspartame, and migraines: a possible connection. Dermatitis. 2008;19(3):E10–1.
48. Koehler SM, Glaros A. The effect of aspartame on migraine headache. Headache. 1988;28(1):10–4.
49. Van den Eeden SK, Koepsell TD, Longstreth WT, Van Belle G, Daling JR, McKnight B. Aspartame ingestion and headaches: a randomized crossover trial. Neurology. 1994;44(10):1787.
50. Schiffman SS, Buckley CE, Sampson HA, Massey EW, Baraniuk JN, Follett JV. Aspartame and susceptibility to headache. N Engl J Med. 1987;317(19):1181–5.
51. Obayashi Y, Nagamura Y. Does monosodium glutamate really cause headache?: a systematic review of human studies. J Headache Pain. 2016;17:54.
52. Tanphaichitr V, Srianujata S, Pothisiri P, Sammasut R, Kulapongse S. Post prandial responses to Thai foods with and without added monosodium L-glutamate. Nutr Rep Int. 1983;28(4):783–92.
53. Tarasoff L, Kelly MF. Monosodium L-glutamate: a double-blind study and review. Food Chem Toxicol. 1993;31(12):1019–35.
54. Prawirohardjono W, Dwiprahasto I, Astuti I, Hadiwandowo S, Kristin E, Muhammad M, et al. The administration to Indonesians of monosodium L-glutamate in Indonesian foods: an assessment of adverse reactions in a randomized double-blind, crossover, placebo-controlled study. J Nutr. 2000;130(4S Suppl):1074S–6S.
55. Rosenblum I, Bradley JD, Coulston F. Single and double blind studies with oral monosodium glutamate in man. Toxicol Appl Pharmacol. 1971;18(2):367–73.
56. Yang WH, Drouin MA, Herbert M, Mao Y, Karsh J. The monosodium glutamate symptom complex: assessment in a double-blind, placebo- controlled, randomized study. J Allergy Clin Immunol. 1997;99(6 Pt 1):757–62.
57. Geha RS, Beiser A, Ren C, Patterson R, Greenberger PA, Grammer LC, et al. Multicenter, double-blind, placebo-controlled, multiple-challenge evaluation of reported reactions to monosodium glutamate. J Allergy Clin Immunol. 2000;106(5):973–80.
58. Baad-Hansen L, Cairns B, Ernberg M, Svensson P. Effect of systemic monosodium glutamate (MSG) on headache and pericranial muscle sensitivity. Cephalalgia. 2010;30(1):68–76.
59. Shimada A, Cairns BE, Vad N, Ulriksen K, Pedersen AM, Svensson P, et al. Headache and mechanical sensitization of human pericranial muscles after repeated intake of monosodium glutamate (MSG). J Headache Pain. 2013;14(1):2.
60. Lebwohl B, Sanders DS, Green PH. Coeliac disease. Lancet (British Edition). 2018;391(10115):70–81.
61. Zelnik N, Pacht A, Obeid R, Lerner A. Range of neurologic disorders in patients with celiac disease. Pediatrics. 2004;113(6):1672–6.
62. Leonard MM, Sapone A, Catassi C, Fasano A. Celiac disease and nonceliac gluten sensitivity: a review. JAMA. 2017;318(7):647–56.
63. Zis P, Julian T, Hadjivassiliou M. Headache associated with coeliac disease: a systematic review and meta-analysis. Nutrients. 2018;10(10):1445.
64. La Mantia L, Pollo B, Savoiardo M, Costa A, Eoli M, Allegranza A, et al. Meningo-cortical calcifying angiomatosis and celiac disease. Clin Neurol Neurosurg. 1998;100(3):209–15.
65. Hadjivassiliou M, Grünewald RA, Lawden M, Davies-Jones GA, Powell T, Smith CM. Headache and CNS white matter abnormalities associated with gluten sensitivity. Neurology. 2001;56(3):385–8.
66. D'Amico D, Rigamonti A, Spina L, Bianchi-Marzoli S, Vecchi M, Bussone G. Migraine, celiac disease, and cerebral calcifications: a new case. Headache. 2005;45(9):1263–7.

67. Currie S, Hadjivassiliou M, Clark MJ, Sanders DS, Wilkinson ID, Griffits PD, et al. Should we be 'nervous' about coeliac disease? Brain abnormalities in patients with coeliac disease referred for neurological opinion. J Neurol Neurosurg Psychiatry. 2012;83(12):1216–21.
68. Gabrielli M, Cremonini F, Fiore G, Addolorato G, Padalino C, Candelli M, et al. Association between migraine and celiac disease: results from a preliminary case-control and therapeutic study [published correction appears in Am J Gastroenterol. 2003;98(7):1674]. Am J Gastroenterol. 2003;98(3):625–9.
69. Terrone G, Parente I, Romano A, Auricchio R, Greco L, Del Giudice E. The pediatric symptom checklist as screening tool for neurological and psychosocial problems in a paediatric cohort of patients with coeliac disease. Acta Paediatr. 2013;102(7):e325–8.
70. Lionetti E, Francavilla R, Maiuri L, Ruggieri M, Spina M, et al. Headache in pediatric patients with celiac disease and its prevalence as a diagnostic clue. J Pediatr Gastroenterol Nutr. 2009;49(2):202–7.
71. Nenna R, Petrarca L, Verdecchia P, Florio M, Pietropaoli N, Mastrogiorgio G, et al. Celiac disease in a large cohort of children and adolescents with recurrent headache: a retrospective study. Dig Liver Dis. 2016;48(5):495–8.
72. Rashid M, Cranney A, Zarkadas M, Graham ID, Switzer C, Case S, et al. Celiac disease: evaluation of the diagnosis and dietary compliance in Canadian children. Pediatrics. 2005;116(6):e754–9.
73. Zarkadas M, Cranney A, Case S, Molloy M, Switzer C, Graham ID, et al. The impact of a gluten-free diet on adults with coeliac disease: results of a national survey. J Hum Nutr Diet. 2006;19(1):41–9.
74. Volta U, Tovoli F, Cicola R, Parisi C, Fabbri A, Piscaglia M, et al. Serological tests in gluten sensitivity (nonceliac gluten intolerance). J Clin Gastroenterol. 2012;46(8):680–5.
75. Steiner UC, Kolliker L, Weber-Chrysochoou C, Schmid-Grendelmeier P, Probst E, Wuillemin WA, et al. Food as a trigger for abdominal angioedema attacks in patients with hereditary angioedema. Orphanet J Rare Dis. 2018;13(1)90.
76. Liu Y, Yan H, Shao F, Li QH, Cui M. Correlation between childhood eczema and specific IgG antibody level. J Biol Regul Homeost Agents. 2018;32(2):341–4.
77. Guo H, Jiang T, Wang J, Chang Y, Guo H, Zhang W. The value of eliminating foods according to food-specific immunoglobulin G antibodies in irritable bowel syndrome with diarrhoea. J Int Med Res. 2012;40(1):204–10.
78. Mullin GE, Swift KM, Lipski L, Turnbull LK, Rampertab SD. Testing for food reactions. Nutr Clin Pract. 2010;25(2):192–8.
79. Nowak-Wegrzyn A, Bloom KA, Sicherer SH, Shreffler WG, Noone S, Wanich N, Sampson HA. Tolerance to extensively heated milk in children with cow's milk allergy. J Allergy Clin Immunol. 2008;122(2):342–7.
80. Pascual J, Oterino A. IgG-mediated allergy: a new mechanism for migraine attacks? Cephalalgia. 2010;30(7):777–9.
81. Aalberse RC, Van Milligen F, Tan KY, Stapel SO. Allergen-specific IgG4 in atopic disease. Allergy. 1993;48(8):559–69.
82. Jansen A, Mandić AD, Bennek E, Frehn L, Verdier J, Tebrügge I, Lutz H, Streetz K, Trautwein C, Sellge G. Anti-food and anti-microbial IgG subclass antibodies in inflammatory bowel disease. Scand J Gastroenterol. 2016;51(12):1453–61.
83. Arroyave Hernandez CM, Echavarria Pinto M, Hernandez Montiel HL. Food allergy mediated by IgG antibodies associated with migraine in adults. Rev Alerg Mex. 2007;54(5):162–8.
84. Rees T, Watson D, Lipscombe S, Speight H, Cousins P, Hadman G, et al. A prospective audit of food intolerance among migraine patients in primary care clinical practice. Headache Care. 2005;2(2):105–10.
85. Alpay K, Ertas M, Orhan EK, Ustay DK, Lieners C, Baykan B. Diet restriction in migraine, based on IgG against foods: a clinical double-blind, randomised, cross-over trial. Cephalalgia. 2010;30(7):829–37.

86. Aydinlar EI, Dikmen PY, Tiftikci A, et al. IgG-based elimination diet in migraine plus irritable bowel syndrome. Headache. 2013;53(3):514–25.
87. Xie Y, Zhou G, Xu Y, He B, Wang Y, Ma R, Chang Y, He D, Xu C, Xiao Z. Effects of diet based on IgG elimination combined with probiotics on migraine plus irritable bowel syndrome. Pain Res Manag. 2019;2019:7890461. https://doi.org/10.1155/2019/7890461.
88. Mitchell N, Hewitt CE, Jayakody S, Islam M, Adamson J, Watt I, Torgerson DJ. Randomised controlled trial of food elimination diet based on IgG antibodies for the prevention of migraine like headaches. Nutr J. 2011;10:85. https://doi.org/10.1186/1475-2891-10-85.
89. Arzani M, Jahromi SR, Ghorbani Z, Vahabizad F, Martelletti P, Ghaemi A, et al. School of Advanced Studies of the European Headache Federation (EHF-SAS). Gut-brain Axis and migraine headache: a comprehensive review. J Headache Pain. 2020;21(1):15.
90. Chang FY, Lu CL. Irritable bowel syndrome and migraine: bystanders or partners? J Neurogastroenterol Motil. 2013;19(3):301–11.
91. Monastero R, Pipia C, Cefalù AB, Liveri ET, Rosano R, Carmada R, et al. Association between plasma lipid levels and migraine in subjects aged > or =50 years: preliminary data from the Zabùt Aging Project. Neurol Sci. 2008;29(Suppl 1):S179–81.
92. Tana C, Santilli F, Martelletti P, di Vincenzo A, Cipollone F, Davi G, et al. Correlation between migraine severity and cholesterol levels. Pain Pract. 2015;15(7):662–70.
93. Gelaye B, Larrabure-Torrealva GT, Qiu C, Luque Fernandez MA, Peterlin BL, Sanchez S, et al. Fasting lipid and lipoproteins concentrations in pregnant women with a history of migraine. Headache. 2015;55(5):646–57.
94. Onderwater GL, Ligthart L, Bot M, Demirkan A, Fu J, van der Kallen CJ, et al. Large-scale plasma metabolome analysis reveals alterations in HDL metabolism in migraine. Neurology. 2019;92(16):e1899–911.
95. Anthony M. Role of individual free fatty acids in migraine. Headache. 1978;6:110–6.
96. Bic Z, Blix GG, Hopp HP, Leslie FM, Schell MJ. The influence of a low-fat diet on incidence and severity of migraine headaches. J Womens Health Gend Based Med. 1999;8(5):623–30.
97. Bunner AE, Agarwal U, Gonzales JF, Valente F, Barnard ND. Nutrition intervention for migraine: a randomized crossover trial. J Headache Pain. 2014;15(1)69.
98. Ferrara LA, Pacioni D, Di Fronzo V, Russo BF, Speranza E, Carlino V, et al. Low-lipid diet reduces frequency and severity of acute migraine attacks. Nutr Metab Cardiovasc Dis. 2015;25(4):370–5.
99. Radulian G, Rusu E, Dragomir A, Posea M. Metabolic effects of low glycaemic index diets. Nutr J. 2009;8:5.
100. Evcili G, Utku U, Öğün MN, Özdemir G. Early and long period follow-up results of low glycemic index diet for migraine prophylaxis. Ağrı. 2018;30(1):8–11.
101. Stafstrom CE, Rho JM. The ketogenic diet as a treatment paradigm for diverse neurological disorders. Front Pharmacol. 2012;3(59):1–8.
102. Paoli A, Mancin L, Giacona MC, Bianco A, Caprio M. Effects of a ketogenic diet in overweight women with polycystic ovary syndrome. J Transl Med. 2020;18(1):104.
103. Moreno B, Bellido D, Sajoux I, Goday A, Saavedra D, Crujeiras AB, et al. Comparison of a very low-calorie-ketogenic diet with a standard low-calorie diet in the treatment of obesity. Endocrine. 2014;47(3):793–805.
104. Paoli A, Rubini A, Volek JS, Grimaldi KA. Beyond weight loss: a review of the therapeutic uses of very-low-carbohydrate (ketogenic) diets. Eur J Clin Nutr. 2013;67(8):789–96.
105. Kossoff E. Ketogenic dietary therapies for the treatment of epilepsy. In: Post TW, editor. UpToDate. Waltham: UpToDate; 2019. Uptodate accessed: April 1, 2020.
106. Sinha SR, Kossoff EH. The ketogenic diet. Neurologist. 2005;11(3):161–70.
107. Huttenlocher PR, Wilbourn AJ, Signore JM. Medium chain triglycerides as a therapy for intractable childhood epilepsy. Neurology. 1971;21(11):1097–103.
108. de Almeida Rabello Oliveira M, da Rocha Ataıde T, de Oliveira SL, de Melo Lucena AL, de Lira CE, Soares AA, Santos de Almeida CB, et al. Effects of short-term and long-term treatment with medium- and long-chain triglycerides ketogenic diet on cortical spreading depression in young rats. Neurosci Lett. 2008;434(1):66–70.

109. Kossoff EH, Rowley H, Sinha SR, Vining EP. A prospective study of the modified Atkins diet for intractable epilepsy in adults. Epilepsia. 2008;49(2):316–9.
110. National Research Council (US) Subcommittee on the Tenth Edition of the Recommended Dietary Allowances. Chapter 6: Protein and amino acids. In: Recommended dietary allowances (10th ed.). Washington, DC: National Academies Press; 1989. Available from: https://www.ncbi.nlm.nih.gov/books/NBK234922/. Accessed on 10 Apr 2020.
111. Di Lorenzo C, Coppola G, Bracaglia M, Di Lenola D, Evangelista M, Sirianni G, et al. Cortical functional correlates of responsiveness to short-lasting preventive intervention with ketogenic diet in migraine: a multimodal evoked potentials study. J Headache Pain. 2016;17:58.
112. Di Lorenzo C, Pinto A, Ienca R, Coppola G, Sirianni G, Di Lorenzo G, et al. A randomized double-blind, cross-over trial of very low-calorie diet in overweight migraine patients: a possible role for ketones? Nutrients. 2019;11(8):1742.
113. Di Lorenzo C, Coppola G, Di Lenola D, Evangelista M, Sirianni G, Rossi P, et al. Efficacy of modified Atkins ketogenic diet in chronic cluster headache: an open-label, single-arm, clinical trial. Front Neurol. 2018;9:64.
114. Bostock EC, Kirkby KC, Taylor BV, Hawrelak JA. Consumer reports of "keto flu" associated with the ketogenic diet. Front Nutr. 2020;7:20.
115. Lin A, Turner Z, Doerrer SC, Stanfield A, Kossoff EH. Complications during ketogenic diet initiation: prevalence, treatment, and influence on seizure outcomes. Pediatr Neurol. 2017;68:35–9.
116. Furth SL, Casey JC, Pyzik PL, Neu AM, Docimo SG, Vining EP, et al. Risk factors for urolithiasis in children on the ketogenic diet. Pediatr Nephrol. 2000;15(1–2):125–8.
117. Kossoff EH, Pyzik PL, Furth SL, Hladky HD, Freeman JM, Vining EP. Kidney stones, carbonic anhydrase inhibitors, and the ketogenic diet. Epilepsia. 2002;43(1):1168–71.
118. Sampath A, Kossoff EH, Furth SL, Pyzik PL, Vining EP. Kidney stones and the ketogenic diet: risk factors and prevention. J Child Neurol. 2007;22(4):375–8.
119. Dekaban AS. Plasma lipids in epileptic children treated with the high fat diet. Arch Neurol. 1966;15(2):177–84.
120. Chesney D, Brouhard BH, Wyllie E, Powaski K. Biochemical abnormalities of the ketogenic diet in children. Clin Pediatr (Phila). 1999;38(2):107–9.
121. Kwiterovich PO, Jr Vining EP, Pyzik P, Skolasky R, Jr Freeman JM. Effect of a high-fat ketogenic diet on plasma levels of lipids, lipoproteins, and apolipoproteins in children. JAMA. 2003;290(7):912–20.
122. Cervenka MC, Patton K, Eloyan A, Henry B, Kossoff EH. The impact of the modified Atkins diet on lipid profiles in adults with epilepsy. Nutr Neurosci. 2016;19(3):131–7.
123. Kang HC, Chung DE, Kim DW, Kim HD. Early- and late-onset complications of the ketogenic diet for intractable epilepsy. Epilepsia. 2004;45(9):1116–23.
124. Stewart WA, Gordon K, Camfield P. Acute pancreatitis causing death in a child on the ketogenic diet. J Child Neurol. 2001;16(9):682.
125. Buse GJ, Riley KD, Dress CM, Neumaster TD. Patient with gemfibrozil-controlled hypertriglyceridemia that developed acute pancreatitis after starting ketogenic diet. Curr Surg. 2004;61(2):224–6.
126. Bergqvist AG, Chee CM, Lutchka L, Rychik J, Stallings VA. Selenium deficiency with cardiomyopathy: a complication of the ketogenic diet. Epilepsia. 2003;44(4):618–20.
127. Sirikonda NS, Patten WD, Phillips JR, Mullett CJ. Ketogenic diet: rapid onset of selenium deficiency-induced cardiac decompensation. Pediatr Cardiol. 2012;33(5):834–8.
128. Arslan N, Kose E, Guzel O. The effect of ketogenic diet on serum selenium levels in patients with intractable epilepsy. Biol Trace Elem Res. 2017;178(1):1–6.
129. Bigal ME, Lipton RB. Obesity is a risk factor for transformed migraine but not chronic tension-type headache. Neurology. 2006;67(2):252–7.
130. Chai N, Scher AI, Moghekar A, Bond DS, Peterlin BL. Obesity and headache: part I–a systematic review of the epidemiology of obesity and headache. Headache. 2014;54(2):219–34.

131. Di Lorenzo C, Coppola G, Sirianni G, Di Lorenzo G, Bracaglia M, Di Lenola D, et al. Migraine improvement during short lasting ketogenesis: a proof-of-concept study. Eur J Neurol. 2015;22(1):170–7.
132. Mulder EJ, Van Baal C, Gaist D, Kallela M, Kaprio J, Svensson DA, et al. Genetic and environmental influences on migraine: a twin study across six countries. Twin Res. 2003;6(5):422–31.
133. Orr SL, Kabbouche MA, O'Brien HL, Kacperski J, Powers SW, Hershey AD. Paediatric migraine: evidence-based management and future directions. Nat Rev Neurol. 2018;14(9):515–27.
134. Sangermani R, Boncimino A. The use of nutraceutics in children's and adolescent's headache. Neurol Sci. 2017;38(Suppl 1):121–4.
135. Nattagh-Eshtivani E, Sani MA, Dahri M, Ghalichi F, Ghavami A, Arjang P, et al. The role of nutrients in the pathogenesis and treatment of migraine headaches. Biomed Pharmacother. 2018;102:317–25.
136. Panetta J, Smith LJ, Boneh A. Effect of high-dose vitamins, coenzyme Q and high-fat diet in paediatric patients with mitochondrial diseases. J Inherit Metab Dis. 2004;27(4):487–98.
137. Gasparini CF, Sutherland HG, Griffiths LR. Studies on the pathophysiology and genetic basis of migraine. Curr Genomics. 2013;14(5):300–15.
138. Taylor FR. Nutraceuticals and headache: the biological basis. Headache. 2011;51(3):484–501.
139. Barbiroli B, Montagna P, Cortelli P, Funicello R, Iotti S, Monari L, et al. Abnormal brain and muscle energy metabolism shown by 31P magnetic resonance spectroscopy in patients affected by migraine with aura. Neurology. 1992;42(6):1209–14.
140. Yorns WR Jr, Hardison HH. Mitochondrial dysfunction in migraine. Semin Pediatr Neurol. 2013;20(3):188–93.
141. Boehnke C, Reuter U, Flach U, Schuh-Hofer S, Einhäupl KM, Arnold G. High-dose riboflavin treatment is efficacious in migraine prophylaxis: an open study in a tertiary care centre. Eur J Neurol. 2004;11(7):475–7.
142. Schoenen J, Jacquy J, Lenaerts M. Effectiveness of high-dose riboflavin in migraine prophylaxis A randomized controlled trial. Neurology. 1998;50(2):466–70.
143. Schoenen J, Lenaerts M, Bastings E. High-dose riboflavin as a prophylactic treatment of migraine: results of an open pilot study. Cephalalgia. 1994;14(5):328–9.
144. Bruijn J, Duivenvoorden H, Passchier J, Locher H, Dijkstra N, Arts WF. Medium-dose riboflavin as a prophylactic agent in children with migraine: a preliminary placebo-controlled, randomised, double-blind, cross-over trial. Cephalalgia. 2010;30(12):1426–34.
145. MacLennan SC, Wade FM, Forrest KM, Ratanayake PD, Fagan E, Antony J. High-dose riboflavin for migraine prophylaxis in children: a double-blind, randomized, placebo-controlled trial. J Child Neurol. 2008;23(11):1300–4.
146. Athaillah A, Dimyati Y, Saing JH, Saing B, Hakimi H, Lelo A. Riboflavin as migraine prophylaxis in adolescents. Paediatr Indones. 2012;52(3):132–7.
147. Sándor PS, Áfra J, Ambrosini A, Schoenen J. Prophylactic treatment of migraine with β-blockers and riboflavin: differential effects on the intensity dependence of auditory evoked cortical potentials. Headache. 2000;40(1):30–5.
148. Nambiar N, Aiyappa C, Srinivasa R. Oral riboflavin versus oral propranolol in migraine prophylaxis: an open label randomized controlled trial. Neurol Asia. 2011;16(3):223–9.
149. Rahimdel A, Zeinali A, Yazdian-anari P, Hajizadeh R, Arefnia E. Effectiveness of vitamin B2 versus sodium valproate in migraine prophylaxis: a randomized clinical trial. Electron Physician. 2015;7(6):1344–8.
150. Gaul C, Diener HC, Danesch U, Migravent Study Group. Improvement of migraine symptoms with a proprietary supplement containing riboflavin, magnesium and Q10: a randomized, placebo-controlled, double-blind, multicenter trial. J Headache Pain. 2015;16(1):32.
151. Lea RA, Ovcaric M, Sundholm J, MacMillan J, Griffiths LR. The methylenetetrahydrofolate reductase gene variant C677T influences susceptibility to migraine with aura. BMC Med. 2004;2(1):3.

152. Isobe C, Terayama Y. A remarkable increase in total homocysteine concentrations in the CSF of migraine patients with aura. Headache. 2010;50(10):1561–9.
153. Shaik MM, Tan HL, Kamal MA, Gan SH. Do folate, vitamins B_6 and B_{12} play a role in the pathogenesis of migraine? The role of pharmacoepigenomics. CNS Neurol Disord Drug Targets. 2014;13(5):828–35.
154. Lippi G, Mattiuzzi C, Meschi T, Cervellin G, Borghi L. Homocysteine and migraine. A narrative review. Clin Chim Acta. 2014;433:5–11.
155. Tietjen GE, Collins SA. Hypercoagulability and migraine. Headache. 2018;58(1):173–83.
156. Liampas I, Siokas V, Aloizou A, Tsouris Z, Metaxia D, Aslanidou P, et al. Pyridoxine, folate and cobalamin for migraine: a systematic review. Acta Neurol Scand. 2020; https://doi.org/10.1111/ane.13251.
157. Lea R, Colson N, Quinlan S, Macmillan J, Griffiths L. The effects of vitamin supplementation and MTHFR (C677T) genotype on homocysteine-lowering and migraine disability. Pharmacogenet Genomics. 2009;19(6):422–8.
158. Menon S, Lea RA, Roy B, Hanna M, Wee S, Haupt LM, et al. Genotypes of the MTHFR C677T and MTRR A66G genes act independently to reduce migraine disability in response to vitamin supplementation. Pharmacogenet Genomics. 2012;22(10):741–9.
159. Menon S, Nasir B, Avgan N, Ghassabian S, Oliver C, Lea R, Smith M, Griffiths L. The effect of 1 mg folic acid supplementation on clinical outcomes in female migraine with aura patients. J Headache Pain. 2016;17(1):60.
160. Di Rosa G, Attinà S, Spanò M, Ingegneri G, Sgrò DL, Pustorino G, et al. Efficacy of folic acid in children with migraine, hyperhomocysteinemia and MTHFR polymorphisms. Headache. 2007;47(9):1342–4.
161. Askari G, Nasiri M, Mozaffari-Khosravi H, Rezaie M, Bagheri-Bidakhavidi M, Sadeghi O. The effects of folic acid and pyridoxine supplementation on characteristics of migraine attacks in migraine patients with aura: a double-blind, randomized placebo-controlled, clinical trial. Nutrition. 2017;38:74–9.
162. Sadeghi O, Nasiri M, Maghsoudi Z, Pahlavani N, Rezaie M, Askari G. Effects of pyridoxine supplementation on severity, frequency and duration of migraine attacks in migraine patients with aura: a double-blind randomized clinical trial study in Iran. Iran J Neurol. 2015;14(2):74.
163. Helde-Frankling M, Björkhem-Bergman L. Vitamin D in pain management. Int J Mol Sci. 2017;18(10):2170.
164. Martin KR, Reid DM. Is there a role for vitamin D in the treatment of chronic pain? Ther Adv Musculoskelet Dis. 2017;9(6):131–5.
165. Holick MF, Binkley NC, Bischoff-Ferrari HA, Gordon CM, Hanley DA, Heaney RP, et al. Evaluation, treatment, and prevention of vitamin D deficiency: an Endocrine Society clinical practice guideline. [Published correction appears in J Clin Endocrinol Metab. 2011;96(12):3908]. J Clin Endocrinol Metab. 2011;96(7):1911–30.
166. Iannacchero R, Costa A, Squillace A, Gallelli L, Cannistrà U, De Sarro G. P060. Vitamin D deficiency in episodic migraine, chronic migraine and medication-overuse headache patients. J Headache Pain. 2015;16(Suppl 1):A184.
167. Kjærgaard M, Eggen AE, Mathiesen EB, Jorde R. Association between headache and serum 25-hydroxyvitamin D; the Tromsø study: Tromsø 6. Headache. 2012;52(10):1499–505.
168. Zandifar A, Banihashemi M, Asgari F, Manouchehri N, Ebrahimi H, Haghdoost F, et al. Vitamin D status in migraine patients: a case-control study. Biomed Res Int. 2014;2014:514782.
169. Donmez A, Orun E, Sonmez FM. Vitamin D status in children with headache: a case-control study. Clin Nutr ESPEN. 2018;23:222–7.
170. Gazerani P, Fuglsang R, Pedersen JG, Sørensen J, Kjeldsen JL, Yassin H, Nedergaard BS. A randomized, double-blinded, placebo-controlled, parallel trial of vitamin D3 supplementation in adult patients with migraine. Curr Med Res Opin. 2019;35(4):715–23.
171. Buettner C, Nir RR, Bertisch SM, Bernstein C, Schain A, Mittleman MA, Burstein R. Simvastatin and vitamin D for migraine prevention: a randomized, controlled trial. Ann Neurol. 2015;78(6):970–81.

172. Mottaghi T, Askari G, Khorvash F, Maracy MR. Effect of vitamin D supplementation on symptoms and C-reactive protein in migraine patients. J Res Med Sci. 2015;20(5):477–82.
173. Knutsen KV, Madar AA, Brekke M, Meyer HE, Natvig B, Mdala I, Lagerløv P. Effect of vitamin D on musculoskeletal pain and headache: a randomized, double-blind, placebo-controlled trial among adult ethnic minorities in Norway. Pain. 2014;155(12):2591–8.
174. Kılıç B, Kılıç M. Evaluation of vitamin D levels and response to therapy of childhood migraine. Medicina (Kaunas). 2019;55(7):321.
175. Cayir A, Turan MI, Tan H. Effect of vitamin D therapy in addition to amitriptyline on migraine attacks in pediatric patients. Braz J Med Biol Res. 2014;47(4):349–54.
176. Dolati S, Rikhtegar R, Mehdizadeh A, Yousefi M. The role of magnesium in pathophysiology and migraine treatment. Biol Trace Elem Res. 2019;5:1–9.
177. Sun-Edelstein C, Mauskop A. Role of magnesium in the pathogenesis and treatment of migraine. Expert Rev Neurother. 2009;9(3):369–79.
178. Altura BT, Altura BM. Withdrawal of magnesium causes vasospasm while elevated magnesium produces relaxation of tone in cerebral arteries. Neurosci Lett. 1980;20(3):323–7.
179. Shahrami A, Assarzadegan F, Hatamabadi HR, Asgarzadeh M, Sarehbandi B, Asgarzadeh S. Comparison of therapeutic effects of magnesium sulfate vs. dexamethasone/metoclopramide on alleviating acute migraine headache. J Emerg Med. 2015;48(1):69–76.
180. Bigal ME, Bordini CA, Tepper SJ, Speciali JG. Intravenous magnesium sulphate in the acute treatment of migraine without aura and migraine with aura. A randomized, double-blind, placebo-controlled study. Cephalalgia. 2002;22(5):345–53.
181. Martinez Cardenas V, Rodriguez M, Burke M, Vasconcellos E. Efficacy and safety of intravenous magnesium sulfate treatment in pediatric patients with headaches. Headache. 2012;52(5):896.
182. Köseoglu E, Talaslıoglu A, Gönül AS, Kula M. The effects of magnesium prophylaxis in migraine without aura. Magnes Res. 2008;21(2):101–8.
183. Peikert A, Wilimzig C, Köhne-Volland R. Prophylaxis of migraine with oral magnesium: results from a prospective, multi-center, placebo-controlled and double-blind randomized study. Cephalalgia. 1996;16(4):257–63.
184. Wang F, Van Den Eeden SK, Ackerson LM, Salk SE, Reince RH, Elin RJ. Oral magnesium oxide prophylaxis of frequent migrainous headache in children: a randomized, double-blind, placebo-controlled trial. Headache. 2003;43(6):601–10.
185. Sândor PS, Di Clemente L, Coppola G, Saenger U, Fumal A, Magis D, et al. Efficacy of coenzyme Q10 in migraine prophylaxis: a randomized controlled trial. Neurology. 2005;64(4):713–5.
186. Rozen TD, Oshinsky ML, Gebeline CA, Bradley KC, Young WB, Shechter AL, Silberstein SD. Open label trial of coenzyme Q10 as a migraine preventive. Cephalalgia. 2002;22(2):137–41.
187. Bentinger M, Tekle M, Dallner G. Coenzyme Q–biosynthesis and functions. Biochem Biophys Res Commun. 2010;396(1):74–9.
188. Shoeibi A, Olfati N, Sabi MS, Salehi M, Mali S, Oryani MA. Effectiveness of coenzyme Q10 in prophylactic treatment of migraine headache: an open-label, add-on, controlled trial. Acta Neurol Belg. 2017;117(1):103–9.
189. Dahri M, Hashemilar M, Asghari-Jafarabadi M, Tarighat-Esfanjani A. Efficacy of coenzyme Q10 for the prevention of migraine in women: a randomized, double-blind, placebo-controlled study. Eur J Integr Med. 2017;16:8–14.
190. Dahri M, Tarighat-Esfanjani A, Asghari-Jafarabadi M, Hashemilar M. Oral coenzyme Q10 supplementation in patients with migraine: effects on clinical features and inflammatory markers. Nutr Neurosci. 2019;22(9):607–15.
191. Slater SK, Nelson TD, Kabbouche MA, LeCates SL, Horn P, Segers A, et al. A randomized, double-blinded, placebo-controlled, crossover, add-on study of CoEnzyme Q10 in the prevention of pediatric and adolescent migraine. Cephalalgia. 2011;31(8):897–905.

192. Hershey AD, Powers SW, Vockell AL, LeCates SL, Ellinor PL, Segers A, Burdine D, Manning P, Kabbouche MA. Coenzyme Q10 deficiency and response to supplementation in pediatric and adolescent migraine. Headache. 2007;47(1):73–80.
193. Sadler C, Vanderjagt L, Vohra S. American Academy of Pediatrics Provisional Section on Complementary, Holistic, and Integrative Medicine. Complementary, holistic, and integrative medicine: butterbur [published correction appears in Pediatr Rev. 2007;28(10):385. Dosage error in article text]. Pediatr Rev. 2007;28(6):235–8. https://doi.org/10.1542/pir.28-6-235.
194. Rajapakse T, Davenport WJ. Phytomedicines in the treatment of migraine. CNS Drugs. 2019;33(5):399–415.
195. Ghasemian M, Owlia S, Owlia MB. Review of anti-inflammatory herbal medicines. Adv Pharmacol Sci. 2016;2016:9130979. https://doi.org/10.1155/2016/9130979.
196. Eaton J. Butterbur, herbal help for migraine. Nat Pharmacother. 1998;2:23–4.
197. Sutherland A, Sweet BV. Butterbur: an alternative therapy for migraine prevention. Am J Health Syst Pharm. 2010;67(9):705–11.
198. Thomet OA, Wiesmann UN, Schapowal A, Bizer C, Simon H. Role of petasin in the potential anti-inflammatory activity of a plant extract of petasites hybridus. Biochem Pharmacol. 2001;61(8):1041–7.
199. Fayyazi A, Khajeh A, Ghazavi A, Sangestani M. Omega 3 in childhood migraines: A double blind randomized clinical trial. Iran J Child Neurol. 2016;10(1):9–13.
200. Danesch U, Rittinghausen R. Safety of a patented special butterbur root extract for migraine prevention. Headache. 2003;43(1):76–8.
201. Diener HC, Rahlfs VW, Danesch U. The first placebo-controlled trial of a special butterbur root extract for the prevention of migraine: reanalysis of efficacy criteria. Eur Neurol. 2004;51(2):89–97.
202. Lipton RB, Göbel H, Einhäupl KM, Wilks K, Mauskop A. Petasites hybridus root (butterbur) is an effective preventive treatment for migraine. Neurology. 2004;63(12):2240–4.
203. Pothmann R, Danesch U. Migraine prevention in children and adolescents: results of an open study with a special butterbur root extract. Headache. 2005;45(3):196–203.
204. Oelkers-Ax R, Leins A, Parzer P, et al. Butterbur root extract and music therapy in the prevention of childhood migraine: an explorative study. Eur J Pain. 2008;12(3):301–13.
205. Anderson N, Borlak J. Hepatobiliary events in migraine therapy with herbs-the case of petadolex, a Petasites hybridus extract. J Clin Med. 2019;8(5):652.

Quick Reference Guides of Commonly Prescribed Drugs and Doses

12

Nathaniel Dusto and Danielle Perret Karimi

Acute Migraine Management

NSAIDs

Nonsteroidal anti-inflammatory drugs (NSAIDs) are available as over-the-counter and prescription medications that can help in the acute phase of migraine management.

Adverse reactions: Anemia and elevated liver function tests are common. Increased risk of cardiovascular thrombotic events including myocardial infarction (MI) and stroke. Increased risk of gastrointestinal inflammation, ulceration, bleeding, and perforation. Increased risk of acute kidney injury. Caution in the elderly, those with hypertension, and those with a history of peptic ulcer disease or gastrointestinal (GI) bleeding. Decreased platelet adhesion and aggregation; caution in patients with blood dyscrasias or those on anticoagulants. Avoid using multiple different NSAIDs concurrently [1].

Contraindications: History of asthma, urticaria, or allergic reaction to aspirin or other NSAIDs. Avoid use in pregnancy after 20 weeks gestation if possible. If NSAID use cannot be avoided between weeks 20 and 30, monitor for oligohydramnios. Avoid NSAID use after week 30 of gestation [2, 3].

Ibuprofen

Brand names: Advil, Motrin, Advil Migraine, Caldolor, and more

Dosage: Oral: 400–600 mg 3–4 times a day as needed. Maximum daily dose of 3200 mg [4, 5]

N. Dusto (✉)
Department of Physical Medicine and Rehabilitation, University of California Irvine, Orange, CA, USA
e-mail: ndusto@hs.uci.edu

D. Perret Karimi
Department of Physical Medicine and Rehabilitation and Department of Anesthesiology, University of California Irvine Health, Orange, CA, USA
e-mail: dperret@hs.uci.edu

© Springer Nature Switzerland AG 2021

S. Shah (ed.), *Migraine*, https://doi.org/10.1007/978-3-030-75239-2_12

Dosage adjustments: Renal impairment: Avoid use in patients with eGFR <60 [1]

Pediatric dosing: For children of ages 6 months to 11 years: Oral: 4–10 mg/kg/dose every 6–8 hours as needed. Maximum single dose: 400 mg. Maximum daily dose: 40 mg/kg/day

For children ≥12 years Oral: 200 mg every 4–6 hours as needed. Can increase to 400 mg single dose if needed. Maximum daily dose 1200 mg [6]

Diclofenac

Brand names: Cambia, Dyloject, Zipsor, Zorvolex

Dosing: Oral: 50–100 mg. Do not exceed 100 mg per day [7–9]

Dosage adjustments: Renal disease – no adjustment for mild to moderate impairment. Avoid use in advanced renal disease [1]

Pediatric dosing: 50 mg single dose for adolescents

Adverse reactions: Edema

Naproxen

Brand names: Aleve, Naprosyn, Anaprox, Mediproxen, Flanax, and more

Dosing: Oral: Initial dose of 750 mg. Additional 250–500 mg given as needed. Maximum 1250 mg per day [10, 11]

Dosing adjustments: Renal failure: Not recommended for CrCl <30 mL/minute

Pediatric dosing: Children <60 kg: 5–6 mg/kg/dose every 12 hours, maximum daily dose 1000 mg/day

Children ≥60 kg: 250–375 mg twice daily, maximum daily dose 1000 mg/day

Notes: For migraine prevention dosing, please refer to the entry for naproxen in the migraine prevention subsection of this chapter

Ketorolac

Brand name: Toradol

Dosing: IV: 30 mg every 6 hours as needed. Do not exceed 120 mg/day. Do not exceed 5 days of use [12]

IM: 60 mg single dose or 30 mg every 6 hours as needed. Do not exceed 120 mg/day. Do not exceed 5 days of use [13]

Dosing adjustment: Low body weight (<50 kg) or mild to moderate renal impairment

IM: 30 mg single dose or 15 mg every 6 hours as needed. Maximum 60 mg/day

IV: 15 mg every 6 hours as needed. Maximum 60 mg/day

Avoid use in advanced renal disease

Pediatric dosing: Ages ≤16 years: IV or IM 0.5 mg/kg/dose every 6 hours. Maximum dose 30 mg

Ages ≥17 follow adult dosing with body weight adjustments if indicated

Adverse reactions: Can cause headache, gastrointestinal pain, dyspepsia, nausea

Indomethacin

Brand names: Indocin, Tivorbex

Dosing: Oral: 20–40 mg 2–3 times daily prn [14]

Dosage adjustment: Avoid in advanced renal disease

Pediatric dosing: No recommended dosing for migraines in pediatric patients

Adverse reactions: Headache, vomiting

Notes: Available in suppository form as well

Aspirin

Brand names: Bayer and others

Dosing: Oral: 900–1000 mg once as needed. Maximum dose 4000 mg/day [15]

Dosage adjustment: Avoid with CrCl <10 mL/minute. Avoid use in severe liver disease [1]

Pediatric dosing: Children <50 kg: 10–15 mg/kg/dose every 4–6 hours as needed. Maximum daily dose 90 mg/kg/day or 4000 mg/day, whichever is less

Children ≥12 years and adolescents weighing ≥50 kg L: 325–650 mg every 4–6 hours as needed. Maximum daily dose 4000 mg/day

Note: Do not use in pediatric patients <18 years who have or are recovering from chickenpox or flu symptoms as this has been associated with Reye syndrome

Acetaminophen

Brand name: Tylenol

Dosing: Oral: 325–650 mg every 4–6 hours as needed or 1 g every 6 hours as needed. Maximum dose 4 g/day [16]

Recommended dose: 1 g every 6 hours as needed

Dosing adjustments: Chronic liver disease or cirrhosis: Maximum dose ≤2 g/day to 3 g/day [17]

Pediatric dosing: 10–15 mg/kg/dose every 4–6 hours as needed. Do not exceed 5 doses Maximum daily dose 75 mg/kg/day or 4 g/day, whichever is less [6]

Adverse reactions: Skin rash, nephrotoxicity with chronic overdose. Increased serum alkaline phosphatase, increased serum bilirubin

Warnings/precautions: Heavy alcohol use, advanced liver disease

Acetaminophen–Aspirin–Caffeine

Brand name: Excedrin

Dosing: Oral: Acetaminophen 250 mg/ aspirin 250 mg/ caffeine 65 mg per tablet. Two tablets once daily. Limit use to no more than 2 days per week [18]

Pediatric dosing: Children >12 years, same as adult dosing

Adverse reactions: Refer to aspirin and acetaminophen sections

Contraindications: Do not use with other products containing acetaminophen or if the patient is allergic to aspirin. Avoid use in pregnancy after week 20 of gestation [3]

Triptans

Adverse reactions: Dizziness, nausea common when administered orally

Contraindications: Avoid in hemiplegic migraines, basilar or hemiplegic migraines, history of ischemic stroke, ischemic heart disease, Prinzmetal's angina, uncontrolled hypertension, pregnancy, arrhythmias associated with cardiac accessory conduction pathway disorders including Wolff–Parkinson–White syndrome [2]

Notes: No more than 10 days of use per month. Overuse can cause headache. Only eletriptan, frovatriptan and naratriptan can be used in combination with a monoamine oxidase inhibitor. Do not use triptans within 24 hours of ergotamine or other triptans. Response to different triptans is variable from patient to patient. The choice of which triptan to use should be individualized. Sumatriptan and rizatriptan may be considered for moderate to severe migraines in pregnancy [19].

Sumatriptan

Brand names: Imitrex, Onzetra, Xsail, Sumavel, Tosymra, Zembrace

Dosing: Oral: 50–100 mg once. May repeat dose after ≥2 hours. Maximum dose 200 mg/day [20]

Intranasal solution: 20 mg once in a single nostril. May repeat dose after ≥2 hours. Maximum dose 40 mg/day

Intranasal powder: 22 mg once given as one 11 mg capsule insufflated in each nostril. May repeat dose after ≥2 hours. Maximum dose 44 mg/day [21]

Intranasal spray: 10 mg once in one nostril. May repeat dose after ≥1 hour. Maximum dose 30 mg per 24 hours [22]

Subcutaneous: 6 mg once. May repeat dose after ≥1 hour. If the initial dose was not tolerated, can decrease subsequent doses to 1–5 mg as tolerated. Maximum dose 12 mg/day [23]

Dosing adjustment: Mild to moderate hepatic impairment: do not exceed single doses of 50 mg

Severe hepatic impairment: Contraindicated

Pediatric dosing:

Intranasal: Ages 5 to ≤17 years: 5 mg, 10 mg, or 20 mg administered in one nostril as a single dose [24]

Oral: Limited data for adolescents ≤17 years. Adolescents ≥18 years: initial single dose 25 mg, 50 mg, or 100 mg. May repeat dose after ≥2 hours. Maximum daily dose 200 mg total

Subcutaneous: Ages ≥6 years and ≤17 years: 3–6 mg single dose

Adolescents ≥18 years: Imitrex and Sumavel: Initial dose 6 mg. May repeat dose after ≥1 hour as needed. Maximum dose 12 mg/day [6]

Zembrace: 3 mg, may repeat dose after ≥1 hour up to 4 total injections separated by 1 hour each. Maximum dose 12 mg/day

Adverse events: Intranasal: Unpleasant taste, nasal discomfort, throat irritation. Subcutaneous: Injection site reaction, chest pressure or heaviness, flushing, weakness, drowsiness, dizziness, malaise, a feeling of warmth, paresthesias. Most resolve spontaneously

Notes: Found to be more effective when combined with naproxen than with monotherapy of either medication

Zolmitriptan

Brand name: Zomig

Dosing: Nasal inhalation: 2.5 mg. Maximum single dose 5 mg. May repeat in ≥2 hours if needed. Maximum dose 10 mg/day [25]

Oral tablet: 1.25–2.5 mg. Maximum single dose 5 mg. May repeat in ≥2 hours if needed Maximum dose 10 mg/day [26]

Oral disintegrating tablet: 2.5 mg. Maximum single dose 5 mg. May repeat in ≥2 hours if needed Maximum dose 10 mg/day [27]

Dosing adjustment: Avoid in moderate to severe hepatic impairment

Pediatric dosing: No adjustment for children ≥12 years [6]

Adverse events: Somnolence, paresthesia, fatigue, tightness in chest or throat

Naratriptan

Brand name: Amerge

Dosing: Oral: 1–2.5 mg. May repeat dose in ≥4 hours. Maximum dose 5 mg/day [28]

Recommended dose: 2.5 mg

Dosing adjustment: Mild to moderate renal or hepatic impairment: 1 mg dose. Maximum dose 2.5 mg/day

Contraindicated in severe renal or hepatic impairment

Pediatric dosing: No recommended dosing for migraines in pediatric patients

Rizatriptan

Brand name: Maxalt

Dosing: Oral: 5–10 mg. May repeat dose after ≥2 hours. Maximum daily dose 30 mg/day [29]

Dosage adjustment: With concomitant propranolol therapy: 5 mg/dose, maximum daily dose 15 mg/day

Pediatric dosing: Children ≥6 years old: <40 kg: 5 mg as a single dose. Do not use if on concomitant propranolol

≥40 kg: 10 mg as a single dose. 5 mg single dose if on concomitant propranolol. Do not repeat dose

Adolescents ≥18 years: 5 mg. May repeat dose after 2 hours. Maximum daily dose 15 mg/day [30]

Notes: Dosage must be adjusted in patients taking propranolol. Propranolol increases levels of rizatriptan by 70%

Almotriptan

Brand name: Axert

Dosing: Oral: 6.25–12.5 mg single dose. May repeat dose after ≥2 hours. No more than 2 doses. Maximum dose: 25 mg/day [31]

Dosage adjustment: If patient is taking a potent CYP3A4 inhibitor: Initial dose 6.25 mg, maximum daily dose 12.5 mg

Severe renal impairment: Initial dose 6.25 mg. Maximum daily dose 12.5 mg

Hepatic impairment: Initial dose 6.25 mg. Maximum daily dose 12.5 mg

Pediatric dosing: Follow adult guidelines for children ≥12 years old. Do not use with renal impairment of any severity if on a potent CYP3A4 inhibitor [32]

Eletriptan

Brand name: Relpax

Dosing: Oral: 20–40 mg. May repeat dose after ≥2 hours. Maximum daily dose 80 mg/day [33]

Dosage adjustments: Do not use with severe hepatic impairment

Pediatric dosing: No recommended dosing for migraines in pediatric patients

Frovatriptan

Brand name: Frova

Dosing: Oral: 2.5 mg. May repeat dose after ≥2 hours. Maximum daily dose 7.5 mg/day [34]

Dosage adjustment: Do not use with severe hepatic impairment

Pediatric dosing: No recommended dosing for migraines in pediatric patients

Antiemetics

Notes: Coadministration of diphenhydramine IV 12.5–25 mg every hour for 2 hours can help prevent side effects of akathisia and acute dystonic reactions. Can alleviate both nausea as well as pain in migraines. Frequently used as adjunctive therapy. Oral formulations should not be used as monotherapy. All are associated with QT interval prolongation and torsades des pointes.

Ondansetron and granisetron both have not been well evaluated, but both have a high incidence of headache as an adverse effect, so they are not recommended.

Metoclopramide

Brand names: Reglan, Metozolv ODT

Dosing: 10 mg as a single dose [35]

Alternative high-dose regimen: IV: 20 mg every 30 minutes, up to 4 times in combination with IV diphenhydramine

Dosing adjustments: Renal impairment CrCl <40 mL/minute: IV: Administer 50% normal dose [36]

Pediatric dosing: No recommended dosing for migraines in pediatric patients

Adverse reactions: Atrioventricular block, bradycardia, drowsiness, dystonic reaction

Notes: IV is preferred, oral and subcutaneous also available. Commonly used as an adjunctive treatment with dihydroergotamine or IV diphenhydramine

Chlorpromazine

Brand name: Thorazine

Dosing: IV or IM: 0.1 mg/kg [37]

Pediatric dosing: No recommended dosing for migraines in pediatric patients

Adverse reactions: Drowsiness, dizziness, dystonic reactions

Notes: IV or IM preferred

Prochlorperazine

Brand name: Compro

Dosing: IV or IM: 10 mg once [35, 38]

Pediatric dosing: Children ≥7 years and adolescents: 0.15 mg/kg as a single dose. Maximum dose 10 mg/dose [39]

Adverse reactions: Agitation, dystonic reactions, dizziness, drowsiness

Notes: IV or IM preferred

Diphenhydramine

Brand names: Benadryl and many more

Dosing: Prophylaxis for dystonic reactions: IV or IM 12.5–25 mg prior to administration of high risk medication [38, 40]

Pediatric dosing: IV or IM: 1–2 mg/kg/dose. Maximum dose 50 mg/dose. May repeat if necessary [39]

Adverse reactions: Confusion, dizziness, drowsiness

Notes: Primarily used as an adjunctive with other antiemetics to reduce the rates of dystonic reactions. Risk factor B in pregnancy [41]

Antipsychotics

Droperidol

Brand names: Droleptan, Dridol, and more

Dosing: IM: 2.75–8.25 mg once [42]

Pediatric dosing: No recommended dosing for migraines in pediatric patients

Adverse reactions: Cardiac arrest, QTc prolongation, akathisia and asthenia

Contraindications: Known or suspected QT prolongation [43]

Notes: Not considered first line. High rates of akathisia and asthenia. Risk factor C in pregnancy, avoid use if possible [44]

Haloperidol

Brand name: Haldol

Dosing: IV: 5 mg once [45, 46]

Pediatric dosing: No recommended dosing for migraines in pediatric patients

Adverse reactions: Sedation, akathisia in 80% of patients. QTc prolongation

Contraindications: Parkinson's disease

Notes: Not considered first line

Lasmiditan

Brand name: Reyvow

Dosing: Oral: 50–200 mg. Do not take more than one dose in 24 hours [47]

Pediatric dosing: No recommended dosing for migraines in pediatric patients

Adverse reactions: Relatively high rates of dizziness, paresthesia, somnolence, fatigue and nausea, driving impairment

Dosing adjustments: Do not take with severe hepatic impairment

Pediatric dosing: No recommended dosing for migraines in pediatric patients

Mechanism of action: Selective serotonin 1F receptor agonist. Lacks vasoconstrictor activity [48]

Notes: May be beneficial in patients with contraindications to triptans due to cardiovascular risk factors. Patient must be able to wait ≥8 hours after dosing to operate heavy machinery or driving

CGRP Antagonists

Calcitonin-gene related peptide. Mediates trigeminovascular pain transmission. Good option for patients with either insufficient response or contraindications to triptan treatment. Used for both acute migraine management and migraine prevention

Rimegepant

Brand name: Nurtec

Dosing: Oral: 75 mg as a single dose [49]

Dosage adjustments: Avoid use in Renal impairment with CrCl <15 mL/minute. Avoid use with severe hepatic impairment

Pediatric dosing: No recommended dosing for migraines in pediatric patients

Adverse reactions: Nausea

Notes: Not preferred during pregnancy [50]

Ubrogepant

Brand name: Ubrelvy

Dosing: Oral: 50–100 mg. May repeat dose after ≥2 hours. Maximum daily dose 200 mg /day [51]

Dose adjustment: Avoid with strong CYP3A4 inhibitors or inducers. Maximum daily dose 50 mg/day with moderate CYP3A4 inhibitors. Maximum daily dose 100 mg/day with weak CYP3A4 inhibitors

Renal impairment with CrCl between 15 and 28 mL/minute. 50 mg single dose, may repeat dose after ≥2 hours. Avoid use with CrCl <15 mL/minute

Severe hepatic impairment: 50 mg as a single dose, may repeat dose after ≥2 hours

Pediatric dosing: No recommended dosing for migraines in pediatric patients

Adverse reactions: Nausea, somnolence, dry mouth

Contraindications: Avoid in pregnancy [52]

Ergots

Ergotamine

Brand name: Ergomar

Dosing: Sublingual: 2 mg, may repeat dose every 30 minutes. Maximum daily dose 6 mg/day Maximum weekly dose 10 mg/week [53]

Dosage adjustment: Contraindicated with impaired renal or hepatic function

Pediatric dosing: Same as adult [54]

Adverse reactions: May worsen nausea and vomiting. Rebound headaches, vascular occlusion noted with doses exceeding 6 tablets per 24 hours. Years of use may be associated with valvular heart disease [55]

Contraindications: Peripheral vascular disease, coronary artery disease, hypertension, breastfeeding, use with strong CYP3A4 inhibitors. Pregnancy is an absolute contraindication [56, 57]

Notes: Dihydroergotamine is the preferred ergot agent

Dihydroergotamine

Brand name: Migranal

Dosing: IM, subcutaneous: 1 mg, repeat hourly to maximum of 3 mg/day, 6 mg/week [58]

IV: 1 mg, repeat hourly to maximum 2 mg/day, 6 mg/week [59]

Intranasal: 1 spray (0.5 mg) in each nostril. Repeat after 15 minutes to a total of 4 sprays (2 mg) [60]

Subcutaneous: 1 mg [61]

Dosage adjustment: Contraindicated with severe renal or severe hepatic impairment

Pediatric dosing: IV: Premedicate with antiemetic

Low-dose IV regimen: Ages 6 to <10 years: 0.1 mg/dose every 6 hours until headache free, up to 8 doses per episode

Ages 10–12 years: 0.15 mg/dose every 6 hours until headache free, up to 8 doses per episode

Ages ≤16 years: 0.2 mg/dose every 6 hours. Continue therapy until headache free, up to 8 doses per episode [62]

High-dose IV regimen: Children 6–9 years or children ≤25 kg: 0.5 mg/dose every 8 hours. If symptoms improve, continue therapy until headache free, maximum of 15 doses per episode

Children ≥10 years weighing >25 kg: 1 mg/dose every 8 hours. If symptoms improve, continue therapy until headache free, maximum of 15 doses per episode

Intranasal: Same as adult dosing. Do not exceed 8 sprays (4 mg) per week [63]

Adverse reactions: Rhinitis (intranasal), taste disorder (intranasal), injection site reaction (IV and IM) [64]

Contraindications: Hypertension, ischemic heart disease, breastfeeding. Do not use in combination with peripheral or central vasoconstrictors. Pregnancy is an absolute contraindication [2]

Note: Often used in conjunction with antiemetic, particularly with IV administration

Do not use within 24 hours of triptans or other ergot-like agents

Dexamethasone

Brand names: Decadron and more

Pharmacologic category: Steroid

Dosing: IV or IM: 10–25 mg [65]

Pediatric dosing: No recommended dosing for migraines in pediatric patients

Adverse reactions: Many adverse reactions with frequent use including adrenal suppression, immunosuppression and more

Warnings: Avoid use in patients with active infection. Use caution in patients with concomitant NSAID use and those with diabetes

Contraindications: Systemic fungal infections

Notes: IV or IM dexamethasone in conjunction with standard acute migraine therapy reduces the rate of early headache recurrence. Frequent use can increase risk of glucocorticoid toxicity, so should be avoided [65]

Migraine Prevention

Antihypertensives

Beta-Blockers

Improvement may not be seen for several weeks. Titrate the dose, use at least for a 3-month evaluation period before the medication response should be considered a failure

Do not use first line for patients over 60 or smokers [66]

Warnings: Use caution in patients with asthma, diabetes mellitus, depression, cardiac conduction disturbances or sinus node dysfunction

Contraindications: Contraindicated in second- or third-degree heart block, uncompensated heart failure, cardiogenic shock, bronchial asthma

Notes: May be used in pregnancy [67]

Metoprolol

Brand name: Lopressor

Dosing: Oral: 50–200 mg total dose daily. Start at 25 mg twice a day. Titrate up every 1–2 weeks [68, 69]

Pediatric dosing: No recommended dosing for migraines in pediatric patients

Adverse reactions: Hypotension, bradycardia, dizziness, decreased libido

Propranolol

Brand name: Inderal

Dosing: Oral: Dose range of 40–160 mg total daily dose (can be IR or ER) [70, 71]

Pediatric dosing: Children ≥3 years age. 0.5–3 mg/kg/day in 2–3 divided doses. Maximum daily dose: 120 mg/day [72]

Adverse reactions: AV conduction disturbances, bradycardia, fatigue, dizziness

Notes: First line

Timolol

Brand names: Betimol, Istalol

Dosing: Oral: 10–30 mg daily, divided into two doses [71]

Pediatric dosing: No recommendations for migraines in pediatric patients

Adverse reactions: Bradycardia, dizziness, fatigue

Atenolol

Brand name: Tenormin

Dosing: Oral: 25–100 mg daily [73]

Pediatric dosing: No recommended dosing for migraines in pediatric patients

Dosage adjustments: For renal disease: CrCl 15–35: Maximum dose 50 mg daily

CrCl <15: Maximum dose 25 mg daily [74]

Adverse reactions: Hypotension, cardiac failure, bradycardia, ventricular tachycardia, supraventricular tachycardia, fatigue

Nadolol

Brand name: Corgard

Dosing: 20–240 mg daily [75]

Pediatric dosing: No recommended dosing for migraines in pediatric patients

Adverse reactions: For renal impairment CrCl 31–50: administer every 24–36 hours

For CrCl 10–30: administer every 24–48 hours

For CrCl <10: administer every 40–60 hours

Calcium Channel Blockers

Commonly used for migraine prevention

Tolerance may develop. If tolerance develops, the medication dose can be increased or the patient can be switched to a different calcium channel blocker

Verapamil

Brand names: Calan, Verelan

Dosing: Oral: 120–240 mg total daily dose. Can be increased to 480 mg total daily dose if no response at lower doses and tolerated well by patient [76, 77]

Dosage adjustments: For renal disease: Start at 100 mg total daily dose

In cirrhosis: Reduce to 20% normal dose and monitor EKG [78]

Pediatric dosing: No recommended dosing for migraines in pediatric patients

Adverse reactions: bradycardia, heart block, particularly at higher doses

Contraindications: Hypotension, second- or third-degree heart block, atrial flutter or fibrillation, accessory pathway conditions like Wolff–Parkinson–White

Notes: Some consider first line for ease of use and low side-effect profile

ACE/ARBs

Lisinopril

Brand names: Prinivil, Zestril

Dosing: Oral: 10 mg daily for 1 week, then 20 mg daily [79]

Dosing adjustments: Renal impairment: CrCl <30: Start with 2.5 mg once daily and titrate up

Pediatric dosing: No recommended dosing for migraines in pediatric patients
Adverse reactions: Hypotension, dizziness, transient increase in creatinine
Contraindications: Idiopathic or hereditary angioedema
Notes: Avoid use in pregnancy due to risk of oligohydramnios [80]

Candesartan

Brand name: Atacand

Dosing: 16 mg daily [81]

Dosing adjustments: Hepatic impairment: For moderate impairment, start with 8 mg daily dose

Pediatric dosing: No recommended dosing for migraines in pediatric patients
Adverse reactions: Hypotension, renal function abnormalities
Notes: Avoid use in pregnancy due to risk of oligohydramnios [82]

Antidepressants

Tricyclics

Adverse reactions are common, mostly sedation. Also, dry mouth, constipation, tachycardia, palpitations, orthostatic hypotension, weight gain, blurred vision, urinary retention, confusion in the elderly

Amitriptyline

Brand name: Elavil

Dosing: Oral: 10–25 mg at bedtime. Titrate up in 10–25 mg increments in intervals of ≥1 week to 150 days. Max dose 150 mg/day but typically 20–50 mg/day is better tolerated [83]

Pediatric dosing: Older children and adults: 0.25 mg/kg/day at bedtime, titrate up by 0.25 mg/kg/day every 2 weeks to 1 mg/kg/day [84]

Warnings: Increased risk of serotonin syndrome in patients taking other serotonergic agents. Lowers seizure threshold, caution in patients with epilepsy or seizure threshold

Contraindications: Coadministration within 14 days of MAOIs, acute recovery phase of myocardial infarction

Notes: First line. The only tricyclic with proven efficacy for migraines. Must titrate down to discontinue. Risk factor C for pregnancy, avoid use during pregnancy if possible [67]

SSRI

Venlafaxine

Brand name: Effexor

Dosing: Oral: Starting dose 37.5 mg daily for 3 days. Increase by 75 mg increments to 75–150 mg once daily [85]

Pediatric dosing: Not approved for pediatric patients

Dosing adjustments: Renal disease: CrCl <30 do not exceed 50% maximum dose. Titrate cautiously [86]

Hepatic impairment: Decrease dose by 50%

Warnings: Increased risk of serotonin syndrome in patients taking other serotonergic agents. Lowers seizure threshold, caution in patients with epilepsy or seizure threshold

Adverse reactions: Insomnia, dizziness, drowsiness, nausea, xerostomia, weakness, diaphoresis

Contraindications: Use within 14 days of MAOIs

Notes: Can be used in patients with comorbid panic disorder, generalized anxiety disorder, or social anxiety disorder. Weak evidence. Risk factor C in pregnancy, avoid use if possible [87]

Anticonvulsants

Valproate

Brand name: Depakote

Dosing: Oral: 500–1000 mg daily. Increase dose in increments of 250 mg/day every >3 days [88, 89]

Pediatric dosing: Children ≥5 years to ≤16 years: Initial 10–15 mg/kg/day, maximum initial dose 250 mg/dose. Titrate up as needed over 4–6 weeks to 40–45 mg/kg/day in two divided doses Maximum daily dose: 1000 mg/day [90]

Adverse reactions: Nausea, somnolence, tremor, dizziness, weight gain, hair loss

Contraindications: Pregnancy or women with childbearing potential are absolute contraindications. Also contraindicated in hepatic disease [91]

Notes: First line. Must be titrated off slowly

Topiramate

Brand name: Topamax

Dosing: Oral: 25 mg daily. Titrate slowly by 50 mg per week. Maximum 100 mg twice a day [92, 93]

Dosing adjustments: Renal disease: CrCl <70. Reduce dose to 50% normal, titrate slower

Pediatric dosing: Children aged 6 to <12 years with weight ≥20 kg: 15 mg once daily for 1 week Increase to 15 mg twice daily for 1 week. Increase to 25 mg twice daily for 1 week. Continue to titrate up to target dose of 2–3 mg/kg/day. Maximum dose 100 mg twice daily

>12 years: Follow adult dosing but recommended maximum dose of 50 mg twice daily [94, 95]

Adverse reactions: Paresthesias, fatigue, dizziness, memory impairment

Contraindications: Pregnancy is an absolute contraindication. Also contraindicated in recent alcohol use for extended release formulation only [91]

Notes: First line. Doses over 100 mg may induce estrogen metabolism and impact efficacy of oral contraception. Must be titrated off slowly

NSAIDs

Naproxen

Brand names: Aleve, Naprosyn, Anaprox, Mediproxen, Flanax and more

Dosing: 250–500 mg twice daily. Continue for at least 2–3 months before assessing clinical benefit. Consider tapering or discontinuing if migraines are well-controlled after 3–6 months [96]

Pediatric dosing: No recommended dosing for migraines in pediatric patients

Adverse reactions: Anemia and elevated liver function tests are common. Increased risk of cardiovascular thrombotic events including MI and stroke. Increased risk of gastrointestinal inflammation, ulceration, bleeding and perforation. Increased risk of acute kidney injury. Caution in the elderly, those with hypertension, and those with a history of peptic ulcer disease or GI bleeding. Decreased platelet adhesion and aggregation; caution in patients with blood dyscrasias or those on anticoagulants. Avoid using multiple different NSAIDs concurrently [1]

Contraindications: History of asthma, urticaria, or allergic reaction to aspirin or other NSAIDs. Avoid use in pregnancy after 20 weeks gestation if possible. If NSAID use cannot be avoided between weeks 20 and 30, monitor for oligohydramnios. Avoid NSAID use after week 30 of gestation [2, 3]

Notes: Best evidence of NSAIDs for prevention of migraines

CGRP Antagonists

Used in both acute migraine management and migraine prevention

Notes: While many of these have not been well studied in pregnancy, their long half-lives makes avoiding use of these medications during pregnancy preferable [97]

Erenumab

Brand name: Aimovig

Dosing: SubQ: 70–140 mg subcutaneous injection monthly [98]

Recommended dose: 70 mg subcutaneous injection monthly

Pediatric dosing: No recommended dosing for migraines in pediatric patients

Adverse reactions: Injection site reactions and constipation

Fremanezumab

Brand name: Ajovy

Dosing: SubQ: 225 mg subcutaneous injection monthly or 675 mg subcutaneous injection every 3 months [99]

Pediatric dosing: No recommended dosing for migraines in pediatric patients

Adverse reactions: injection site reactions

Galcanezumab

Brand name: Emgality

Dosing: SubQ: Loading dose of 240 mg, followed by 120 mg monthly [100]

Pediatric dosing: No recommended dosing for migraines in pediatric patients

Adverse reactions: Injection site reactions, angioedema, anaphylaxis

Eptinezumab

Brand name: Vyepti

Dosing: IV: 100 mg infusion over 30 minutes every 3 months. Can be increased to 300 mg/dose [101]

Pediatric dosing: No recommended dosing for migraines in pediatric patients

Adverse reactions: Upper respiratory tract infections, hypersensitivity, fatigue

Other Agents

Petasites/Butterbur

Dosing: Oral: 75 mg twice a day [102]

Adverse reactions: GI upset, burping

Contraindications: Pregnancy and breastfeeding are absolute contraindications [103]

Notes: A perennial shrub, herbal medicine and marketed as a food supplement.

Butterbur has hepatotoxic and potentially carcinogenic components that are removed from petasites root extract, but there is minimal long-term safety data and being marketed as a food supplement that is not subject to strict safety regulation like medications, means that caution should be used [102].

Riboflavin

Brand name: B-2-400

Dosing: Oral: 400 mg daily [104]

Pediatric dosing: Children ≥8 years old: 200–400 mg daily

Adverse reactions: Yellow-orange urine discoloration

Notes: Benefits may take up to 3 months to be noticed

Coenzyme Q

Dosing: Oral: 100 mg three times a day [105]

Pediatric dosing: No recommended dosing for migraines in pediatric patients

Simvastatin & Vitamin D Co-treatment

Brand names: FloLipid, Zocor

Recommended dose: Oral: Simvastatin 20 mg twice daily, Vitamin D3 1000 units twice daily [106]

Pediatric dosing: No recommended dosing for migraines in pediatric patients

Adverse reactions: Atrial fibrillation, constipation, headache, upper respiratory infection, bronchitis

Contraindications: Pregnancy is an absolute contraindication, pregnancy risk factor X. Also contraindicated in women who may become pregnant, breastfeeding, and active liver disease [107]

Botulinum Toxin/OnabotulinumtoxinA

Brand name: Botox

Dosing: IM: 5 units/0.1 mL per site. Recommended total dose is 155 units once every 12 weeks Divide the units equally bilaterally into 31 total sites [108]

Pediatric dosing: For adolescents ≥18 years old, follow adult dosing

Adverse reactions: Headache, neck pain, myasthenia, stiffness

Notes: Not recommended for prevention of episodic migraine, but is effective for chronic migraine

References

1. Risser A, Donovan D, Heintzman J, Page T. NSAID prescribing precautions. Am Fam Physician [Internet]. 2009;80(12):1371–8. Available from: http://www.ncbi.nlm.nih.gov/pubmed/20000300.
2. Becker WJ. Acute Migraine Treatment in Adults. Headache J Head Face Pain [Internet]. 2015;55(6):778–93. Available from: http://doi.wiley.com/10.1111/head.12550.
3. Dathe K, Hultzsch S, Pritchard LW, Schaefer C. Risk estimation of fetal adverse effects after short-term second trimester exposure to non-steroidal anti-inflammatory drugs: a literature review. Eur J Clin Pharmacol [Internet]. 2019;75(10):1347–53. Available from: http://link.springer.com/10.1007/s00228-019-02712-2.
4. Codispoti JR, Prior MJ, Fu M, Harte CM, Nelson EB. Efficacy of nonprescription doses of ibuprofen for treating migraine headache. A randomized controlled trial. Headache. 2001;41(7):665–79.
5. Kellstein DE, Lipton RB, Geetha R, Koronkiewicz K, Evans FT, Stewart WF, et al. Evaluation of a novel solubilized formulation of ibuprofen in the treatment of migraine headache: a randomized, double-blind, placebo-controlled, dose-ranging study. Cephalalgia. 2000;20:233–43.
6. Lewis D, Ashwal S, Hershey A, Hirtz D, Yonker M, Silberstein S. Practice Parameter: Pharmacological treatment of migraine headache in children and adolescents: Report of the American Academy of Neurology Quality Standards Subcommittee and the Practice Committee of the Child Neurology Society. Neurology [Internet]. 2004;63(12):2215–24. Available from: http://www.neurology.org/cgi/doi/10.1212/01.WNL.0000147332.41993.90.
7. Vécsei L, Gallacchi G, Sági I, Semjén J, Tajti J, Szok D, et al. Diclofenac epolamine is effective in the treatment of acute migraine attacks. A randomized, crossover, double blind, placebo-controlled, clinical study. Cephalalgia. 2007;27(1):29–34.
8. Bussone G, Grazzi L, D'Amico D, Manzoni C, Granella F, Cortelli P, et al. Acute treatment of migraine attacks: Efficacy and safety of a nonsteroidal anti-inflammatory drug, diclofenac-potassium, in comparison to oral sumatriptan and placebo. Cephalalgia. 1999;19(4):232–40.
9. Lipton RB, Grosberg B, Singer RP, Pearlman SH, Sorrentino J V, Quiring JN, et al. Efficacy and tolerability of a new powdered formulation of diclofenac potassium for oral solution for the acute treatment of migraine: Results from the International Migraine Pain Assessment Clinical Trial (IMPACT). Cephalalgia. 2010;30(11):1336–45.

10. Wentz AL, Jimenez TB, Dixon RM, Aurora SK, Gold M. A double-blind, randomized, placebo-controlled, single-dose study of the cyclooxygenase-2 inhibitor, GW406381, as a treatment for acute migraine. Eur J Neurol. 2008;15(4):420–7.
11. Smith TR, Sunshine A, Stark SR, Littlefield DE, Spruill SE, Alexander; W James, et al. Sumatriptan and Naproxen Sodium for the Acute Treatment of Migraine. Headache. 2005;45(8):983–91.
12. Meredith JT, Wait S, Brewer KL. A prospective double-blind study of nasal sumatriptan versus IV ketorolac in migraine. Am J Emerg Med [Internet]. 2003;21(3):173–5. Available from: https://linkinghub.elsevier.com/retrieve/pii/S0735675702422565.
13. Harden RN, Gracely RH, Carter T, Warner G. The Placebo Effect in Acute Headache Management: Ketorolac, Meperidine, and Saline in the Emergency Department. Headache J Head Face Pain [Internet]. 1996;36(6):352–6. Available from: http://doi.wiley.com/10.1046/j.1526-4610.1996.3606352.x.
14. Pareja JA, Sjaastad O. Chronic Paroxysmal Hemicrania and Hemicrania Continua. Interval Between Indomethacin Administration and Response. Headache J Head Face Pain [Internet]. 1996;36(1):20–3. Available from: http://doi.wiley.com/10.1046/j.1526-4610.1996.3601020.x.
15. Lipton RB, Goldstein J, Baggish JS, Yataco AR, Sorrentino J V., Quiring JN. Aspirin Is Efficacious for the Treatment of Acute Migraine. Headache J Head Face Pain [Internet]. 2005;45(4):283–92. Available from: https://onlinelibrary.wiley.com/doi/abs/10.1111/j.1526-4610.2005.05065.x.
16. Lipton RB, Baggish JS, Stewart WF, Codispoti JR, Fu M. Efficacy and Safety of Acetaminophen in the Treatment of Migraine. Arch Intern Med [Internet]. 2000;160(22):3486. Available from: http://archinte.jamanetwork.com/article.aspx?doi=10.1001/archinte.160.22.3486.
17. Bosilkovska M, Walder B, Besson M, Daali Y, Desmeules J. Analgesics in Patients with Hepatic Impairment. Drugs [Internet]. 2012;72(12):1645–69. Available from: http://link.springer.com/10.2165/11635500-000000000-00000.
18. Lipton RB, Stewart WF, Ryan RE, Saper J, Silberstein S, Sheftell F. Efficacy and Safety of Acetaminophen, Aspirin, and Caffeine in Alleviating Migraine Headache Pain. Arch Neurol [Internet]. 1998;55(2):210. Available from: http://archneur.jamanetwork.com/article.aspx?doi=10.1001/archneur.55.2.210.
19. Evans EW, Lorber KC. Use of 5-HT 1 Agonists in Pregnancy. Ann Pharmacother [Internet]. 2008;42(4):543–9. Available from: http://journals.sagepub.com/doi/10.1345/aph.1K176.
20. Jelinski SE, Becker WJ, Christie SN, Ahmad FF, Pryse-Phillips W, Simpson SD. Pain Free Efficacy of Sumatriptan in the Early Treatment of Migraine. Can J Neurol Sci [Internet]. 2006;33(01):73–9. Available from: http://www.journals.cambridge.org/abstract_S031716710000473X.
21. Djupesland P, Dočekal P. Intranasal sumatriptan powder delivered by a novel breath-actuated bi-directional device for the acute treatment of migraine: A randomised, placebo-controlled study. Cephalalgia [Internet]. 2010;30(8):933–42. Available from: http://journals.sagepub.com/doi/10.1177/0333102409359314.
22. Boureau F, Kappos L, Schoenen J, Esperanca P, Ashford E. A clinical comparison of sumatriptan nasal spray and dihydroergotamine nasal spray in the acute treatment of migraine. Int J Clin Pract [Internet]. 2000;54(5):281–6. Available from: http://www.ncbi.nlm.nih.gov/pubmed/10954953.
23. Sang C, Ramadan N, Wallihan R, Chappell A, Freitag F, Smith T, et al. LY293558, a Novel AMPA/GluR5 Antagonist, is Efficacious and Well-Tolerated in Acute Migraine. Cephalalgia [Internet]. 2004;24(7):596–602. Available from: http://journals.sagepub.com/doi/10.1111/j.1468-2982.2004.00723.x.
24. Ahonen K, Hamalainen ML, Rantala H, Hoppu K. Nasal sumatriptan is effective in treatment of migraine attacks in children: A randomized trial. Neurology [Internet]. 2004;62(6):883–7. Available from: http://www.neurology.org/cgi/doi/10.1212/01.WNL.0000115105.05966.A7.

25. Dodick D, Brandes J, Elkind A, Mathew N, Rodichok L. Speed of Onset, Efficacy and Tolerability of Zolmitriptan Nasal Spray in the Acute Treatment of Migraine. CNS Drugs [Internet]. 2005;19(2):125–36. Available from: http://link.springer.com/10.2165/00023210-200519020-00003.
26. Rapoport AM, Ramadan NM, Adelman JU, Mathew NT, Elkind AH, Kudrow DB, et al. Optimizing the dose of zolmitriptan (Zomig,* 311C90) for the acute treatment of migraine. Neurology [Internet]. 1997;49(5):1210–8. Available from: http://www.neurology.org/lookup/doi/10.1212/WNL.49.5.1210.
27. Loder E, Freitag FG, Adelman J, Pearlman S, Abu-Shakra S. Pain-free rates with zolmitriptan 2.5 mg ODT in the acute treatment of migraine: results of a large double-blind placebo-controlled trial. Curr Med Res Opin [Internet]. 2005;21(3):381–9. Available from: http://www.tandfonline.com/doi/full/10.1185/030079905X28926.
28. Mathew NT, Asgharnejad M, Peykamian M, Laurenza A. Naratriptan is effective and well tolerated in the acute treatment of migraine: Results of a double-blind, placebo-controlled, crossover study. Neurology [Internet]. 1997;49(6):1485–90. Available from: http://www.neurology.org/cgi/doi/10.1212/WNL.49.6.1485.
29. Ahrens S, Farmer M, Williams D, Willoughby E, Jiang K, Block G, et al. Efficacy and Safety of Rizatriptan Wafer for the Acute Treatment of Migraine. Cephalalgia [Internet]. 1999;19(5):525–32. Available from: http://journals.sagepub.com/doi/10.1046/j.1468-2982.1999.019005525.x.
30. Ahonen K, Hamalainen ML, Eerola M, Hoppu K. A randomized trial of rizatriptan in migraine attacks in children. Neurology [Internet]. 2006;67(7):1135–40. Available from: http://www.neurology.org/cgi/doi/10.1212/01.wnl.0000238179.79888.44.
31. Dahlof C, Tfelt-Hansen P, Massiou H, Fazekas A. Dose finding, placebo-controlled study of oral almotriptan in the acute treatment of migraine. Neurology [Internet]. 2001;57(10):1811–7. Available from: http://www.neurology.org/cgi/doi/10.1212/WNL.57.10.1811.
32. Linder SL, Mathew NT, Cady RK, Finlayson G, Ishkanian G, Lewis DW. Efficacy and Tolerability of Almotriptan in Adolescents: A Randomized, Double-Blind, Placebo-Controlled Trial. Headache J Head Face Pain [Internet]. 2008;48(9):1326–36. Available from: http://doi.wiley.com/10.1111/j.1526-4610.2008.01138.x.
33. Goadsby PJ, Ferrari MD, Olesen J, Stovner LJ, Senard JM, Jackson NC, et al. Eletriptan in acute migraine: A double-blind, placebo-controlled comparison to sumatriptan. Neurology [Internet]. 2000;54(1):156–156. Available from: http://www.neurology.org/cgi/doi/10.1212/WNL.54.1.156.
34. Ryan R, Géraud G, Goldstein J, Cady R, Keywood C. Clinical Efficacy of Frovatriptan: Placebo-Controlled Studies. Headache J Head Face Pain [Internet]. 2002;42(s2):84–92. Available from: https://onlinelibrary.wiley.com/doi/abs/10.1046/j.1526-4610.42.s2.6.x.
35. Jones J, Pack S, Chun E. Intramuscular prochlorperazine versus metoclopramide as single-agent therapy for the treatment of acute migraine headache. Am J Emerg Med [Internet]. 1996;14(3):262–4. Available from: https://linkinghub.elsevier.com/retrieve/pii/S0735675796901710.
36. Lehmann CR, Heironimus JD, Collins CB, O'Neil TJ, Pierson WP, Crowe JT, et al. Metoclopramide kinetics in patients with impaired renal function and clearance by hemodialysis. Clin Pharmacol Ther [Internet]. 1985;37(3):284–9. Available from: http://doi.wiley.com/10.1038/clpt.1985.41.
37. Bigal ME, Bordini CA, Speciali JG. Intravenous chlorpromazine in the Emergency Department treatment of migraines: a randomized controlled trial. J Emerg Med [Internet]. 2002;23(2):141–8. Available from: https://linkinghub.elsevier.com/retrieve/pii/S0736467902005024.
38. Friedman BW, Irizarry E, Solorzano C, Latev A, Rosa K, Zias E, et al. Randomized study of IV prochlorperazine plus diphenhydramine vs IV hydromorphone for migraine. Neurology [Internet]. 2017;89(20):2075–82. Available from: http://www.neurology.org/lookup/doi/10.1212/WNL.0000000000004642.

39. Dupuis LL, Nathan PC. Options for the Prevention and Management of Acute Chemotherapy-Induced Nausea and Vomiting in Children. Pediatr Drugs [Internet]. 2003;5(9):597–613. Available from: http://link.springer.com/10.2165/00148581-200305090-00003.
40. Kostic MA, Gutierrez FJ, Rieg TS, Moore TS, Gendron RT. A Prospective, Randomized Trial of Intravenous Prochlorperazine Versus Subcutaneous Sumatriptan in Acute Migraine Therapy in the Emergency Department. Ann Emerg Med [Internet]. 2010;56(1):1–6. Available from: https://linkinghub.elsevier.com/retrieve/pii/S0196064409017946.
41. Anderka M, Mitchell AA, Louik C, Werler MM, Hernández-Diaz S, Rasmussen SA. Medications used to treat nausea and vomiting of pregnancy and the risk of selected birth defects. Birth Defects Res Part A Clin Mol Teratol [Internet]. 2012;94(1):22–30. Available from: http://doi.wiley.com/10.1002/bdra.22865.
42. Silberstein SD, Young WB, Mendizabal JE, Rothrock JF, Alam AS. Acute migraine treatment with droperidol: A randomized, double-blind, placebo-controlled trial. Neurology [Internet]. 2003;60(2):315–21. Available from: http://www.neurology.org/cgi/doi/10.1212/01.WNL.0000042477.63516.B2.
43. Marmura MJ, Silberstein SD, Schwedt TJ. The Acute Treatment of Migraine in Adults: The American Headache Society Evidence Assessment of Migraine Pharmacotherapies. Headache J Head Face Pain [Internet]. 2015;55(1):3–20. Available from: http://doi.wiley.com/10.1111/head.12499.
44. ACOG Practice Bulletin No. 189: Nausea And Vomiting Of Pregnancy. Obstet Gynecol [Internet]. 2018;131(1):e15–30. Available from: https://journals.lww.com/00006250-201801000-00039.
45. Honkaniemi J, Liimatainen S, Rainesalo S, Sulavuori S. Haloperidol in the Acute Treatment of Migraine: A Randomized, Double–Blind, Placebo-Controlled Study. CME. Headache J Head Face Pain [Internet]. 2006;46(5):781–7. Available from: http://doi.wiley.com/10.1111/j.1526-4610.2006.00438.x.
46. McCoy JJ, Aldy K, Arnall E, Petersen J. Treatment of Headache in the Emergency Department: Haloperidol in the Acute Setting (THE-HA Study): A Randomized Clinical Trial. J Emerg Med [Internet]. 2020;59(1):12–20. Available from: https://linkinghub.elsevier.com/retrieve/pii/S0736467920303498.
47. Kuca B, Silberstein SD, Wietecha L, Berg PH, Dozier G, Lipton RB. Lasmiditan is an effective acute treatment for migraine. Neurology [Internet]. 2018;91(24):e2222–32. Available from: http://www.neurology.org/lookup/doi/10.1212/WNL.0000000000006641.
48. Nelson DL, Phebus LA, Johnson KW, Wainscott DB, Cohen ML, Calligaro DO, et al. Preclinical pharmacological profile of the selective 5-HT 1F receptor agonist lasmiditan. Cephalalgia [Internet]. 2010;30(10):1159–69. Available from: http://journals.sagepub.com/doi/10.1177/0333102410370873.
49. Croop R, Goadsby PJ, Stock DA, Conway CM, Forshaw M, Stock EG, et al. Efficacy, safety, and tolerability of rimegepant orally disintegrating tablet for the acute treatment of migraine: a randomised, phase 3, double-blind, placebo-controlled trial. Lancet [Internet]. 2019;394(10200):737–45. Available from: https://linkinghub.elsevier.com/retrieve/pii/S014067361931606X.
50. Burch R. Headache in Pregnancy and the Puerperium. Neurol Clin [Internet]. 2019;37(1):31–51. Available from: https://linkinghub.elsevier.com/retrieve/pii/S0733861918312532.
51. Dodick DW, Lipton RB, Ailani J, Lu K, Finnegan M, Trugman JM, et al. Ubrogepant for the Treatment of Migraine. N Engl J Med [Internet]. 2019;381(23):2230–41. Available from: http://www.nejm.org/doi/10.1056/NEJMoa1813049.
52. Lasmiditan (Reyvow) and ubrogepant (Ubrelvy) for acute treatment of migraine. Med Lett Drugs Ther [Internet]. 2020;62(1593):35–9. Available from: http://www.ncbi.nlm.nih.gov/pubmed/32555120.
53. Miljković S, Smajlović D, Tirić Campara M, Jurina R, Duranović Vinković L, Janković SM, et al. The first comparative double-blind trial on efficacy and safety of ergotamine based five-component combination and sumatriptan in migraine without aura. Hippokratia [Internet]. 22(1):17–22. Available from: http://www.ncbi.nlm.nih.gov/pubmed/31213753.

54. Geraud G, Lantri-Minet M, Lucas C, Valade D. French guidelines for the diagnosis and management of migraine in adults and children. Clin Ther [Internet]. 2004;26(8):1305–18. Available from: https://linkinghub.elsevier.com/retrieve/pii/S0149291804801619.
55. Tfelt-Hansen P, Saxena P, Dahlof C, Pascual J, Lainez M, Henry P, et al. Ergotamine in the acute treatment of migraine: A review and European consensus. Brain [Internet]. 2000;123(1):9–18. Available from: https://academic.oup.com/brain/article-lookup/doi/10.1093/brain/123.1.9.
56. MaassenVanDenBrink A, Reekers M, Bax WA, Ferrari MD, Saxena PR. Coronary Side-Effect Potential of Current and Prospective Antimigraine Drugs. Circulation [Internet]. 1998;98(1):25–30. Available from: https://www.ahajournals.org/doi/10.1161/01.CIR.98.1.25.
57. Bánhidy F, Ács N, Puhó E, Czeizel AE. Ergotamine treatment during pregnancy and a higher rate of low birthweight and preterm birth. Br J Clin Pharmacol [Internet]. 2007;64(4):510–6. Available from: http://doi.wiley.com/10.1111/j.1365-2125.2007.02901.x.
58. González-Espinosa LE, Gómez-Viera N, Olivera-Leal I, Reyes-Lorente R. [Treatment of acute attack of migraine with sumatriptan]. Rev Neurol [Internet]. 1997;25(147):1672–5. Available from: http://www.ncbi.nlm.nih.gov/pubmed/9484515.
59. Bell R, Montoya D, Shuaib A, Lee MA. A comparative trial of three agents in the treatment of acute migraine headache. Ann Emerg Med [Internet]. 1990;19(10):1079–82. Available from: https://linkinghub.elsevier.com/retrieve/pii/S0196064405815070.
60. Serio FJ. Efficacy, Safety, and Tolerability of Dihydroergotamine Nasal Spray as Monotherapy in the Treatment of Acute Migraine. Headache J Head Face Pain [Internet]. 1995;35(4):177–84. Available from: http://doi.wiley.com/10.1111/j.1526-4610.1995.hed3504177.x.
61. Winner P, Ricalde O, Le Force B, Saper J, Margul B. A Double-blind Study of Subcutaneous Dihydroergotamine vs Subcutaneous Sumatriptan in the Treatment of Acute Migraine. Arch Neurol [Internet]. 1996;53(2):180–4. Available from: http://archneur.jamanetwork.com/article.aspx?articleid=593860.
62. Linder SL. Treatment of Childhood Headache with Dihydroergotamine Mesylate. Headache J Head Face Pain [Internet]. 1994;34(10):578–80. Available from: http://doi.wiley.com/10.1111/j.1526-4610.1994.hed3410578.x.
63. Kabbouche MA, Powers SW, Segers A, LeCates S, Manning P, Biederman S, et al. Inpatient Treatment of Status Migraine With Dihydroergotamine in Children and Adolescents. Headache J Head Face Pain [Internet]. 2009;49(1):106–9. Available from: http://doi.wiley.com/10.1111/j.1526-4610.2008.01293.x.
64. Colman I, Brown MD, Innes GD, Grafstein E, Roberts TE, Rowe BH. Parenteral metoclopramide for acute migraine: meta-analysis of randomised controlled trials. BMJ [Internet]. 2004;329(7479):1369. Available from: https://www.bmj.com/lookup/doi/10.1136/bmj.38281.595718.7C.
65. Colman I, Friedman BW, Brown MD, Innes GD, Grafstein E, Roberts TE, et al. Parenteral dexamethasone for acute severe migraine headache: meta-analysis of randomised controlled trials for preventing recurrence. BMJ [Internet]. 2008;336(7657):1359–61. Available from: https://www.bmj.com/lookup/doi/10.1136/bmj.39566.806725.BE.
66. Limmroth V, Michel MC. The prevention of migraine: a critical review with special emphasis on β-adrenoceptor blockers. Br J Clin Pharmacol [Internet]. 2001;52(3):237–43. Available from: http://doi.wiley.com/10.1046/j.0306-5251.2001.01459.x.
67. Pringsheim T, Davenport WJ, Mackie G, Worthington I, Aubé M, Christie SN, et al. Canadian Headache Society guideline for migraine prophylaxis. Can J Neurol Sci [Internet]. 2012; 39(2 Suppl 2):S1–59. Available from: http://www.ncbi.nlm.nih.gov/pubmed/22683887.
68. Pringsheim T, Davenport WJ, Becker WJ. Prophylaxis of migraine headache. Can Med Assoc J [Internet]. 2010;182(7):E269–76. Available from: http://www.cmaj.ca/cgi/doi/10.1503/cmaj.081657.
69. Kangasniemi P, Andersen A, Andersson P, Gilhus N, Hedman C, Hultgren M, et al. Classic Migraine: Effective Prophylaxis with Metoprolol. Cephalalgia [Internet]. 1987;7(4):231–8. Available from: http://journals.sagepub.com/doi/10.1046/j.1468-2982.1987.0704231.x.

70. Linde K, Rossnagel K. Propranolol for migraine prophylaxis. In: Hobson A, editor. Cochrane Database of Systematic Reviews [Internet]. Chichester, UK: John Wiley & Sons, Ltd; 2004. Available from: http://doi.wiley.com/10.1002/14651858.CD003225.pub2.
71. Tfelt-Hansen P, Standnes B, Kangasneimi P, Hakkarainen H, Olesen J. Timolol vs propranolol vs placebo in common migraine prophylaxis: a double-blind multicenter trial. Acta Neurol Scand [Internet]. 1984;69(1):1–8. Available from: http://doi.wiley.com/10.1111/j.1600-0404.1984.tb07772.x.
72. Eidlitz-Markus T, Dlugatch Y, Haimi-Cohen Y, Goldberg-Stern H, Zeharia A. Nonpharmacologic Treatment of Migraine With Low-Dose Propranolol or Amitriptyline. Pediatr Neurol [Internet]. 2012;46(6):345–9. Available from: https://linkinghub.elsevier.com/retrieve/pii/S0887899412001555.
73. Forssman B, Lindblad CJ, Zbornikova V. Atenolol for Migraine Prophylaxis. Headache J Head Face Pain [Internet]. 1983;23(4):188–90. Available from: http://doi.wiley.com/10.1111/j.1526-4610.1983.hed2304188.x.
74. Kirch W, Kohler H, Mutschler E, Schafer M. Pharmacokinetics of atenolol in relation to renal function. Eur J Clin Pharmacol [Internet]. 1981;19(1):65–71. Available from: http://link.springer.com/10.1007/BF00558387.
75. Freitag FG, Diamond S. Nadolol and placebo comparison study in the prophylactic treatment of migraine. J Am Osteopath Assoc [Internet]. 1984;84(4):343–7. Available from: http://www.ncbi.nlm.nih.gov/pubmed/6150909.
76. Markley HG, Cheronis JCD, Piepho RW. Verapamil in prophylactic therapy of migraine. Neurology [Internet]. 1984;34(7):973–973. Available from: http://www.neurology.org/cgi/doi/10.1212/WNL.34.7.973.
77. Solomon GD, Steel JG, Spaccavento LJ. Verapamil prophylaxis of migraine. A double-blind, placebo-controlled study. JAMA [Internet]. 1983;250(18):2500–2. Available from: http://www.ncbi.nlm.nih.gov/pubmed/6355533.
78. Somogyi A, Albrecht M, Kliems G, Schafer K, Eichelbaum M. Pharmacokinetics, bioavailability and ECG response of verapamil in patients with liver cirrhosis. Br J Clin Pharmacol [Internet]. 1981;12(1):51–60. Available from: http://doi.wiley.com/10.1111/j.1365-2125.1981.tb01854.x.
79. Schrader H, Stovner L, Helde G, Sand T, Bovim G. Prophylactic treatment of migraine with angiotensin converting enzyme inhibitor (lisinopril): randomised, placebo controlled, crossover study. BMJ [Internet]. 2001;322(7277):19–19. Available from: https://www.bmj.com/lookup/doi/10.1136/bmj.322.7277.19.
80. Regitz-Zagrosek V, Roos-Hesselink JW, Bauersachs J, Blomström-Lundqvist C, Cífková R, De Bonis M, et al. 2018 ESC Guidelines for the management of cardiovascular diseases during pregnancy. Eur Heart J [Internet]. 2018;39(34):3165–241. Available from: https://academic.oup.com/eurheartj/article/39/34/3165/5078465.
81. Tronvik E, Stovner LJ, Helde G, Sand T, Bovim G. Prophylactic Treatment of Migraine With an Angiotensin II ReceptorBlocker. JAMA [Internet]. 2003 Jan 1;289(1):65. Available from: http://jama.jamanetwork.com/article.aspx?doi=10.1001/jama.289.1.65.
82. Cabiddu G, Castellino S, Gernone G, Santoro D, Moroni G, Giannattasio M, et al. A best practice position statement on pregnancy in chronic kidney disease: the Italian Study Group on Kidney and Pregnancy. J Nephrol [Internet]. 2016;29(3):277–303. Available from: http://link.springer.com/10.1007/s40620-016-0285-6.
83. Bank J. A Comparative Study of Amitriptyline and Fluvoxamine in Migraine Prophylaxis. Headache J Head Face Pain [Internet]. 1994;34(8):476–8. Available from: http://doi.wiley.com/10.1111/j.1526-4610.1994.hed3408476.x.
84. Hershey AD, Powers SW, Bentti A-L, DeGrauw TJ. Effectiveness of Amitriptyline in the Prophylactic Management of Childhood Headaches. Headache J Head Face Pain [Internet]. 2000;40(7):539–49. Available from: http://doi.wiley.com/10.1046/j.1526-4610.2000.00085.x.
85. Ozyalcin SN, Talu GK, Kiziltan E, Yucel B, Ertas M, Disci R. The Efficacy and Safety of Venlafaxine in the Prophylaxis of Migraine. Headache J Head Face Pain [Internet]. 2005;45(2):144–52. Available from: http://doi.wiley.com/10.1111/j.1526-4610.2005.05029.x.

86. Troy SM, Schultz RW, Parker VD, Chiang ST, Blum RA. The effect of renal disease on the disposition of venlafaxine. Clin Pharmacol Ther [Internet]. 1994;56(1):14–21. Available from: http://doi.wiley.com/10.1038/clpt.1994.95.
87. ACOG Practice Bulletin No. 92: Use of Psychiatric Medications During Pregnancy and Lactation. Obstet Gynecol [Internet]. 2008;111(4):1001–20. Available from: https://journals.lww.com/00006250-200804000-00039.
88. Hering R, Kuritzky A. Sodium Valproate in The Prophylactic Treatment of Migraine: A Double-Blind Study Versus Placebo. Cephalalgia [Internet]. 1992;12(2):81–4. Available from: http://journals.sagepub.com/doi/10.1046/j.1468-2982.1992.1202081.x.
89. Jensen R, Brinck T, Olesen J. Sodium valproate has a prophylactic effect in migraine without aura. Neurology [Internet]. 1994;44(4):647–647. Available from: http://www.neurology.org/lookup/doi/10.1212/WNL.44.4.647.
90. Gunner KB, Smith HD, Ferguson LE. Practice Guideline for Diagnosis and Management of Migraine Headaches in Children and Adolescents: Part Two. J Pediatr Heal Care [Internet]. 2008;22(1):52–9. Available from: https://linkinghub.elsevier.com/retrieve/pii/S0891524507004038.
91. Harden CL, Meador KJ, Pennell PB, Hauser WA, Gronseth GS, French JA, et al. Practice Parameter update: Management issues for women with epilepsy--Focus on pregnancy (an evidence-based review): Teratogenesis and perinatal outcomes: Report of the Quality Standards Subcommittee and Therapeutics and Technology Assessment Subcommittee. Neurology [Internet]. 2009;73(2):133–41. Available from: http://www.neurology.org/cgi/doi/10.1212/WNL.0b013e3181a6b312.
92. Brandes JL, Saper J, Diamond M, Couch J, Lewis D, Schmitt J, et al. Topiramate for Migraine Prevention<SUBTITLE>A Randomized Controlled Trial</SUBTITLE>. JAMA [Internet]. 2004;291(8):965. Available from: http://jama.jamanetwork.com/article.aspx?doi=10.1001/jama.291.8.965.
93. Silberstein SD, Neto W, Schmitt J, Jacobs D. Topiramate in Migraine Prevention. Arch Neurol [Internet]. 2004;61(4):490. Available from: http://archneur.jamanetwork.com/article.aspx?doi=10.1001/archneur.61.4.490.
94. Oskoui M, Pringsheim T, Billinghurst L, Potrebic S, Gersz EM, Gloss D, et al. Practice guideline update summary: Pharmacologic treatment for pediatric migraine prevention. Neurology [Internet]. 2019;93(11):500–9. Available from: http://www.neurology.org/lookup/doi/10.1212/WNL.0000000000008105.
95. Winner P, Pearlman EM, Linder SL, Jordan DM, Fisher AC, Hulihan J. Topiramate for Migraine Prevention in Children: A Randomized, Double-Blind, Placebo-Controlled Trial. Headache J Head Face Pain [Internet]. 2005;45(10):1304–12. Available from: http://doi.wiley.com/10.1111/j.1526-4610.2005.00262.x.
96. Ziegler DK, Ellis DJ. Naproxen in Prophylaxis of Migraine. Arch Neurol [Internet]. 1985;42(6):582–4. Available from: http://archneur.jamanetwork.com/article.aspx?articleid=584255.
97. Tepper SJ. History and Review of anti-Calcitonin Gene-Related Peptide (CGRP) Therapies: From Translational Research to Treatment. Headache J Head Face Pain [Internet]. 2018 Nov;58:238–75. Available from: http://doi.wiley.com/10.1111/head.13379.
98. Goadsby PJ, Reuter U, Hallström Y, Broessner G, Bonner JH, Zhang F, et al. A Controlled Trial of Erenumab for Episodic Migraine. N Engl J Med [Internet]. 2017;377(22):2123–32. Available from: http://www.nejm.org/doi/10.1056/NEJMoa1705848.
99. Dodick DW, Silberstein SD, Bigal ME, Yeung PP, Goadsby PJ, Blankenbiller T, et al. Effect of Fremanezumab Compared With Placebo for Prevention of Episodic Migraine. JAMA [Internet]. 2018;319(19):1999. Available from: http://jama.jamanetwork.com/article.aspx?doi=10.1001/jama.2018.4853.
100. Stauffer VL, Dodick DW, Zhang Q, Carter JN, Ailani J, Conley RR. Evaluation of Galcanezumab for the Prevention of Episodic Migraine. JAMA Neurol [Internet]. 2018;75(9):1080. Available from: http://archneur.jamanetwork.com/article.aspx?doi=10.1001/jamaneurol.2018.1212.

101. Ashina M, Saper J, Cady R, Schaeffler BA, Biondi DM, Hirman J, et al. Eptinezumab in episodic migraine: A randomized, double-blind, placebo-controlled study (PROMISE-1). Cephalalgia [Internet]. 2020;40(3):241–54. Available from: http://journals.sagepub.com/doi/10.1177/0333102420905132.
102. Lipton RB, Gobel H, Einhaupl KM, Wilks K, Mauskop A. Petasites hybridus root (butterbur) is an effective preventive treatment for migraine. Neurology [Internet]. 2004;63(12):2240–4. Available from: http://www.neurology.org/cgi/doi/10.1212/01.WNL.0000147290.68260.11.
103. Rapoport AM, Bigal ME. Migraine preventive therapy: current and emerging treatment options. Neurol Sci [Internet]. 2005;26(S2):s111–20. Available from: http://link.springer.com/10.1007/s10072-005-0422-9.
104. Schoenen J, Jacquy J, Lenaerts M. Effectiveness of high-dose riboflavin in migraine prophylaxis A randomized controlled trial. Neurology [Internet]. 1998;50(2):466–70. Available from: http://www.neurology.org/cgi/doi/10.1212/WNL.50.2.466.
105. Sandor PS, Di Clemente L, Coppola G, Saenger U, Fumal A, Magis D, et al. Efficacy of coenzyme Q10 in migraine prophylaxis: A randomized controlled trial. Neurology [Internet]. 2005;64(4):713–5. Available from: http://www.neurology.org/cgi/doi/10.1212/01.WNL.0000151975.03598.ED.
106. Buettner C, Nir R-R, Bertisch SM, Bernstein C, Schain A, Mittleman MA, et al. Simvastatin and vitamin D for migraine prevention: A randomized, controlled trial. Ann Neurol [Internet]. 2015;78(6):970–81. Available from: http://doi.wiley.com/10.1002/ana.24534.
107. Godfrey LM, Erramouspe J, Cleveland KW. Teratogenic Risk of Statins in Pregnancy. Ann Pharmacother [Internet]. 2012;46(10):1419–24. Available from: http://journals.sagepub.com/doi/10.1345/aph.1R202.
108. Diener H, Dodick D, Aurora S, Turkel C, DeGryse R, Lipton R, et al. OnabotulinumtoxinA for treatment of chronic migraine: Results from the double-blind, randomized, placebo-controlled phase of the PREEMPT 2 trial. Cephalalgia [Internet]. 2010;30(7):804–14. Available from: http://journals.sagepub.com/doi/10.1177/0333102410364677.

Index

© Springer Nature Switzerland AG 2021
S. Shah (ed.), *Migraine*, https://doi.org/10.1007/978-3-030-75239-2

R

S

MIX
Papier aus verantwortungsvollen Quellen
Paper from responsible sources
FSC® C105338

If you have any concerns about our products,
you can contact us on
ProductSafety@springernature.com

In case Publisher is established outside the EU,
the EU authorized representative is:
Springer Nature Customer Service Center GmbH
Europaplatz 3, 69115 Heidelberg, Germany

Printed by Libri Plureos GmbH
in Hamburg, Germany